Human Cancer Markers

Contemporary Biomedicine

HUMAN CANCER MARKERS

Edited by

STEWART SELL
University of California, San Diego

and

BRITTA WAHREN
Karolinska Hospital, Stockholm, Sweden

Humana Press · Clifton, New Jersey

Library of Congress Cataloging in Publication Data

Main entry under title:

Human cancer markers.

(Contemporary biomedicine)
Includes bibliographies and index.
1. Tumor antigens. 2. Cancer—Diagnosis. I. Sell,
Stewart. II. Wahren, Britta. III. Title: Cancer
markers. IV. Series. [DNLM: 1. Neoplasms—Diagnosis.
2. Neoplasms—Classification. 3. Antigens, Neoplasms.
QZ 241 H918]
RC268.3.H85   616.99′40756   81-80902
ISBN 0-89603-029-6   AACR2

©1982 the HUMANA Press Inc.
Crescent Manor
P.O. Box 2148
Clifton, NJ 07015

PREFACE

The ability to diagnose cancer by simple measurement of a serum or tissue "marker" has been a goal of medical science for many years. There is ample evidence that tumor cells are different from normal cells and produce substances that can be detected by currently available immunochemical or biochemical methods. These "cancer markers" may be secreted proteins, enzymes, hormones, fetal serum components, monoclonal immunoglobulins, cell surface components, or cytoplasmic constituents. The purpose of this book is to present the current status of our knowledge of such cancer markers.

The first tumor marker identified by laboratory means was Bence-Jones protein. In a series of lectures delivered to the Royal College of Physicians in London in 1846, Dr. H. Bence Jones described studies on a urine sample sent to him with the following note: "Dear Dr. Jones—The tube contains urine of very high specific gravity. When boiled it becomes slightly opaque. . . . etc." Dr. Jones found that heating of the urine after addition of nitric acid resulted in formation of a heavy precipitate; acid addition may have been required to bring the urine to pH 4–6 at which Bence Jones proteins are more likely to precipitate when heated. This urinary precipitate was associated with a bone disease termed "mollities ossium." [H. Bence Jones, Papers on Chemical Pathology, Lecture III. *Lancet* **2,** 269–274 (1847)]. It is now known that this precipitate represents immunoglobulin light chains passed into the urine of many patients with multiple myeloma [Edelman and Galley, *J. Exp. Med.* **116,** 207 (1962)]. A definitive chapter on monoclonal immunoglobulins as biomarkers of cancer was written for the first volume of this series (Sell, S., *Cancer Markers,* Humana Press, Clifton, NJ, 1980) by Alan Solomon and this subject is therefore not treated in the present volume.

The second era of cancer markers started in 1963 with the discovery of alphafetoprotein (AFP) by the noted Soviet scientist Garri I. Abelev. Abelev identified this protein in the sera of fetal mice and in the sera of adult mice with hepatocellular cancer, but not in normal adult mice. With the development of more sensitive assays, AFP has now also been found in normal adult sera, but in very small amounts. Thus AFP, like other "cancer markers," is not uniquely produced by cancer, but is normally produced during development and in small amounts by mature adult tissue. It is rapidly secreted into the blood so that measurement in serum accurately reflects the synthesis rate.

A second relatively well-studied cancer marker is carcinoembryonic antigen (CEA), discovered by Gold and Freedman in 1965. CEA is a normal cell surface glycoprotein found in the cells lining the gastrointestinal tract, particularly in the large intestine. Normally very small amounts of this cell surface glycoprotein appear in the circulation. The cells that make CEA usually secrete most of the CEA produced into the gastrointestinal tract. With the development of tumors of the gastrointestinal lining cells, the secretory polarity of the cells is changed so that CEA is secreted into the blood, where it may be detected by immunochemical techniques.

Unfortunately, elevations of the serum concentrations of both AFP and CEA are not limited to cancer, but are also found in non-neoplastic inflammatory conditions such as hepatitis and cirrhosis (AFP) or ulcerative colitis (CEA), as well as other diseases. Thus these markers do not fulfill the ultimate goal of being diagnostic markers unique for cancer. However, determination of the serum concentrations of these markers is an important part of the diagnostic and prognostic evaluation of patients with suspected cancer. Elevations of serum AFP above 1000 ng/mL (normal 5–10 ng/mL) are essentially diagnostic of hepatocellular or yolk sac tumors (see Chapter 6). Although elevation of CEA above normal cannot by itself be considered diagnostic of cancer, the serum concentrations of CEA after treatment of a CEA-producing tumor may be extremely useful in following the effects of therapy. If the CEA level falls to normal and stays there, it is almost certain that the patient has been successfully treated; if the CEA remains elevated or becomes re-elevated after falling to normal, recurrence or metastasis is likely.

Other "cancer markers" include hormones or enzymes whose abnormal production may aid in the diagnosis of cancer, particularly that of endocrine organs. These markers may be extremely useful for a small number of individuals, but have had little impact on the diagnosis of cancer in general. Although active investigation continues on many other serum cancer markers that might be used diagnostically, none has been convincingly shown to be useful to the point of general application at this time. However, surveys now underway may well provide the clinical oncologist with important new diagnostic and prognostic serologic markers for cancer.

Markers that are not found in the blood may be useful for the identification of tumor tissue. Pathologists are often faced with the problem of determining the origin of a metastatic lesion. Using immunohistologic techniques, CEA and AFP localization in metastatic lesions has already been widely used to identify the tissue origin of the primary lesion. Other markers for breast, pancreatic, and prostatic cancer are now being evaluated with promising preliminary results.

Cancer markers have also been used to detect sites of tumor growth in vivo. Antibody to the marker is radiolabeled, injected into the patient and localization determined by radioscintigraphy. This technique, "radioimmunoscintigraphy," is considered by some to have great promise for detecting occult tumors, but as yet has been successful in only a few selected patients screened for CEA-producing tumors. Application of other markers for this purpose is expected in the future.

Immune reactants may also be used to direct chemotherapeutic agents or suitable isotopes to cancer cells in vivo. Therapy with anti-AFP alone has produced marginal results in experimental models, but conjugation of chemotherapeutic agents, such as daunomycin, to antibodies to a cancer marker might provide more effective therapy.

The application of hybridoma technology and enzyme immunoassay to the identification and quantitation of tumor markers signals a third era in cancer markers. These techniques have the promise of providing a new generation of cancer markers. In Chapter 1, Dr. William Raschke summarizes hybridoma techniques, while in Chapter 2, Dr. Robert Fox and his colleagues provide a more detailed description of the application of hybridoma reagents to markers of lymphoproliferative diseases. In Chapter 3, Dr. Reisfeld and his colleagues describe the molecular approach to identification and charactization of a tumor antigen. These three chapters set the tone for the remainder of the volume, articles that not only review the present status of tumor markers for various organ sites, but that also, in most instances, point out prospects for the future.

Thus, this volume on cancer markers appears at an exciting and potentially critical time. Although the clinical applications of CEA and AFP have not fulfilled the optimistic expectations that many predicted, these markers do have a place in cancer diagnosis and management. Will new cancer markers be as good or better? Many of the new markers will almost certainly not be as useful as their uncritical proponents argue. Claims of a universal cancer marker have been made repeatedly in the past and have gone unsubstantiated. New cancer markers usually generate high enthusiasm from those that find them [see, for instance, Maugh, T. H., *Science* **24**, 909 (1981)], but unfortunately most have not performed as advertised when subjected to critical evaluation. However, the availability of new technology may justify some of the current enthusiam! A continued search for new tumor markers is more than justified by the tremendous potential for clinical application. It is hoped that this book will help stimulate and focus the quest for cancer markers.

CONTRIBUTORS

STEPHEN BAIRD · *University of California, San Diego, California*

STEPHEN B. BAYLIN · *Oncology Center and the Department of Medicine, The Johns Hopkins University School of Medicine and Hospital, Baltimore, Maryland*

DARRELL D. BIGNER · *Department of Pathology, Duke University Medical Center, Durham, North Carolina*

JEAN-CLAUDE BYSTRYN · *Department of Dermatology, New York University School of Medicine, New York, New York*

T. MING CHU · *Department of Diagnostic Immunology Research and Biochemistry, Roswell Park Memorial Institute, Buffalo, New York*

THOMAS S. EDGINGTON · *Department of Molecular Immunology, Research Institute of Scripps Clinic, La Jolla, California*

EVA ENGVALL · *La Jolla Cancer Research Foundation, La Jolla, California*

ROBERT FOX · *Department of Clinical Research, Scripps Clinic and Research Foundation, La Jolla, California*

D. R. GALLOWAY · *Department of Molecular Immunology, Scripps Clinic and Research Foundation, La Jolla, California*

JOHN R. HOBBS · *Department of Chemical Pathology, Westminster Medical School, London, Great Britain*

TREVOR R. JONES · *Department of Pathology, Duke University Medical Center, Durham, North Carolina*

CARL S. KILLIAN · *Department of Diagnostic Immunology Research and Biochemistry, Roswell Park Memorial Institute, Buffalo, New York*

PATRICK KUNG · *Ortho Pharmaceutical Corporation, Raritan, New Jersey*

MANABU KURIYAMA · *Department of Diagnostic Immunology Research and Biochemistry, Roswell Park Memorial Institute, Buffalo, New York*

PAUL H. LANGE · *Department of Urologic Surgery, University of Minnesota College of Health Sciences, Minneapolis, Minnesota*

CHING-LI LEE · Department of Diagnostic Immunology Research and Biochemistry, Roswell Park Memorial Institute, Buffalo, New York

RON LEVY · Stanford University Medical Center, Stanford, California

K. ROBERT McINTIRE · Diagnosis Branch, Division of Cancer Biology and Diagnosis, National Cancer Institute, Bethesda, Maryland

GEOFFREY MENDELSOHN · Oncology Center and the Department of Pathology, The Johns Hopkins University School of Medicine and Hospital, Baltimore, Maryland

GERALD P. MURPHY · Department of Diagnostic Immunology Research and Biochemistry, Roswell Park Memorial Institute, Buffalo, New York

ROBERT M. NAKAMURA · Department of Molecular Immunology, Research Institute of Scripps Clinic, La Jolla, California

LAWRENCE D. PAPSIDERO · Department of Diagnostic Immunology Research and Biochemistry, Roswell Park Memorial Institute, Buffalo, New York

PETER PERLMANN · Department of Immunology, University of Stockholm, Stockholm, Sweden

WILLIAM C. RASCHKE · Developmental Biology Laboratory, The Salk Institute, San Diego, California

R. A. REISFELD · Department of Molecular Immunology, Scripps Clinic and Research Foundation, La Jolla, California

IVOR ROYSTON · University of California, San Diego, California

STEWART SELL · Department of Pathology, University of California Medical School, San Diego, La Jolla, California

MARKKU SEPPÄLÄ · Department of Obstetrics and Gynecology, University Central Hospital, Helsinki, Finland

HANS O. SJÖGREN · The Wallenberg Laboratory, University of Lund, Lund, Sweden

TORGNY STIGBRAND · Department of Physiological Chemistry, University of Umeå, Umeå, Sweden

LUIS A. VALENZUELA · Department of Diagnostic Immunology Research and Biochemistry, Roswell Park Memorial Institute, Buffalo, New York

BRITTA WAHREN · Radiumhemmet, Karolinska Hospital, Stockholm, Sweden

MING C. WANG · Department of Diagnostic Immunology Research and Biochemistry, Roswell Park Memorial Institute, Buffalo, New York

CONTENTS

CHAPTER 3

An Immunochemical Approach to the Isolation
of Human Melanoma-Associated Antigens
D. A. Galloway and A. A. Reisfeld

CHAPTER 6
Hepatocellular Carcinoma Markers
Stewart Sell

CHAPTER 7
Pancreatic Tumor Markers
John A. Hobbs

CHAPTER 10
Ovarian and Uterine Cancer Markers
Markku Seppälä

CHAPTER 11
Testicular Cancer Markers
Paul H. Lange

CHAPTER 12
Placental Proteins as Tumor Markers
Torgny Stigbrand and Eva Engvall

CHAPTER 13
Bladder and Renal Tumor Markers
Britta Wahren and Peter Perlmann

CHAPTER 14

Endocrine Markers of Cancer: The Biological and Clinical
Implications of Polypeptide Hormones

Geoffrey Mendelsohn and Stephen B. Baylin

CHAPTER 15

Lung Cancer Markers

K. Robert McIntire

CHAPTER 16

Central Nervous System Tumor Markers
Trevor R. Jones and Darrell D. Bigner

1

Monoclonal Antibodies to Human Tumor Antigens

William C. Raschke

Developmental Biology Laboratory, The Salk Institute, San Diego, California

1. Introduction

Human tumors are diagnosed and classified by a variety of criteria, one of which is serological analysis of cell surface antigens. In this chapter, a major recent development in serological classification, the production of monoclonal antibodies, will be evaluated.

Tumor cells express two types of surface markers that are potentially useful in clinical and therapeutic applications. Normal differentiation antigens characteristic of the stage of development of the normal cell counterpart provide one type of useful surface antigens on tumor cells. The presence of such antigens presumably represents the normal alteration of the genetic program accompanying maturation. Different forms of leukemia, for example, can now be distinguished to a great extent on the basis of surface antigens characteristic of well-defined stages of lymphocyte differentiation. The second type are tumor specific antigens that are characteristic of a particular tumor class. These antigens undoubtedly represent an abnormal alteration of the genetic program that accompanies oncogenic transformation.

Until recently, conventional antisera, typically raised in rabbits or goats, have been used to detect these antigens. Although considerable progress has been made in defining differentiation and tumor-specific antigens using these antisera, drawbacks in their preparation and use are evident. Since species-specific antigens are abundant, if not predominant, many unwanted specificities in the antisera are obtained. Only after extensive absorption regimens can the desired specificities be adequately measured. Antisera raised in nonhuman primates in order to minimize species differences have not significantly alleviated this problem. Even after extensive absorptions and a "specific" antiserum by one criterion is obtained, multiple specificities as measured in other assays often remain. Since the preparation of a specific antiserum may be tedious and difficult, the chances are good that different preparations will vary in quality, especially if prepared in different laboratories. The standardization of antiserum reagents, therefore, is indeed a difficult task.

The recent development of two techniques for the production of monoclonal antibody to preselected antigens offers an escape from many of the problems plaguing conventional antisera. The most widely used procedure is the production of hybridomas that are somatic cell hybrids resulting from the fusion of plasmacytoma tissue culture cells with antigen-specific normal cells of the B lymphocyte lineage. The second procedure involves the in vitro transformation of antigen-specific human cells by Epstein-Barr virus. Both of these techniques will be described in detail later. The fundamental importance of both procedures is the production of cloned cell lines, each of which produces a single antibody that specifically recognizes the preselected antigen. The problems accompanying extensive absorption of conventional antisera are therefore alleviated. Large scale production of the monoclonal reagents is also available, and with the widespread distribution of the cell lines or the monoclonal antibodies, every laboratory is assured of working with standardized reagents.

Since the introduction of monoclonal antibody technology in 1975, the production and usage of these reagents has expanded dramatically as many laboratories around the world became engaged in preparing the monoclonal antibodies suitable for their needs. The growth and variety of this research effort can be estimated by noting the monoclonal antibodies reported at a NIH hybridoma conference in 1978 (Melchers et al, 1978) and a review on the subject prepared in 1979 (Raschke, 1980). The seemingly exponential growth of the number of reports of new monoclonal antibody reagents and their use would make a comprehensive cataloguing of such reagents today a monumental and an unenviable task. The range of usage of this technology is equally impressive and encompasses virtually all areas of the biological sciences.

The serological analysis of human tumors clearly has need of suitable monoclonal antibody reagents. The capability for the production of reagents that can subdivide existing categories of tumors on the basis of specific surface markers will provide more accurate treatment for those with different prognoses. The possibilities for therapeutic as well as clinical applications hold great promise and will be described in a later section. At present, the field is still in its infancy since relatively few monoclonal antibodies useful in the analysis of human tumors have been developed. However, with the rapidly increasing attention to this area of research, the expectations are great.

This chapter will attempt to describe not only the monoclonal antibodies to human tumors developed to date, but also the potential usefulness of these reagents in medicine and the potential problems in their use. Similar to having one's car repaired, the replacement of one troublesome part with a better one often reveals quite glaringly the next weakest components.

2. Monoclonal Antibodies to Preselected Antigens—Technology

2.1. Hybridomas

The production of monoclonal antibodies by cell–cell hybridization is predicated on the finding that the fusion of two plasmacytoma cell lines yields a hybrid that secretes both parental immunoglobulins (Cotton and Milstein, 1973). The extension of that result predicts that the fusion of a normal plasma cell with a plasmacytoma would produce a hybrid secreting the plasma cell immunoglobulin. From other somatic cell hybrid studies, the transformed phenotype of the plasmacytoma was expected to be dominant in the hybrid over the normal (nontransformed) phenotype (Coffino et al., 1971). If the plasma cell came from an animal immunized to a particular antigen, the hybrid might secrete the specific monoclonal antibody that recognized this antigen.

The first successful hybridomas (hybrids between a plasmacytoma cell line and spleen cells) secreting immunoglobulin specific for antigen were obtained using spleen cells from a mouse immunized with sheep erythrocytes and a mouse plasmacytoma cell line (Köhler and Milstein, 1975). Approximately 10% of the hybrid clones secreted immunoglobulin with anti-sheep erythrocyte activity. Thus, a portion of the anti-sheep erythrocyte response of the mouse was immortalized through hybridization with the plasmacytoma cells.

The production of specific hybridomas utilizes the principles established by the somatic cell geneticists. Both Sendai virus and polyethylene glycol have been used as fusing agents, with the latter finding broader use owing to its universal effectiveness. The selective growth of hybrid cells out of the mixture, which contains both parent cell populations, utilizes the HAT selection method (Fig. 1). The plasmacytoma parent line must have a drug resistance genetic marker, either 8-azaguanine resistance (loss of hypoxanthine–guanine phosphoribosyl transferase activity) or 5-bromodeoxyuridine resistance (loss of thymidine kinase activity) for this selec-

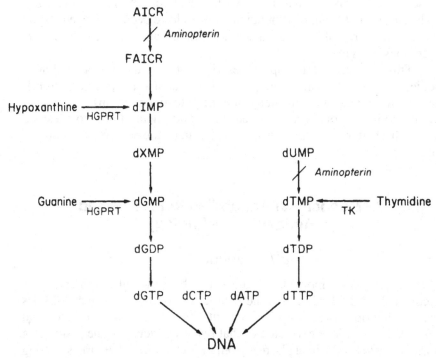

Fig. 1. The basis of HAT selection. Mutant cells lacking a functional hypoxanthine–guanine phosphoribosyl transferase (HGPRT) gene, in order to synthesize DNA, are forced to use exclusively the second pathway of deoxyguanosine triphosphate (dGTP) synthesis utilizing 5-aminoimidazole-4-carboximide ribonucleotide (AICR). Similarly, mutant cells lacking a functional thymidine kinase (TK) gene must use an alternative pathway of thymidine triphosphate (dTTP) synthesis for generating new DNA. Aminopterin, a competitive inhibitor of folate, blocks both of these alternative pathways at the steps shown. Normal cells survive in the presence of aminopterin if supplied with hypoxanthine and thymidine, but the mutants die since HGPRT⁻ cells cannot synthesize dGTP from hypoxanthine and TK ⁻ cells cannot utilize thymidine. The hybrid between a HGPRT ⁻ cell and a TK⁻ cell carries functional genes for both HGPRT and TK and is able to grow in medium containing hypoxanthine, aminopterin, and thymidine (HAT medium) (Szybalski et al., 1962; Littlefield, 1964). Hybridomas are prepared by fusing normal lymphocytes with cells of a mutant plasmacytoma line which is either HGPRT⁻ or TK ⁻. Only hybridomas will survive in the HAT selection medium, since the lymphocytes will not grow for extended periods in culture and HAT medium will kill the parental plasmacytoma line. Other terms abbreviated are 5-formamidoimidazole-4-carboximide ribonucleotide (FAICR); the monophosphates of inosine (dIMP), xanthine (dXMP), deoxyguanosine (dGMP), and thymidine (dTMP), the diphosphates of deoxyguanosine (dGDP) and thymidine (dTDP), and the triphosphates of deoxycytidine (dCTP) and deoxyadenosine (dATP).

tion procedure. After fusion, the unfused drug-resistant plasmacytoma cells then die in HAT medium, the unfused normal cells do not survive extended periods in culture, and only the hybrids, which have acquired the growth potential of the plasmacytoma and the functional enzyme for nucleotide metabolism from the normal cell genome, are able to survive (Fig. 2).

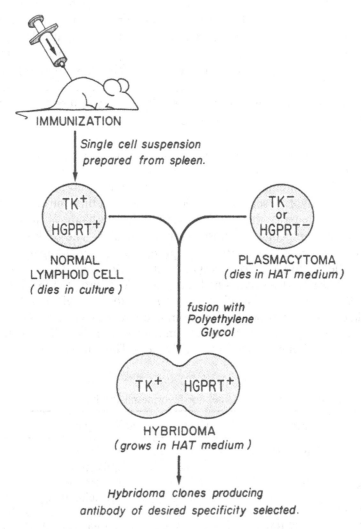

Fig. 2. The production and selection of antigen-specific hybridomas. The selection of hybrids by HAT medium is described in Fig. 1. The screening of hybridoma clones secreting the desired immunoglobulin products is described in the text.

The normal cell participating in a fusion yielding an antigen-specific hybrid undoubtedly comes from the B cell lineage. Since several workers have observed an unexpectedly high proportion of antigen-specific hybridomas, antigenically activated B cells seem to have a selective advantage over resting B cells in the hybridization process (Köhler and Milstein, 1975, 1976; Köhler and Shulman, 1978). Although the assumption is usually made that an immunoglobulin-secreting plasmablast or plasma cell is the cell type involved in specific hybridoma formation, recent evidence from fusions of B lymphoma lines with plasmacytomas indicates that the nonsecreting B lymphocyte bearing surface immunoglobulin receptors may also yield hybridomas secreting antigen-specific immunoglobulins (Raschke et al., 1979; Laskov et al., 1979; Levy and Dilley, 1978). The latter finding may have considerable signficance since the selective purification of antigen-specific B cells by available procedures may provide the means for obtaining high frequencies of hybrids with the desired characteristics.

Several advances and refinements have been made since the original reports. A number of murine plasmacytoma lines have now been selected that synthesize no immunoglobulin chains themselves (Table 1 and Fig. 3). The resulting hybrids secrete only the immunoglobulin contributed by the normal cell parent, thereby eliminating the problem of inactive immunoglobulin molecules composed of mixed chains. The finding that rat immune cells can be fused with mouse plasmacytomas yielding hybrids that secrete the rat immunoglobulin (Galfre et al., 1977) and the development of a rat plasmacytoma line suitable for hybridoma production (Galfre et al., 1979), extended the specificities available to those of the rat.

To date, hybridoma production is limited exclusively to the use of mouse and rat plasmacytoma lines and to immunized normal cells from the same two species (but see note at end of chapter). Thus, monoclonal anti-

Table 1
Plasmacytoma Cell Lines for Hybridoma Production

Cell line	Strain	Chains secreted	Reference
P3-X63-Ag8	BALB/c (mouse)	κ, γ_1	Köhler and Milstein (1975)
P3-NSI-1-Ag4-1	BALB/c	κ^a	Köhler and Milstein (1976)
P3-X63-Ag8.653	BALB/c	None	Kearney et al. (1979)
MPC11-45.6TG1.7	BALB/c	κ, γ_{2b}	Margulies et al. (1976)
SP2/O-Ag14	BALB/c	None	Shulman et al. (1978)
S194/5.XXO.BU.1	BALB/c	None	Trowbridge (1978)
210.RCY3.Ag.1.2.3	Lou (rat)	κ	Galfre et al. (1979)

[a]Light chain is intracellular in NS-1, but secreted in hybridomas.

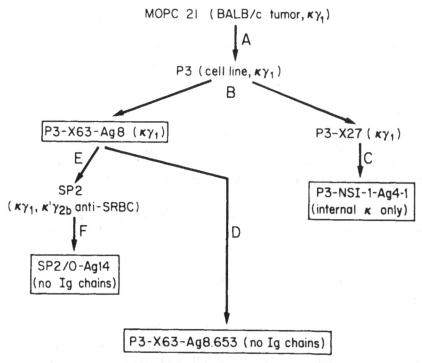

Fig. 3. History of one plasmacytoma line used to make hybridomas. The tumor MOPC 21, has been adapted to cell culture (step A) and two subclones selected (step B) (Horibata and Harris, 1970). A further subclone of one of the lines (step C) was found to have lost immunoglobulin secretion while still synthesizing light chain intracellularly (Köhler and Milstein, 1976). In step D a subclone was specifically selected for lack of immunoglobulin expression (Kearney et al., 1979) and synthesizes no immunoglobulin chains. In step E, a hybridoma, SP2, between P3-X63-Ag8 and an antisheep erythrocyte (SRBC) spleen cell was selected and found to secrete all four immunoglobulin chains of both parents (Köhler and Milstein, 1976). A subclone of this hybridoma synthesizes no immunoglobulin chains, presumably due to chromosomal segregation (Shulman et al., 1978). Each cell line that has been used to make hybridomas is boxed in the figure. Each has been seleced for loss of HGPRT gene expression (see Fig. 1) and therefore dies in HAT medium.

bodies presumably can be prepared against any determinant capable of eliciting an antibody response in these species. The extension of the technique to species more distantly related than mice and rats has so far failed. For example, immune cells from the rabbit, a species in which antibodies are commonly generated, fuse successfully with mouse plasmacytomas but the hybrids do not secrete complete rabbit immunoglobulin molecules (Köhler and Shulman, 1978). The establishment of a rabbit plasmacytoma cell line may possibly alleviate this obstacle. Human plasmacytomas in culture have been reported (Krueger et al., 1976; Burk et al., 1978;

Ralph, 1979) but have yet to be shown useful for making human hybridomas (see note at end of chapter). Human monoclonal reagents will presumably be the most useful in some cases, such as in vivo administration and the study of those antigenic determinants recognized by the human immune system. Transformation of human lymphocytes by Epstein-Barr virus is an alternative to hybridomas for the generation of human monoclonal antibodies and is discussed further in a later section.

Perhaps the most troublesome aspect of antigen-specific monoclonal antibody production has been the screening of large numbers of hybrids for the few that are secreting the product of interest. A wide variety of relatively quick and easy methods have recently been devised that greatly ease this problem.

In human tumor antigen research the precise determinants being studied often are not known and are many times hypothetical. One typically hopes to find a monoclonal antibody specificity that will discriminate between tumor types without knowing for sure beforehand that such a determinant exists. Therefore, a quick and definitive assay is particularly important in the preparation of monoclonal antibodies to human tumors since they must be screened against a large panel of cells. First, the clones producing antibody that bind the cell used for immunization must be selected out of the many clones typically produced in an experiment. These must then be screened against normal cell types and a statistically significant number of tumors of a variety of classes to determine the pattern of reactivity. This pattern of reactivity will ultimately determine the usefulness of each monclonal antibody. Clearly, maximizing efficiency in specificity testing has earned considerable attention.

Most of the assays for reactivity of monoclonal antibodies simply measure binding to the antigen since this is usually the only property required. Sensitive radioimmunoassays have been developed for the rapid screening of large numbers of monoclonal antibodies (Parkhouse and Guarnotta, 1978; Nowinski et al., 1979; Stocker and Heusser, 1979; Schneider and Eisenbarth, 1979; Brown et al., 1979). Similarly, an enzyme-linked immunosorbant assay (ELISA) utilizing a binding assay system coupled to the action of alkaline phosphatase on p-nitrophenyl-phosphate provides a colorimetric determination of reactivity (Kearney et al., 1979). Some innovations have made use of fluorescence techniques (Guesdon et al., 1979; Phillips et al., 1980) while others have provided means of testing the products of hybridoma colonies grown in soft agar (Sharon et al., 1979). A particularly elegant technique selects antigen-specific hybrids from the original mixture of fusion products and clones them in one step (Parks et al., 1979). For this procedure, HAT-resistant hybrids are incubated with fluorescent-labeled antigen and single fluorescent cells are sorted directly into separate microwells by a fluorescence-activated cell sorter.

For some purposes, monoclonal antibodies with special properties are required. For example, an antibody that is cytotoxic for the target cell in the presence of complement can be detected by a plaque assay (Marshak-Rothstein et al., 1979). The plaque assay has broad usage since it may be used with non-erythrocyte target cells. Biochemical analysis of antigens often requires monoclonal antibody that precipitates the antigen from detergent lysates of labeled cells. An efficient method of cross-pooling hybridoma products, immunoprecipitation and gel analysis is now available for analyzing hybridomas (Brown et al., 1980).

Not all of the advances have occurred in screening procedures. Preselection and enrichment of antigen-specific cells prior to fusion have been shown to increase the proportion of specific hybridomas. The induction of tolerance to unwanted specificities (Middleton et al., 1980), the use of blocking antibodies to unwanted specificities at the time of immunization (Kennett and Gilbert, 1979) and the immunization regimen itself (Stähli et al., 1980) have each been effective. In a preliminary report, the direct attachment of antigen to the plasmacytoma cell surface prior to fusion was shown to significantly increase the yield of antigen-specific hybrids (Hodach and Winkelhake, 1980).

2.2. Epstein-Barr Virus Transformation of Human Lymphocytes

Although responses to human antigens can be generated by xenogeneic immunizations of mice and rats, many specificities, particularly those to human alloantigens (e.g., histocompatibility and blood group antigens), have been defined using human antisera. Thus, the human humoral immune response in the form of human monoclonal antibodies is particularly desirable. The prospects for the production of human hybridomas seem dim at present since no plasmacytoma cell line has yet proved useful for this purpose (see note at end of chapter).

An alternative means of producing antigen-specific human monoclonal antibodies has now been succesfully explored (Steinitz et al., 1977). The approach is based on the finding that the Epstein-Barr virus (EBV) transforms human B lymphocytes in vitro to generate permanent immunoglobulin-secreting cell lines. Although most human B lymphocytes have cell surface receptors for EBV (Jondal and Klein, 1973), the subpopulation of B lymphocytes that has already begun to secrete immunoglobulin seems to contain the cells susceptible to EBV transformation (Steel et al., 1977). By using peripheral blood lymphocytes from donors with high natural antibody levels to a particular antigen and using cells bearing the antigen to rosette and enrich the antigen-binding lymphocytes, the transformation of antigen-specific lymphocytes with EBV has been achieved (Steinitz et al., 1977). The resulting cell cultures not only

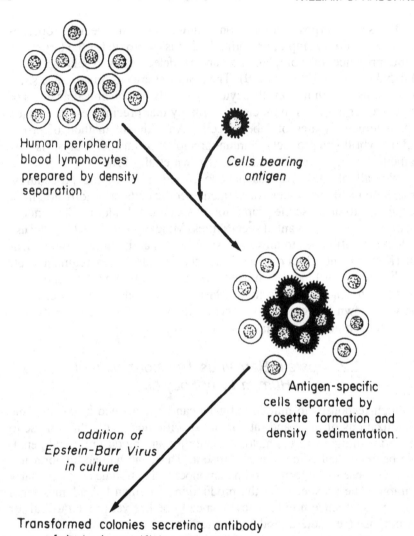

Human peripheral
blood lymphocytes
prepared by density
separation.

*Cells bearing
antigen*

Antigen-specific
cells separated by
rosette formation and
density sedimentation.

*addition of
Epstein-Barr Virus
in culture*

Transformed colonies secreting antibody
of desired specificity selected

Fig. 4. Transformation of antigen-specific human lymphocytes by Epstein-Barr virus for the production of human monoclonal antibodies (Steinitz et al., 1977).

form rosettes with the proper target cell, but secrete sufficient levels of immunoglobulin to give plaques in a plaque-forming cell assay. The secreted immunoglobulin also agglutinates cells expressing the antigen.

The critical condition for production of specific antibody-forming human cell lines by this procedure is the selection of an enriched B lymphocyte population having affinity for the chosen antigen. In cultures where the preselection had not been performed, no antigen-specific cell lines were derived. This result is expected since the possibility of finding a cell that binds a single determinant in a "non-immunized" lymphocyte population is certainly low.

Owing to the ease of production of hybridomas and the handy accessibility and flexibility of using immunized laboratory animals, the production of monoclonal antibodies by EBV transformation has not been nearly as prolific as the production of the reagents by hybridoma research. Specificities to only four antigens have been produced to date. Two of them, NNP (Steinitz et al., 1977) and TNP (Kozbor et al., 1979), are synthetic haptens that were used to establish the technology. Human monoclonal antibodies to tetanus toxoid (Zurawski et al., 1978) and Rh-antigen (Koskimies, 1979) mark the first efforts to make medically useful reagents. The former is the forerunner of human monoclonal reagents to human pathogens and the latter to tissue typing antigens. At this point in the early history of this technology, its eventual usefulness in the study of human tumor antigens is not certain.

3. Monoclonal Antibodies to Human Tumors

Although hybridoma technology has been a relatively recent development, a variety of monoclonal antibodies to human tumors have been produced. Specificities to both normal differentiation antigens and tumor-associated antigens are potentially useful in the detection, classification, and the subsequent assignments of prognosis and treatment. The properties of monoclonal antibodies to both types of antigens are described below and represent the beginning effort in a burgeoning field.

3.1. Leukemia Antigens

The leukemias provide an excellent example of the usefulness of both normal differentiation antigens and tumor-associated antigens for the discrimination of different tumor types. The hematopoietic system contains a vast assortment of cell types, the full complexity of which is still being unraveled. Within each lineage, whether it be T lymphocyte, B lymphocyte, monocyte, etc., a number of different stages of differentiation have been identified. Neoplasms of each stage of maturation are conceivably possible, and some have vastly different prognoses with correspondingly different treatments. Therefore, differentiation antigens that distinguish the cell types will also be of great assistance in assigning classifications of tumors. A thorough description of normal antigens and tumor antigens associated with leukemias is presented in Chapter 2. Only a brief summary of the monoclonal antibodies produced that discriminate between forms of leukemia will be presented here and the reader is directed to Chapter 2 for greater detail on this subject.

Each of 20 monoclonal antibodies specific for T lymphocytes seems to recognize a different determinant and thus a different portion of the spectrum of normal cells and leukemic cells (Table 2) (Fox et al., 1981). These first hybridomas undoubtedly only scratch the surface of lymphocyte subset antigens. Some of the specificities correlate with known functional properties of T lymphocyte subsets. Others have already been shown to distinguish between T cell leukemias. One study has initiated the diagnostic application of monoclonal antibodies by using the reactivity profile of three monoclonal specificities to distinguish high risk T cell leukemias from those with standard risk (Zipf et al., 1980).

Four B cell monoclonal specificities have been reported. One monoclonal antibody binds to all B cell lines and B cell CLL tumors, but not to a myeloma line, a T cell line, null cell lines, acute myelomonocytic leukemias, and acute lymphocytic leukemias of the T or null cell type (Brooks et al., 1980). Of normal cells all T lymphocytes are negative, but only 9–21% of peripheral B lymphocytes are positive, indicating that this hybridoma reacts with a subset of B lymphocytes. Interestingly, another hybridoma specificity recognizes an antigen that is linked to the HLA locus, is also found on mouse and rat B cells and is linked to the mouse and rat histocompatibility loci as well (Gasser et al., 1979). A preliminary report describes a hybridoma antibody that binds to all pre-B cell lines and surface immunoglobulin positive (B cell) ALL and CLL tumor cells (Abramson et al., 1980). Only a subset of B lymphocytes is detected by this reagent. Another monoclonal specificity recognizes B lymphoblastic lines, B cell tumors, and some null cell ALL tumors (Chan et al., 1980). Such specificities, which overlap existing classifications, may yield more accurate groupings with regard to prognosis and treatment assignment.

A monoclonal antibody specific for peripheral blood monocytes and granulocytes has been reported (Breard et al., 1980). Most acute myelomonocytic leukemias are also recognized by this antibody, although thymocytes, lymphocytes, and lymphoid (both B and T cell) tumors and cell lines are negative. However, two myeloid lines are also negative. The adherent population of monocytes is preferentially recognized by this specificity, providing further evidence that a subpopulation of myeloid cells and tumors express this determinant.

3.2. Melanoma Antigens

Melanoma tumors are known to express cell surface antigens to which the melanoma patients can mount an immune response (Hellström and Brown, 1979). Both humoral and cell-mediated responses to these antigens have been demonstrated in these patients (Hellström et al., 1971; Lewis et al., 1969). Considerable evidence indicates the responses are directed against two classes of melanoma-associated antigens. Antigens of one class are restricted in expression to a single melanoma, or at most, to a

Table 2

Monoclonal Antibodies to Human Tumor-Associated Antigens

Name	Immunogen	Characteristics		Antigen	References
		Binds	Does not bind		
		Leukemia Antigens—T cell[a]			
17F12	T-ALL	Peripheral T cells Thymocytes T-ALLs	B cells B cell lines Monocytes	67,000	Engleman et al. (1980) Fox et al. (1980)
12E7	T-ALL cell line	Cortical thymocytes T-ALLs Some null ALLs	B cell leukemias B lymphoblastoid lines Myeloid tumors	28,000	Levy et al. (1979)
T101	T cell line	Peripheral T cells T-ALLs T-CLLs B-CLLs	B cells Lymphosarcoma cell leukemias Hairy cell leukemias, myelomas Burkitt's lymphoma	65,000	Royston et al. (1980)
3A1	T cell line	65% Peripheral T cells	B cells Monocytes Polymorphonuclear leukocytes	ND[b]	Haynes et al. (1979) Eisenbarth et al. (1980)
9.3(HuLyt-1)	T cell line	50–80% Peripheral T cells 20–50% Thymocytes 4 of 6 Leukemia lines	B cells Monocytes B cell lines	44,000	Hansen et al. (1980)
OKT1	Peripheral T cells	10% Thymocytes All peripheral T cells T-CLLs	B cells Null cells Monocytes Granulocytes T-ALLs	67,000	Reinherz et al. (1979a)

(continued)

Table 2 (*cont.*)

| Name | Immunogen | Characteristics | | | References |
		Binds	Does not bind	Antigen	
OKT3	Peripheral T cells	10% Thymocytes All peripheral T cells	B cells Null cells Monocytes Granulocytes 20 of 21 T-ALLs	20,000	Kung et al. (1979)
OKT4	Peripheral T cells	80% Thymocytes 55% Peripheral T cells Helper T cells	B cells Null cells Monocytes Granulocytes 19 of 21 T-ALLs	62,000	Reinherz et al. (1979b) Terhorst et al. (1980)
α-Leu1	Peripheral T cells	80–95% Peripheral T cells Thymocytes 11 of 14 B-CLLs	B cells B lymphoblastoid cells	69,000 and 71,000	Wang et al. (1980)
OKT5	Thymocytes	80% Thymocytes 20% Peripheral T cells Cytotoxic/suppressor T cells	B cells Null cells Monocytes Granulocytes 20 of 21 T-ALLs	30,000 and 32,000	Reinherz et al. (1980b) Terhorst et al. (1980)
OKT6	Thymocytes	70% Thymocytes	Peripheral T cells B cells 16 of 21 T-ALLs	ND	Reinherz et al. (1980a)
OKT8	Thymocytes	80% Thymocytes 30% Peripheral T cells	B cells 17 of 21 T-ALLs	ND	Reinherz et al. (1980a)
OKT9	Thymocytes	10% Thymocytes	Peripheral T cells B cells 12 of 21 T-ALLs	ND	Reinherz et al. (1980a)

Antibody	Immunogen	Reactivity		MW	Reference
OKT10	Thymocytes	95% Thymocytes 21 of 22 T-ALLs	Peripheral T cells	ND	Reinherz et al. (1980a)
NA1/34(HTA-1)	Thymocytes	85% Thymocytes 1 of 1 T cell line	Peripheral lymphocytes (B and T) 1 B lymphoblastoid line	45,000	McMichael et al. (1979)
			Leukemia Antigens—B cell		
HC11A	B cell line	60–70% B cells in blood B lymphoblastoid lines CLLs	T cells Null cells A myeloma line T cell lines Null cell lines	ND	Brooks et al. (1980)
MB-1	Pre-B line	5–20% PBLs Pre-B-ALLs B-ALLs B-CLLs	T-ALL tumors and cell lines AMLs	ND	Abramson et al. (1980)
G4F8	(Not reported)	B cell tumors and cell lines Some null ALLs	T cell lines	ND	Chan et al. (1980)
H76	Rat lymphocytes	B cells B cell lines 1 of 1 Null cell line	T cells T cell lines	ND	Gasser et al. (1979)
			Leukemia Antigens—Monocyte		
OKM1	Mononuclear cells	Granulocytes AMLs	Thymocytes Lymphocytes T or B cell tumors Lymphoblastoid lines 2 of 2 myeloid lines	ND	Breard et al. (1980)

(continued)

Table 2 (cont.)

Name	Immunogen	Characteristics Binds	Characteristics Does not bind	Antigen	References
Melanoma Antigens					
4.1	Melanoma cell line	90% of melanomas 55% of other tumors	Skin fibroblasts B lymphoblastoid lines	97,000	Woodbury et al. (1980)
3.1, 3.2, and 3.3	Melanoma tumor	Immunizing melanoma only out of 12 melanomas	PBL Fibroblasts Carcinomas Sarcomas CLLs Lymphoblastoid lines	ND	Yeh et al. (1979)
691-13-17	Melanoma tumor	8 of 9 melanomas (both primary superficial spreading tumors and metastatic tumors)	Fibroblasts A giant hairy nevus Colorectal carcinomas	ND	Koprowski et al. (1978) Steplewski et al. (1979)
691-19-19	Melanoma tumor	7 of 8 melanomas (both primary superficial spreading tumors and metastatic tumors)	Fibroblasts A giant hairy nevus	ND	Koprowski et al. (1978) Steplewski et al. (1979)
Colorectal Carcinoma Antigens					
1116NS-3d 1116NS-33a	Group I CRC cell lines	8 of 8 CRCs	Normal colonic mucosa Lung and breast carcinomas Melanomas Astrocytomas Sarcomas	180,000(CEA) ND	Koprowski et al. (1979)
1116NS-22				ND	
1116NS-29				ND	

Antibody	Antigen/specificity	Molecular weight	Reference
1116-56-2	Sarcomas	32,000 and 39,000	
1083-17-1A			
1116NS-33b	Same as group I, except binds to 2 of 10 melanomas	ND	
1116NS-20	Same as group I, except binds to 9 of 10 melanomas, a breast carcinoma, and an astrocytoma	180,000(CEA), 130,000, and 60,000	
1116NS-38e	Same as Group I, except binds to only 7 of 8 CRCs	ND	
1116NS-43	Same as Group I, except binds to 7 of 8 CRCs and 1 of 10 melanomas	ND	
1116NS-10		ND	
1116NS-3a	Same as Group I, except binds to 6 of 8 CRCs	ND	
1116NS-38a		ND	
1116NS-38b	Same as Group I, except binds to 5 of 8 CRCs	ND	
1116NS-38c		ND	
1116NS-3b		ND	
1116NS-19		ND	
1116NS-36	Same as Group I, except binds to 5 of 8 CRCs and 1 of 10 melanomas	ND	
1116NS-52a		ND	
1116NS-52b	Same as Group I, except binds to 4 of 8 CRCs	ND	
1116NS-15	Pure CEA CEA Colorectal carcinomas	ND	
VII-23	CEA-crossreacting antigen (NGP) Colonic mucosa Normal lung	180,000(CEA)	Accolla et al. (1980)

(continued)

Table 2 (*cont.*)

Name	Immunogen	Characteristics			References
		Binds	Does not bind	Antigen	
VII-37	Pure CEA	CEA Colorectal carcinomas	CEA-crossreacting antigen (NGP) Colonic mucosa Normal lung	180,000(CEA)	Accolla et al. (1980)
41/9 50/3 73/3 73/8	Pure AFP	Amniotic fluid Hepatoma serum Teratocarcinoma serum	*Alphafetoprotein* Normal adult serum	70,000(AFP)	Uotila et al. (1980)
PII53/3	Neuroblastoma cell line	Fetal brain 1 of 2 retinoblastomas A glioblastoma	*Neuroblastoma Antigens* Adult brain Fetal fibroblast line	ND	Kennett and Gilbert (1979)

[a]See also Fox and Baird (1980).
[b]Not determined.

very small number (Lewis et al., 1969; Shiku et al., 1976). Those of the other class are shared by most melanomas and some other tumors (Shiku et al., 1976; Cornain et al., 1975).

Hybridoma antibodies, which represent part of the mouse antihuman melanoma response, exhibit specificities that fall in the same two classes (Table 2). Several studies have reported monoclonal antibodies that react either exclusively with the melanoma used for immunization or with that tumor plus at most only a few other melanomas (Koprowski et al., 1978; Steplewski et al., 1979; Yeh et al., 1979). The various reports have used different tumor cells from nonmelanoma neoplasms and different normal cell populations to determine specificity. The overall conclusion is that these antibodies do not react with a wide variety of carcinomas and leukemias. Normal skin fibroblasts, cells from a giant hairy nevus, as well as peripheral blood lymphocytes have also been found negative with monoclonal antibodies of this class. The implication from these findings is that many melanoma-associated antigens exist and that each melanoma expresses only a small number of them. A small number of antimelanoma specificities were tested against primary superficial spreading melanomas and metastatic melanomas. None could distinguish between the two forms of the disease (Steplewski et al., 1979).

Monoclonal antibodies with the second class of reactivity with melanomas recognize most melanomas and approximately 50% of a wide spectrum of carcinomas and sarcomas (Woodbury et al., 1980). Positive nonmelanoma tumors include carcinomas of the bladder, breast, colon, kidney, lung, and ovary as well as liposarcomas and an osteogenic sarcoma. Not all tumors of each type were positive, however, so these specificities do not at this point offer clear discrimination among any of the tumor types, including melanomas.

The reactivity of this second class of antimelanoma monoclonal antibodies illustrates brilliantly one of the problems faced in the study of tumor antigens as specific markers of tumor cells. These antigens, which are recognized and defined by monospecific reagents, not only appear on various tumor types, but among the melanoma tumors tested, they appear in quantitatively different amounts (Woodbury et al., 1980). With one monoclonal antibody, for example, the binding to the immunizing melanoma was set at 100%. The remaining 24 melanomas tested had binding levels ranging from 75 to 0.3% with virtually all levels of intermediate values observed. Determination of cutoff levels for positive binding and the interpretation of this marker as a melanoma-associated antigen is certainly not as definitive as one would like. Further complicating the issue is the report that a few normal cell lines show positive binding with this class of antimelanoma monospecific antibodies (Herlyn et al., 1979), although a large number of normal human fibroblast and lymphoblastoid lines were negative as were peripheral blood lymphocytes and normal tissues of skin, muscle, fascia, lung, placenta, ovary, fallopian tube, and uterus (Woodbury et al., 1980; Herlyn et al., 1979).

A 97,000 dalton cell surface protein (p97) is immunoprecipitated from labeled cell extracts by one monoclonal antibody with the broad range specificity (Woodbury et al., 1980). This molecule was immunoprecipitated from extracts of two of four melanomas and the single carcinoma (breast) tested. All normal human tissues tested for p97 were negative. (See Chapter 3 for 94K and 240K antigens.)

The usefulness of the monoclonal antimelanoma specificities in clinical applications is limited at present. The specificities unique to a particular melanoma will not be of general use until a large number of these specificities corresponding to most of the variations in these melanoma-associated antigens are produced or until it becomes practical to prepare this type of monoclonal reagent on a case by case basis. The broad-specificity monoclonal antibodies may prove to be more useful for possible clinical or therapeutic uses since a melanoma patient is unlikely to have a second tumor and the number of normal cell types bearing these determinants appears to be small.

Of possible therapeutic interest is the recent finding that an antimelanoma monoclonal antibody suppressed the growth of a human melanoma in nude mice (Koprowski et al., 1978; Herlyn et al., 1979). In vitro analysis of this phenomenon showed that the rejection probably resulted from antibody-dependent cell-mediated cytotoxicity and not complement-mediated lysis.

3.3. Colorectal Carcinoma Antigens

One of the most common malignant tumors in man is colorectal carcinoma. Many studies have been directed toward identifying and characterizing tumor-specific antigens of these tumors, with the result that no antigens of this type are universally agreed upon (Goldenberg, 1976; Gold et al., 1979). The carcinoembryonic antigen (CEA), for example, is present on the cell surface of colorectal carcinomas and cells from digestive organs of fetuses of 2- to 6-month gestation (Gold et al., 1979; Pritchard and Todd, 1979). Since CEA is also found on some noncolorectal tumors and on a small proportion of cells from the normal human colon mucosa, the classification of CEA both as a specific marker for a subset of fetal cells and as a tumor-specific antigen is inaccurate (Goldenberg, 1976; Shively et al., 1978; Pusztaszeri and Mach, 1973). However, the presence of CEA in the blood and on lingering tumor cells is potentially very useful in the monitoring of colorectal carcinoma patients in various stages of treatment or remission (Fuks et al., 1980). Other antigenic markers will possibly allow further definition of the stages or forms of this disease.

Monoclonal antibodies have been prepared against colorectal carcinoma cells and against purified CEA (Table 2). Out of approximately 20 anticolorectal carcinoma hybridomas (Koprowski et al.,1979) six reacted exclusively with all eight of these tumors tested. Lung and breast carcinomas, melanomas, astrocytomas, sarcomas, leukemias, and lymphoblastoid lines were negative, as were normal fibroblasts, brain cells, and erythrocytes. The other monoclonal antibodies produced in this study reacted with only a portion, 50–88%, of the colorectal carcinomas tested.

At least five different tumor-associated determinants were identified on the tumor cells using the hybridomas specificities in competition binding (Koprowski et al., 1979). In some cases the molecular species bearing these determinants were identified. One antibody immunoprecipitates 32,000 and 39,000 dalton proteins from an extract of biosynthetically labeled carcinoma cells. Not known is whether these molecules share the same determinant, exist as a complex, or have a precursor–product relationship. Two other monoclonal antibodies with specificities for different determinants immunoprecipitate a 36,000 dalton protein. Different determinants on the same molecule or different molecules of the same size are both possibilities. Other monoclonal antibodies do not immunoprecipitate any proteins from extracts of labeled cells. Some of the possible explanations for this finding are that either the determinant or the immunoglobulin binding site may be unstable in the presence of detergent, that the determinant is a carbohydrate and present on glycolipids, or that the labeling procedure did not label the protein bearing the determinant.

Of the anticolorectal carcinoma hybridoma antibodies described in this study, two were found to react with CEA. One recognizes a determinant shared by other cell surface molecules and is present on a variety of tumor types. The other exclusively recognizes the 180,000-dalton CEA molecule.

Another group of investigators using purified CEA for the immunization of mice for hybridoma production has prepared two monoclonal antibodies specific for CEA (Accolla et al., 1980). In competitive binding experiments the hybridoma products were also shown to recognize different determinants on the CEA molecules. Both determinants are absent on cells from normal colon mucosa and normal lung, and also distinct from the crossreacting antigen present in large quantities in normal adult tissues (Shively and Todd, 1980). Both antibodies react with frozen sections and cell lines of CEA-positive colon carcinomas.

The possibility exists that the tumor-associated antigens other than CEA detected on colorectal carcinoma cells by hybridoma antibodies also represent re-expression of other embryonic antigens. The antigens could be responsible for the perception of division-initiating signals, which may well be the common parameter between tumor cells exhibiting unrestrained growth and fetal cells proliferating in the normal maturation process. In support of this possibility is the finding that four hybridomas putatively specific for colorectal carcinomas and negative for a wide variety of other tumors and normal cells show positive reactivity with teratocarcinomas (Koprowski et al., 1979).

3.4. Alphafetoprotein

Alphafetoprotein (AFP), like carcinoembryonic antigen, is a gene product normally expressed in embryonal and fetal stages of development and reexpressed in restricted classes of tumors in adults (Ruoslahti and Seppälä, 1979; Sell, 1980). AFP is predominantly produced by cells of the yolk sac and by hepatocytes of the fetal liver. Abnormally high AFP levels in amniotic fluid or maternal serum have proved to be a valuable prenatal diagnostic tool for a variety of fetal abnormalities including aberrant pregnancies, neural tube defects, and congenital nephrosis. Increased levels of AFP are also often observed in adults with liver injury or disease and in these conditions may be associated with regeneration efforts by hematocytes.

Analogous with the embryonal sites of AFP synthesis, tumors of adult hematocytes (primary hepatocarcinomas) and yolk sac cells of the ovary and testis (teratocarcinomas) produce AFP and result in elevated levels in the serum. Approximately 70–80% of all hepatocarcinomas (hepatocellular and cholangiocellular) and essentially all multipotent embryonal carcinomas containing elements analogous to the yolk sac (endodermal sinus tumors, choriocarcinomas, and teratocarcinomas) produce AFP (Ruoslahti and Seppälä, 1979; Sell, 1980).

Rising or prolonged elevation of AFP levels have been used diagnostically for monitoring hepatocarcinoma and teratocarcinoma tumor burden as well as liver disease and abnormal pregnancies. In an effort to standardize the radioimmunoassay for AFP, an international standard preparation consisting of pooled human cord blood has been prepared and an international unit of AFP defined (Sizaret et al., 1975). Since differences between normal and pathological levels of AFP are often small, the accuracy of the radioimmunoassay is critical. Monospecific antibody reagents could reduce some of the variables introduced by a polyspecific antiserum and thus increase the accuracy of the assay.

To standardize the anti-AFP reagent and to study the antigenic determinants of AFP, monoclonal antibodies have been prepared to AFP (Uotila et al., 1980). Using spleen cells from mice immunized with purified AFP, four hybridomas have been produced with anti-AFP specificity (Table 2). Two have relatively high affinity for AFP. When tested against a variety of AFP samples, including normal adult serum, amniotic fluid, teratocarcinoma serum, hepatocarcinoma serum, and the international standard, the monoclonal antibodies gave essentially identical results with a conventional anti-AFP serum. Thus, the monoclonal antibodies exhibit similar specificity in the AFP radioimmunoassay to that of the conventional assay.

AFP exists as molecular variants on the basis of concanavalin A binding (Ruoslahti et al., 1978). These variants are diagnostically significant in pregnancies where the fetus has anencephaly, spina bifida, or congenital nephrosis and in patients with teratocarcinomas (Ruoslahti et al., 1979; Smith et al., 1979). Neither conventional antisera nor the monoclonal antibodies to AFP prepared so far distinquish between these variants. The future selection of hybridomas specific for the variant forms of AFP will undoubtedly be of considerable clinical usefulness.

3.5. Neuroblastoma Antigens

A hybridoma prepared against a human neuroblastoma recognizes an antigen present on all eight neuroblastomas tested, a retinoblastoma, and a glioblastoma (Table 2) (Kennett and Gilbert, 1979). All three classes of tumors are of cell types that are embryologically derived from the neuroectoderm. Since the antigen is also found on cells of the fetal brain, but not the adult brain, the antigen recognized by this monoclonal antibody represents yet another example of an embryonal differentiation antigen reexpressed on tumors of the corresponding cell type in the adult. This hybridoma antibody does not react with peripheral blood lymphocytes, T and B lymphoblastoid cell lines, HeLa cells, a fibroblast line, a fibrosarcoma line, and a hepatoma line.

The production of a larger repertoire of antineuroblastoma hybridomas will hopefully provide a classification scheme for these tumors. These reagents would not only provide useful reagents for clinical use in tumor cases, but also for research into the cell lineages and architecture in the nervous system.

4. Potential Diagnostic and Therapeutic Uses of Monoclonal Antibodies

The advantages of antibodies produced by hybridomas and transformed human lymphocytes over conventional antisera stem from the homogeneity of the reagent. The homogeneity, and thus monospecificity, of each reagent is insured by the clonal origin of the cultured cell lines. With the elimination of unwanted specificities and variations in preparations of conventional antisera, standard antibody reagents will be possible on an international basis for a wide range of diagnostic, prognostic, and therapeutic uses.

The diagnostic uses of monoclonal antibodies are already evident from studies of leukemias. The wide variety of hematopoietic cell types and their malignant states makes accurate diagnosis of the tumors on morphological and histological grounds difficult and in many cases inadequate. The serological identification of subsets of hematopoietic malignancies having a poor prognosis and those having a better prognosis is feasible on the basis of studies using conventional antisera (Lister et al., 1979; Pesando et al., 1979; Reinherz et al., 1979c). Monoclonal antibodies have been used to identify three subsets of T cell acute lymphoblastic leukemias that correspond to three normal thymocyte maturation stages (Reinherz and Schlossman, 1980). Of particular significance is a study on the use of similar monoclonal antibodies to subdivide all acute lymphoblastic leukemias into distinct groups, one of which contains exclusively those carrying a poor prognosis (Zipf et al., 1980). With this information, those patients requiring a more rigorous treatment can be identified. Those with a less severe form of disease may then be spared unnecessarily devastating treatments.

Another diagnostic use of monoclonal antibody reagents is the monitoring of patients during remission for the reappearance of tumor cells. The appearance of CEA and AFP in the sera of patients not only accompanies the initial onset of the associated tumor, but also accompanies the reappearance of tumor cells after remission. Regular monitoring of sera from the patients can provide evidence of relapse before morphological appearance of tumor cells is observed. Similarly, serological detection of leukemia-associated antigens in the bone marrow of patients with acute myeloblastic leukemia provided evidence of relapse an average of 3.7 months before standardly used morphological criteria (Baker et al., 1979). Since overt relapse of the disease is usually fatal in spite of reinduction efforts by chemotherapy, the significantly earlier detection of relapse may allow effective therapy before the disease becomes beyond control.

Several therapeutic approaches have been suggested for the use of monoclonal antibodies to eliminate tumor cells. Among these are the physical separation (Stocker et al., 1979) and direct killing by in vitro complement-mediated lysis (Thierfelder et al., 1979) of tumor cells of the hematopoietic lineages using the appropriate tumor-specific antibody. In such cases, the normal cells could be reinfused into the patient. The arrest of tumor growth in model systems has also been reported. Human melanoma and colorectal carcinomas, which grow and produce tumors in nude mice, do not produce tumors if these mice are given a hybridoma antibody specific for a tumor antigen on the corresponding tumor (Koprowski et al., 1978; Herlyn et al., 1979). The inhibition of tumor growth in these cases appears to owe to antibody-dependent cell-mediated cytotoxicity. A second mechanism for inhibiting tumor development is the direct blockage of tumor cell division, as has been demonstrated in an in vitro murine lymphoma model system (McGrath et al., 1980). Select monoclonal antibodies to cell surface molecules on these cells reversibly inhibit cell division, indicating that these tumor cells and possibly all tumor cells are under cell surface regulation for stimulation and cessation of DNA synthesis.

Finally, the unique specificities of antibodies recognizing tumor-associated antigens for tumor cells has inspired the use of these antibodies to carry covalently bound toxic agents directly to the tumor cells. This "poisoned arrow" strategy is especially appealing since the toxic agent can be delivered to all areas of the body normally reached by antibody. A variety of toxic agents (Gregoriadis, 1977) have been employed including toxins, such as diphtheria toxin (Philpott et al., 1973; Moolten et al., 1972); radioisotopes (McGaughey, 1974), which would irradiate the target cells to death; and drugs, such as alkylating agents [chlorambucil (Flechner, 1973), Trenimon (Linford et al., 1974) and nitrogen mustards (Davies and O'Neill, 1974)], intercalating agents [adriamycin and daunomycin (Levy et al., 1975)] and metabolic inhibitors [methotrexate (Robinson et al., 1973)]. The "poisoned arrow" approach has been tested in several in vitro and in vivo systems with generally encouraging results.

5. Potential Problems with Monoclonal Antibody Usage

The introduction of monoclonal antibody technology has alleviated one of the major headaches of polyspecific antisera, the removal of unwanted specificities by extensive and tedious absorptions. Remaining, however, are most of the other problems encountered by serological techniques. In fact, some of the problems are worse with monoclonal antibodies since the many different specificities and immunoglobulin types present in an antiserum can cover the peculiarities of any single antibody. In the headlong rush to develop and use these reagents that sometimes accompanies the enthusiasm for a new and potentially revolutionary technology, these limitations may be incorrectly judged unimportant or forgotten altogether.

The monospecificity accompanying a monoclonal antibody means reactivity with a single antigenic determinant. Although it is possible to imagine a single antibody binding site recognizing structures that vary to a limited extent, such as slightly different sequences of amino acids in different proteins, this has turned out not to be one of the problems of monoclonal antibody technology. However, the measurement of the level of expression of a determinant on a cell surface by monoclonal reagent does reflect a complex mixture of variables including the assay used, the affinity of the antibody, the accessibility of the determinant, and the total number of determinants on the cell. Not only do different assays (for example, radioimmunoassays, fluorescence assays, cytotoxic assays, and immunoprecipitation assays) have different levels of sensitivity, but variations within a single assay procedure can yield dramatically different results. The binding of one monoclonal antibody was enhanced approximately 100-fold by the addition of a second monoclonal antibody of a different specificity (Goodfliesch et al., 1980). Furthermore, not all immunoglobulin classes fix complement and not all monoclonal antibodies that recognize a given molecule will precipitate that molecule in detergent extracts. The possibility exists that a negative cell will become positive if a different assay is used.

The antimelanoma hybridomas provide a good example of the problems in the interpretation of positive versus negative binding. With the assay conditions constant, one antibody reacts with most of the 25 melanomas tested with the degree of reactivity ranging in a near continuum from high to low (Woodbury et al., 1980). Not only is it difficult to discriminate definitively between high and low binding melanomas, but also to assess the significance of intermediate to low level binding to other cell types.

Two additional problems reflect differences in behavior between monoclonal and polyclonal antibodies. Some monoclonal antibodies may recognize a different site on an antigenic molecule than that recognized by the bulk of the antibodies of a standard antiserum. Thus, the assumption that a monoclonal specificity is the same as that defined by an antiserum can only be validated by extensive testing. The second of these problems concerns the possibility of microheterogeneity or genetic variants of the antigen. A polyclonal antiserum has specificities for a variety of determinants and probably will still react with these variant molecules. However, different ways of processing or modifying an antigen or a single amino acid change introduced by a point mutation can distort a determinant to an extent that the monoclonal antibody will no longer recognize the antigen. The production of monoclonal specificities to a variety of determinants on the antigen would help alleviate these types of problems.

The tumor cell represents a normal cell that has escaped normal regulation of growth. Genetic changes that result in the expression of tumor antigens and chromosomal changes that produce aneuploidy often accompany oncogenic transformation. Aneuploidy can potentially produce a loss of antigen expression owing to segregation of the chromosome encoding either the structural gene for the antigen or a gene regulating expression of the antigen. For example, it is difficult to determine whether the odd colorectal carcinoma out of eight that does not react with a particular anticolorectal carcinoma hybridoma (Koprowski et al., 1979) is such an example of chromosomal segregation or whether this hybridoma antibody delineates a true, clinically relevant subset of carcinomas.

The likelihood that tumor-specific antigens do not exist creates another problem that is not unique to monoclonal antibodies. The presence of putative tumor-specific antigens on a small proportion of normal cells appears to be the rule, not the exception. AFP and CEA, as discussed in earlier sections, represent clear examples (Sell, 1980). Therefore, these antigens have been referred to as tumor-associated rather than tumor-specific antigens throughout this chapter, and should be considered normal antigens present on a highly restricted number of nonmalignant cells and select classes of tumors. This acknowledgment does not preclude the clinical usefulness of antibody specificities to these antigens. However, therapeutic uses, such as those involving in vivo cytotoxic principles, must be viewed with extra caution since a rare population of essential normal cells may be eliminated along with tumor cells.

A further possible consequence of oncogenic transformation, that tumor cells continue to differentiate while exhibiting unrestrained growth, has been elegantly demonstrated in several examples of multiple myeloma (Abdou and Abdou, 1975; Mellstedt et al., 1976; Kubagawa et al., 1979), macroglobulinemia (Wernet et al., 1972) and chronic lymphocytic leukemia associated with monoclonal gammopathy (Salsano et al., 1974; Schroer et al., 1974). In each of these cases an anti-idiotype serum that reacts with unique binding site determinants on the monoclonal immunoglobulin protein isolated from the patient's serum was prepared and used to locate cells in the hematopoietic tissues bearing the idiotypic determinants. Virtually all stages of B lymphocyte development bearing the idiotypic marker could be identified in these tissues, implying that an early stage of B lymphocyte differentiation was oncogenically transformed. However, in these particular cases of multiple myeloma, the disease presented as a malignant plasma cell, the end stage of B lymphocyte maturation, presumably since the tumor cells continued differentiation and accumulated at this dead end. The exclusive use of antibody reagents specific for a myeloma-associated antigen would miss the stem cell source of the tumor, while reagents specific for each B lymphocyte differentiation step might well give a more accurate picture of the disease by indicating the presence of several tumor cell types. These examples may not be typical of all tumors, but must be considered a possibility.

6. Final Comments

The production of monoclonal antibodies to human tumor antigens has only begun. The clinical usefulness of these reagents is highly promising, but will ultimately be judged on the grounds of whether any additional information is gained that is important in making a medical decision and whether a patient will receive different treatment based on this information. Since diagnostic decisions are critical to the proper treatment of a patient, a long and careful look at this technology is mandatory.

The potential problems associated with monoclonal antibody usage are numerous, but not insurmountable. Virtually all can be adequately addressed through the preparation of sufficiently large numbers of the reagents and the systematic screening of their specificities and clinical usages. The vast potential of the technology indicates at present that this effort is worthwhile.

Based on the rapid growth of hybridoma research in the last five years, the medical importance of monoclonal antibodies in cancer research and the number of laboratories initiating research in this field, a treatise similar to this one in 1990 may well take up a volume by itself. The expectation is that many enlightening and life-saving subjects will highlight those pages.

Note Added in Proof

The production of human hybridomas has now been reported [Olsson, L., and H.S. Kaplan (1980), *Proc. Natl. Acad. Sci.*, **77**, 5429–5431.]. A HAT-sensitive human myeloma cell line, U-266, was fused with splenic lymphoid cells obtained from a patient with Hodgkin's disease who had been sensitized with 2-dinitrochlorobenzene, a potent chemical allergen. The HAT-resistant hybridomas were screened for antidinitrophenyl antibodies and clones were selected that secrete human antibodies specific for this hapten. With the extension of hybridoma technology to human antibodies, the human immune response to antigens, including tumor antigens, is now accessible in monoclonal form. An additional limitation, however, accompanies human hybridoma technology in comparison with that of mouse or rat hybridomas, since immunization to a number of antigens may not be possible on ethical grounds. Thus, difficulty in obtaining human immune lymphoid cells may prove to be a principal obstacle.

Acknowledgments

The research of the author and the preparation of this manuscript has been supported by National Cancer Institute grant CA 21531.

References

Abdou, N.I., and N.L. Abdou (1975), *Ann. Intern. Med.* **83**, 42.

Abramson, C.S., J.H. Kersey, and T.W. LeBien (1980), *Fed. Proc.* **39**, 926.

Accolla, R.S., S. Carrel, and J.P. Mach (1980), *Proc. Natl. Acad. Sci.* **77**, 563.

Baker, M.A., J.A. Falk, W.H. Carter, R.N. Taub, and Toronto Leukemia Study Group (1979), *New England J. Med.* **301**, 1353.

Breard, J., E.L. Reinherz, P.C. Kung, G. Goldstein, and S.F. Schlossman (1980), *J. Immunol.* **124**, 1943.

Brooks, D.A., I. Beckman, J. Bradley, P.J. McNamara, M.E. Thomas, and H. Zola (1980), *Clin. Exptl. Immunol.* **39**, 477.

Brown, J.P., J.D. Tamerius, and I. Hellström (1979), *J. Immunol. Methods* **31**, 201.

Brown, J.P., P.W. Wright, C.E. Hart, R.G. Woodbury, K.E. Hellström, and I. Hellström (1980), *J. Biol. Chem.* **225**, 4980.

Burk, K.H., B. Drewinko, J.M. Trujillo, and M.J. Ahearn (1978), *Cancer Res.* **38**, 2508.

Chan, W.C., I.J. Check, and R.L. Hunter (1980), *Fed. Proc.* **39**, 926.

Coffino, P., B. Knowles, S.G. Nathenson, and M.D. Scharff (1971), *Nature New Biol.* **231**, 87.

Cornain, S., J.E. DeVries, J. Collard, C. Vennegoor, I.V. Wingerden, and P. Rümke (1975), *Int. J. Cancer* **16**, 981.

Cotton, R.G.H., and C. Milstein (1973), *Nature* **224**, 42.

Davies, D.A.L., and G.J. O'Neill (1974), *Proc. Int. Cancer Congress* **1**, 218.

Eisenbarth, G.S., B.F. Haynes, J.A. Schroer, and A.S. Fauci (1980), *J. Immunol.* **124**, 1237.

Engleman, E., R. Fox, R. Warnke, and R. Levy (1981), *Proc. Natl. Acad. Sci.*, in press.

Flechner, I. (1973), *Eur. J. Cancer* **9**, 741.

Fox, R., S. Baird, et al. (1982), in *Human Cancer Markers* (Sell, S., and B. Wahren eds.), Humana, Clifton, New Jersey.

Fuks, A., J. Shuster, and P. Gold (1980), in *Cancer Markers* (Sell, S., ed.), Humana, Clifton, New Jersey, p. 315.

Galfre, G., S.C. Howe, C. Milstein, G.W. Butcher, and J.C. Howard (1977), *Nature* **226**, 550.

Galfre, G., C. Milstein, and B. Wright (1979), *Nature* **277**, 131.

Gasser, D.L., B.A. Winters, J.B. Haas, T.J. McKearn, and R.H. Kennett (1979), *Proc. Natl. Acad. Sci.* **76**, 4636.

Gold, P., S.O. Freedman, and J. Shuster (1979), in *Immunodiagnosis of Cancer, Part I* (Herberman, R.B., and K.R. McIntire, eds.), Dekker, New York, p. 147.

Goldenberg, D.M. (1976), *Curr. Top. Pathol.* **63**, 289.

Goodfliesch, R., S.V. Hunter, Z. Maciorowski, and M.D. Poulik (1980), *Fed. Proc.* **39**, 919.

Gregoriadis, G. (1977), *Nature* **265**, 407.

Guesdon, J., T. Ternynck, and S. Avrameas (1979), *J. Histochem. Cytochem.* **27**, 1131.

Hansen, J.A., P.J. Martin, and R.C. Nowinski (1980), *Immunogenetics* **10**, 247.

Haynes, B.F., G.S. Eisenbarth, and A.S. Fauci (1979), *Proc. Natl. Acad. Sci.* **76**, 5829.

Hellström, K.E., and J.P. Brown (1979), in *The Antigens* (Sela, M., ed.), Vol. 5, Academic, New York, p. 1.

Hellström, I., K.E. Hellström, H.O. Sjögren, and G.A. Warner (1971), *Int. J. Cancer* **7**, 1.

Herlyn, D., Herlyn, M., Z. Steplewski, and H. Koprowski (1979), *Eur. J. Immunol.* **9**, 657.

Hodach, A.E., and J.L. Winklehake (1980), *Fed. Proc.* **39**, 927.

Horibata, K., and A.W. Harris (1970), *Exptl. Cell. Res.* **60**, 61.

Jondal, M., and G. Klein (1973), *J. Exptl. Med.* **138**, 1365.

Kearney, J.F., A. Radbruch, B. Liesegang, and K. Rajewsky (1979), *J. Immunol.* **123**, 1548.

Kennett, R.H., and F. Gilbert (1979), *Science* **203**, 1120.

Köhler, G., and C. Milstein (1975), *Nature* **256**, 495.

Köhler, G., and C. Milstein (1976), *Eur. J. Immunol.* **6**, 511.

Köhler, G., and M.J. Shulman (1978) *Current Topics Microbiol. Immunol.* **81**, 143.

Koprowski, H., Z. Steplewski, D. Herlyn, and M. Herlyn (1978), *Proc. Natl. Acad. Sci.* **75**, 3405.

Koprowski, H., Z. Steplewski, K. Mitchell, M. Herlyn, D. Herlyn, and P. Fuhrer (1979), *Somatic Cell Genetics* **5**, 957.

Koskimies, S. (1979), *Scand. J. Immunol.* **10**, 371.

Kozbor, D., M. Steinitz, G. Klein, S. Koskimies, and O. Mäkelä (1979), *Scand. J. Immunol.* **10**, 187.

Krueger, R.G., L.D. Staneck, and J.M. Boehlecke (1976), *J. Natl. Cancer Inst.* **56**, 711.

Kubagawa, H., L.B. Vogler, J.D. Capra, M.E. Conrad, A.R. Lawton, and M.D. Cooper (1979), *J. Exptl. Med.* **150**, 792.

Kung, P.C., G. Goldstein, E.L. Reinherz, and S.F. Schlossman (1979), *Science,* **206**, 347.

Laskov, R., K.J. Kim, and R. Asofsky (1979), *Proc. Natl. Acad. Sci.* **76**, 915.

Levy, R., and J. Dilley (1978), *Proc. Natl. Acad. Sci.* **75**, 2411.

Levy, R., J. Dilley, R.I. Fox, and R. Warnke (1979), *Proc. Natl. Acad. Sci.* **76**, 6552.

Levy, R., E. Hurwitz, R. Maron, R. Arnon, and M. Sela (1975), *Cancer Res.* **35**, 1182.

Lewis, M.G., R.L. Ikonopisov, R.C. Nairn, T.M. Phillips, G. Hamilton-Fairly, D.C. Bodenham, and P. Alexander (1969), *Brit. Med. J.* **3**, 547.

Linford, J.H., G. Froese, I. Berczi, and L.G. Israels (1974), *J. Natl. Cancer Inst.* **52**, 1665.

Littlefield, J.W. (1964), *Science* **145**, 709.

Lister, T.A., M.M. Roberts, R.L. Brearley, R.K. Woodruff, and M.F. Greaves (1979), *Cancer Immunol. Immunother.* **6**, 227.

Margulies, D.H., W.M. Kuehl, and M.D. Scharff (1976), *Cell* **8**, 405.

Marshak-Rothstein, A., P. Fink, T. Gridley, D.H. Raulet, M.J. Bevan, and M.J. Gefter (1979), *J. Immunol.* **122**, 2491.

McGaughey, C. (1974), *Oncology* **29**, 302.

McGrath, M., E. Pillemer, and I.L. Weissman (1980), *Nature* **285**, 259.

McMichael, A.J., J.R. Pilch, G. Galfre, D.Y. Mason, J.W. Fabre, and C. Melchers, F., M. Potter, and N. Warner (1978), *Current Topics Microbiol. Immunol.* **81**.

Mellstedt, H., D. Pettersson, and G. Holm (1976), *Scand. J. Haematol.* **16**, 112.

Milstein (1979), *Eur. J. Immunol.* **9**, 205.

Middleton, S., S.A. Andrew, and A.J. Strelkauskas (1980), *Fed. Proc.* **39**, 926.

Moolten, F.L., N.J. Capparell, and S.R. Cooperband (1972), *J. Natl. Cancer Inst.* **49**, 1057.

Nowinski, R.C., M.E. Lostrom, M.R. Tam, M.R. Stone, and W.N. Burnette (1979), *Virology* **93**, 111.

Parkhouse, R.M.E., and G. Guaranotta (1978), *Current Topics Microbiol. Immunol.* **81,** 142.

Parks, D.R., V.M. Bryan, V.T. Oi, and L.A. Herzenberg (1979), *Proc. Natl. Acad. Sci.* **76,** 1962.

Pesando, J.M., J. Ritz, H. Lazarus, S.B. Costello, S. Sallan, and S.F. Schlossman (1979), *Blood* **54,** 1240.

Phillips, D.G., A.P. Kendal, R.G. Webster, and C.B. Reimer (1980), *Fed. Proc.* **39,** 929.

Philpott, G.W., R.J. Bower, and C.W. Parker (1973), *Surgery* **73,** 928.

Pritchard, D.G., and C.W. Todd (1979), in *Immunodiagnosis of Cancer,* Part I (Herberman, R.B., and K.R. McIntire, eds.), Dekker, New York, p. 165.

Pusztaszeri, G., and J.P. Mach (1973), *Immunochemistry* **10,** 197.

Ralph, P. (1979), *Immunol. Rev.* **48,** 107.

Raschke, W.C. (1980), *Biochem. Biophys. Acta* **605,** 113.

Raschke, W.C., B. Mather, and M. Koshland (1979), *Proc. Natl. Acad. Sci.* **76,** 3469.

Reinherz, E.L., P.C. Kung, G. Goldstein, and S.F. Schlossman (1979a), *J. Immunol.* **123,** 1312.

Reinherz, E.L., P.C. Kung, G. Goldstein, and S.F. Schlossman (1979b), *J. Immunol.* **123,** 2894.

Reinherz, E.L., P.C. Kung, G. Goldstein, R.H. Levey, and S.F. Schlossman (1980a), *Proc. Natl. Acad. Sci.* **77,** 1588.

Reinherz, E.L., P.C. Kung. G. Goldstein, and S.F. Schlossman (1980b), *J. Immunol.* **124,** 1301.

Reinherz, E.L., L.M. Nadler, D.S. Rosenthal, W.C. Moloney, and S.F. Schlossman (1979c), *Blood* **53,** 1066.

Reinherz, E.L., and S.F. Schlossman (1980), *Cell* **19,** 821.

Robinson, D.A., J.M. Whitely, and N.G.L. Harding (1975), *Biochem. Soc. Trans.* **1,** 722.

Royston, I., J. Majda, S. Baird, G. Yamamoto, B. Meserve, C. Ivor, and J. Griffiths (1980), *J. Immunol.,* **125,** 725.

Ruoslahti, E., E. Engvall, A. Pekkala, and M. Seppälä (1978), *Int. J. Cancer* **22,** 515.

Ruoslahti, E., and A. Pekkala, D.E. Comings, and M. Seppälä (1979), *Brit. Med. J.* **2,** 768.

Ruoslahti, E., and M. Seppälä (1979), *Adv. Cancer Res.* **29,** 275.; 1 Salsano, F., S.S. Frøland, J.B. Natvig, and T.E. Michaelsen (1974), *Scand. J. Immunol.* **3,** 841.

Schneider, M.D., and G.S. Eisenbarth (1979), *J. Immunol. Methods* **29,** 331.

Schroer, K.R., D.E. Briles, J.A. Van Boxel, and J.M. Davie (1974), *J. Exptl. Med.* **140,** 1416.

Sell, S. (1980), in *Cancer Markers* (Sell, S., ed.), Humana, Clifton, New Jersey, p. 249.

Sharon, J., S.L. Morrison, and E.A. Kabat (1979), *Proc. Natl. Acad. Sci.* **76,** 1420.

Shiku, H., T. Takashashi, H.F. Oettgen, and L.J. Old (1976), *J. Exptl. Med.* **144,** 873.

Shively, J.E., and C.W. Todd (1980), in *Cancer Markers* (Sell, S., ed .). Humana, Clifton, New Jersey, p. 295.

Shively, J.E., C.W. Todd, V.L.W. Go, and M.L. Egan (1978), *Cancer Res.* **38**, 503.

Shulman, M., C.D. Wilde, and G. Köhler (1978), *Nature* **276**, 269.

Sizaret, P., N. Breslow, and S.G. Anderson (1975), *J. Biol. Stand.* **3**, 201.

Smith, C.J., P.C. Kelleher, L. Belanger, and L. Dallaire (1979), *Brit. Med. J.* **1**, 920.

Stähli, C., T. Staehelin, V. Miggiano, J. Schmidt, and P. Häring (1980), *J. Immunol. Methods* **32**, 297.

Steel, C.M., J. Philipson, E. Arthur, S.E. Gardiner, M.S. Newton, and R.V. McIntosh (1977), *Nature* **270**, 729.

Steinitz, M., G. Klein, S. Koskimies, and O. Makela (1977), *Nature* **269**, 420.

Steplewski, Z., M. Herlyn, D. Herlyn, W.H. Clark, and H. Koprowski (1979), *Eur. J. Immunol.* **9**, 94.

Stocker, J.W., G. Garotta, B. Hausmann, M. Trucco, and R. Ceppellini (1979), *Tissue Antigens* **13**, 212.

Stocker, J.W., and C.H. Heusser (1979), *J. Immunol. Methods* **26**, 87.

Szybalski, W., N.H. Szybalski, and G. Ragni (1962), *Natl. Cancer Inst. Monograph* **7**, 75.

Terhorst, C., A. van Agthoven, E. Reinherz, and S. Schlossman (1980), *Science* **209**, 520.

Thierfelder, S., H. Rodt, E. Thiel, G. Hoffmann-Fezer, B. Netzel, R.J. Haas, G.F. Wündisch, and C. Bender-Götze (1979), *Rec. Res. Cancer Res.* **69**, 41.

Trowbridge, I.S. (1978), *J. Exptl. Med.* **148**, 313.

Uotila, M., E. Engvall, and E. Ruoslahti (1980), *Mol. Immunol.* **17**, 791.

Wang, C., R. Good, P. Ammirati, G. Dymbort, and R. Evans (1980), *J. Exptl. Med.* **151**, 1539.

Wernet, P., T. Feizi, and H.G. Kunkel (1972), *J. Exptl. Med.* **136**, 650.

Woodbury, R.G., J.P. Brown, M. Yeh, I. Hellström and K.E. Hellström (1980), *Proc. Natl. Acad. Sci.* **77**, 2183.

Yeh, M., I. Hellström, J.P. Brown, G.A. Warner, J.A. Hansen, and K.E. Hellström (1979), *Proc. Natl. Acad. Sci.* **76**, 2927.

Zipf, T.F., R.I. Fox, J. Dilley, and R. Levy (1980), *Cancer Treatment Reports, in press.*

Zurawski, V.R., E. Haber, and P.H. Black (1978), *Science* **199**, 1439.

2

Cell Surface Antigens on Normal and Neoplastic Human Lymphoid Cells

Robert Fox,[1] Stephen Baird,[2] Patrick Kung,[3] Ron Levy,[4] and Ivor Royston[2]

Department of Clinical Research, Scripps Clinic and Research Foundation, La Jolla, California[1]; University of California, San Diego, California[2]; Ortho Pharmaceutical Corporation, Raritan, New Jersey[3]; and Stanford University Medical Center, Stanford California[4]

In the last 20 years, we have learned a great deal about the structure and function of the normal lymphoid system. In parallel, we have also learned much more about tumors of the lymphoid system. Frequently, information developed through experiments on lymphomas has been helpful to our understanding of normal lymphoid cells and vice versa. The irresistible tendency to draw parallels between the normal and malignant lymphoid system is illustrated by the current ways of classifying lymphomas. It is postulated that different types of malignant lymphoid cells reflect a particular stage of development of a normal lymphoid cell. For example, not only do we now classify some lymphomas as B cell-derived, but also attempt an even further refinement and describe the surface markers of the malignant cells as characteristic of pre B cells, mature B cells, or plasma cells (Greaves and Janossy, 1978; Greaves et al., 1980.) For physicians, the ultimate goals of such classification attempts are to describe accurately a patient's disease in order to give a reliable prognosis and predict which therapy will be most effective. In addition, the biological scientist hopes that a careful comparison of the properties of malignant and normal cells will help in understanding their fundamental differences.

In this chapter we will first review different techniques used to characterize human lymphocyte subsets, including the ability to form rosettes with sheep cells, the binding to receptors for the Fc portion of immunoglobulin, and the study of their reactivity with particular antibodies against cell surface antigens. We will concentrate on the use of monoclonal antibodies since these reagents can potentially provide an unlimited supply of a standardized reagent that can be easily used to determine human lymphocyte subsets (Kung et al., 1979).

Many groups of investigators have reported production of monoclonal antibodies that recognize human lymphocytes. This proliferation of monoclonal antibodies may lead to confusion since a side-by-side comparison of different reagents has not yet been published. For example, different monoclonal antibodies have been reported that react with all peripheral blood "T" cells (pan-T cell), but that differ in their reactivity with human T-acute lymphoblastic leukemia (T-ALL)* cells and T-ALL derived cell lines (Reinherz, 1979a; Zipf, 1980; Engleman, 1980; Royston, 1980a). Basic questions about the nature of the antigens detected by these different antibodies must be resolved to allow comparison of results obtained using different antibodies. Therefore, we will present a side-by-side comparison of pan-T antibodies prepared by several different groups. Finally we will discuss other monoclonal antibodies that are reactive with lymphocyte subsets or leukemic cells or both.

1. Three Major Classes of Immunocompetent Lymphocytes

In the 1960s, lymphocytes were divided into thymus- (T) and bursa- (B) derived cells in animal systems (reviewed by Katz, 1977). A class of bone marrow cells appear to migrate to the thymus where these small lymphocytes differentiate to become specific subsets by virtue of some critical influence of the thymus. These thymus-derived lymphocytes are referred to as T cells; they are responsible for various phenomena of cell mediated immunity (such as delayed-type hypersensitivity and cell-mediated resistance to infection) and regulation of other lymphoid cells in the immune system. The second lymphocyte type, B cells, also arises in the bone marrow and ultimately settles in distinct anatomical sites in peripheral lymphoid tissues where they give rise to the precursors of antibody secreting cells (Claman and Chaperon, 1969). Finally, a third class of lymphocytes lacks

*Abbreviations used in this manuscript: T-ALL, T-lymphocyte acute lymphocytic leukemia; SRBC, sheep red blood cell, ADCC, antibody dependent cellular cytotoxicity; Tγ, T-cells with a receptor for the Fc fragment of IgG; Tμ, T-cells with a receptor for the Fc fragment of IgM; PBL, peripheral blood lymphocyte; PHA, phytohemaglutinin; CALLA, common acute lymphocytic leukemia antigen, CLL, chronic lymphocytic leukemia; CML, chronic myelogenous leukemia; SDS, sodium dodecyl sulfate; SaCI, *staphylcoccus aureus* Cowan Strain I; Ig, immunoglobulin.

markers characteristic of T or B cells and thus are referred to as non T-non B cells (Niaudet and Greaves, 1980).

In animal systems, the availability of inbred strains has made possible the production of particular antibodies to delineate these lymphoid subsets. Adoptive transfer and in vitro assays have allowed functional characterization (Katz and Benacerraf, 1972). For example, differentiation antigens such as TL, Thy 1, and Ly-1,2,3 are cell surface markers that have helped identify particular subsets of lymphoid T cells (Cantor et al., 1976). It has been the aim of many research groups to devise methods that could delineate similar subsets in the human lymphoid system.

1.1. Subsets of Lymphocytes Defined by Rosetting with Sheep Red Blood Cells

In humans, obvious limitations have prevented an approach similar to that used in mice, where inbred strains and the ability to perform immunizations allowed the production of specific antibodies to lymphoid cells. Separation of human lymphoid cells was initially accomplished based on the ability to form rosettes with sheep red blood cells (SRBC), leading to separation of SRBC positive and negative subpopulations of peripheral blood lymphocytes (Jondal et al., 1972). Since thymocytes were also able to form rosettes, the presence of this marker indicated apparent thymic origin of the SRBC rosette-positive lymphocytes in peripheral blood (Minowada et al., 1972; Brown et al., 1974; Seligman et al., 1973). Thus the SRBC rosette-positive cells appeared analogous to the T cells defined in animal systems; the simplicity of the rosetting procedure led to widespread clinical use of this method to enumerate T cells.

Initial studies using SRBC rosettes demonstrated a dependence of this technique on temperature (Wybran and Fudenberg, 1973) and the concentration of serum employed (Wybran et al., 1973). These factors can significantly alter the fraction of lymphocytes that are enumerated as SRBC rosette-positive. For example, approximately 65% of normal peripheral blood lymphocytes (PBL) form rosettes at 4°C, but only 25% form rosettes at 37°C (Wybran et al., 1973). Cells that are able to rosette at the elevated temperature (29 or 37°C) have been referred to as possessing "high-affinity" SRBC receptor, and this property may characterize particular lymphocyte subpopulation(s) (Mackler et al., 1980).

Modifications of the SRBC rosette technique have been proposed that involve *prior treatment of the SRBC* with neuraminidase (Weiner et al., 1973) or AET, a sulfhydryl compound (Pellegrino et al., 1975). Such treatments increase the percentage of PBL able to form rosettes; it has been suggested that this increase results in part from "increased stability" of the rosettes so that they are more stable to mechanical manipulation. Additional modifications of the rosetting technique have involved *prior treatment of the lymphocytes* with agents such as neuraminidase (Bentwich et al., 1973) or phospholipase (Hanaumi et al., 1976). With both treatments, lymphocytes that had previously been SRBC rosette negative now could form rosettes. Such treatments appear to "uncover" a receptor for SRBC that had previously been "hidden". Finally, recent studies have demonstrated that theophylline, which alters $3',5'$-cyclic AMP levels, can affect the ability of lymphocytes to form rosettes with SRBC (Limatibul et al., 1978). Some lymphocyte subsets are resistant to the action of theophylline whereas other subsets are susceptible.

B cells, defined by the presence of membrane immunoglobulin (Ig), are separated into the SRBC rosette-negative fraction. Quantitation of B cells is usually performed using immunofluorescent techniques to detect surface Ig. False-positive staining results may occur because of the presence of Ig bound to the Fc receptors on T cells or monocytes (Kumagi et al., 1975). Incubation of PBL at 37°C or brief exposure to acid pH prior to testing allows "shedding" of this cytophilic Ig so that only cells bearing membrane Ig will be enumerated as B cells.

In addition to T cells (i.e., those able to form SRBC rosettes) and B cells (i.e., membrane Ig+), there are lymphocytes that lack these properties and are referred to as "null lymphocytes." Much attention has recently been focused on the "null" lymphocytes since they appear to mediate antibody-dependent cytotoxicity (ADCC) (Cordier et al., 1976; Shore et al., 1977). "Null" cells are heterogeneous with respect to surface antigens and functions. Most null cells express Fc receptors for Ig (Niaudet and Greaves, 1979), react with monoclonal antibody OKM1 (Breard et al., 1980), are negative for Ia-like antigens (Ozer et al., 1979) and express T-cell differentiation antigens as defined by heteroantisera reactive with thymocytes (Balch et al., 1980). There is some evidence that "null" cells may have low-affinity SRBC receptors (West et al., 1978) and may be further induced to express "more" SRBC receptors after in vitro culture with thymic extracts (Touraine, 1978). Finally, a minority of null cells (25%) are reported to bear Ia-like antigens; they may represent B cell or monocyte precursors (Ozer et al., 1979).

In summary, a variety of rosetting techniques have been employed to define T cells; B cells can be enumerated based on the presence of surface Ig molecules, after "shedding" at 37°C to remove Ig bound via Fc receptors. Finally, a non-T, non-B fraction of mononuclear cells contains macrophage-like cells and "null" lymphocytes. Each of these fractions can be further subdivided into subfractions that perform distinct functions and have characteristic cell surface antigens.

1.2. T Cell Subsets Defined by Membrane Receptors for Immunoglobulin

Initial studies by Moretta et al. (1976) suggested that T cell subsets could be identified by their expression of the Fc receptor for immunoglobulin. T cells that bear the receptor for the Fc fragment of IgM (T_μ) were shown in certain *in vitro* assays to function as helper cells, while T cells bearing the receptor for the Fc fragment of IgG (T_γ) appear to express predominantly suppressor activity (Moretta et al., 1977; Mingari et al., 1978). Approximately 10% of normal T_μ cells also bear T_γ receptors (Merrill et al., 1980). In addition, receptors have been reported for the Fc portion of IgA and IgE (Lum et al., 1979; Gonzalez and Speigelberg, 1977).

Since the presence of Fc receptors provided an initial means to study T lymphocyte subsets, extensive (and sometimes conflicting) literature has recently been generated. At this time, it appears that the assignment of function as T helper or T suppressor according to Fc receptors for Ig is not absolute (Moriya et al., 1980; Hayard et al., 1978). With increasing studies being performed using Fc receptors to characterize subsets, difficulties in the standardization of reagents and techniques have become apparent. In part, different results obtained by differerent workers may result from the fact that detection of these receptors varies with different in vitro culture conditions (Ferrarini et al., 1977). Furthermore, interpretation of functional data may be complicated by the fact that a single subset may bear either Fc-$_\mu$ or Fc-$_\gamma$ receptors at different stages of its functional development (Pichler and Broder, 1978).

Alterations in T_μ and T_γ populations have been reported in various diseases such as immunodeficiency and autoimmune syndromes (Moretta et al., 1977; Broder et al., 1978; Haynes et al., 1979; Schuster et al., 1980) as well as lymphoproliferative diseases (Noorloos et al., 1980). Additionally, in patients with multiple sclerosis, there is an increased number of lymphocytes that bear both Fc-$_\gamma$ and Fc-$_\mu$ receptors (Merrill et al., 1980).

1.3. Cell Surface Markers
Defined by Heteroantisera

In humans, the analysis of B cell lymphocytes has proceeded with greater speed than analysis of T cells owing to our ability to purify immunoglobulin products and make specific antisera (Unanue, 1971). The study of immunoglobulins as cell surface markers has provided insight into both normal and abnormal stages and pathways of B cell differentiation. For example, tumors may involve accumulation of cells with cytoplasmic Ig (as in some acute lymphatic leukemias), cells with surface Ig (some acute lymphocytic leukemias, most non-Hodgkin's lymphomas), and cells secreting Ig (multiple myeloma). Antibodies directed against immunoglobulin determinants associated with the antigen-binding site (idiotypes) can serve to identify affected members of a particular myeloma clone (Preud'homme, 1977). Such anti-idiotypic antibodies have been used to trace the extent of involvement of myeloma clones back to their earliest recognizable differentiation (Cooper, 1979). Antisera have also been reported that detect B cell antigens that are neither immunoglobulin nor Ia-like molecules (Balch et al., 1978).

In recent years, investigators have tried to produce heteroantisera that are specific for T lymphocytes. A few antisera were made specific for human T cell subpopulations by extensive absorptions (Evans et al., 1977; Evans et al., 1978; Brouet and Seligman, 1976). Ades et al. (1980) prepared an antiserum (anti-p25) that recognizes a 25,000-dalton glycoprotein molecule that is possibly a homolog of murine Thy 1. This antibody reacts with 95% of human thymocytes and PBL T-cells. Pratt et al. (1980) have produced a rabbit anti-human T cell heteroantiserum (Serum A99) that reacts specifically with T-ALL and peripheral blood T cells. Immunoprecipitation with serum A99 demonstrated five antigens of molecular weights 52,000, 96,000, 120,000, 152,000, and 195,000 daltons (Pratt et al., 1980). Immunoprecipitations with other T lymphocyte-specific antisera have identified proteins of 25,000, 30,000, 40,000, 48,000, 55,000, 60,000, 80,000, 135,000, 160,000, and 220,000 daltons from various human T cell preparations (Friedman et al., 1976; Ades et al., 1978; Checkik et al., 1978; Anderson and Metzgar, 1978; Niaudet and Greaves, 1980; Owen et al., 1976). Although such antisera have proven useful in demonstrating the existence of lymphocyte subsets and antigens, they are available in only limited quantity and thus are not suitable as standardized reagents.

To summarize the first section of this chapter, a number of cell surface markers have been identified that help to categorize both normal and malignant lymphocytes. These are summarized in Tables 1 and 2. Table 1 lists the markers commonly used to differentiate T cells, B cells, monocytes and their subclasses. Table 2 presents markers on lymphomas and leukemias. Both have been completely reviewed in Sell's *Cancer Markers: Diagnostic and Developmental Significance* (1980). There is significant variability for these markers between different cases with the same histologic diagnosis, particularly the receptors for IgM, IgG, and C3.

2. Cell Surface Markers Defined by Monoclonal Antibodies

The hybridoma technique of Köhler and Milstein (1975) provides a new approach whereby large amounts of individual antibodies can be obtained, each of which recognizes only one of the determinants recognized by a broadly reactive conventional heteroantiserum. The current approach involves immunizing mice with human lymphoid cells, removing the spleens and making a cell suspension that is then fused with a mouse myeloma cell line. The resulting "hybridomas" are then distributed into multi-well dishes by a limiting dilution method to insure that each reactive culture was derived from a single hybridoma cell. The resulting clones produce a single antibody, and by screening the supernatant of each well

Table 1
Surface Markers on Normal Human Lymphoid Cells[a]

Cell	SRBC rosette	Surface Ig	Cytoplasmic Ig	Fc IgG	Fc IgM	C'3 receptor	Ia	Phagocytosis
T$_{helper}$	+	−	−	−	+	−	−	−
T$_{suppressor}$	+	−	−	+	−	−	−	−
T$_{cytotoxic}$	+	−	−	+	−	−	−	−
Thymocyte	+	−	−	−	−	−	−	−
B cell	−	+	−	+	+	+	+	−
Plasma cell	−	±	+	−	−	+	−	−
B precursor	−	−	+	−	−	−	+	−
Monocyte	−	−	−	+	−	±	−	+

[a]Fc IgG is the Fc receptor specific for IgG; Fc IgM is the Fc receptor specific for IgM: C'3 receptor is that receptor specific for the third component of complement; Ia is that antigen associated with immune response genes; SRBC is the sheep red blood cell.

Table 2

Surface Markers on Lymphoid Leukemias and Lymphomas

Cell	SRBC rosette	Surface Ig	Cytoplasmic Ig	Fc IgG	Fc IgM	C'3 receptor	Ia	Common ALL antigen
T-ALL	+	−	−	+	+	±	−	−
B-ALL	−	+	−			+	+	−
Common-ALL	−	−	−	+	+		+	+
Pre-B ALL	−	−	+				+	−
CLL	−	+	−	+	+	+	+	−
HCL	−	+	−	+	+	−	−	−
B lymphomas								
Nodular	−	+				+	+	−
Diffuse								
WDL	−	+				+	+	−
PDL	−	+				+	+	−
Undifferentiated	−	+				−		−

aWDL, well-differentiated lymphocytic (small round) cells; PDL, poorlydifferentiated lymphocytic (small irregularlyshaped) cells; HCL, hairy cell leukemia.

specific clones are selected for antibody with the desired reactivity. This procedure is described by William Raschke in another chapter of this book.

2.1. Antigens That Potentially May Be Detected by Monoclonal Antibodies

Before discussing some of the monoclonal antibodies that have been reported, a list of the various types of antigens that could be found on lymphoid cells is presented in Table 3. Some antigens will be shared by all T cells, analogous to Thy antigen in mice or characteristic of subsets such as Lyt antigens (Cantor et al., 1976; Ledbetter and Herzenberg, 1980). There also exist antigens on T cells characteristic of their particular subsets (Kung et al., 1979; Reinherz et al., 1979a-g). In addition, antigens may be present on activated T cells that are not detectable on non-stimulated T cells; e.g., the appearance of "Ia"-like antigens (HLA-D) on T cells after stimulation with mitogens (Reinherz et al., 1979c; Evans et al., 1978; Ko et al., 1979; Winchester and Kunkel, 1980). Finally peripheral blood T cells will bear antigens shared by other cells (including lymphoid) such as HLA-A, -B, -C. In a similar manner, human B cells can be expected to share antigens characteristic of their common B cell lineage (Brooks et al., 1980; Bowman et al., 1980), or representing B cell subsets (Nadler et al., 1981). Obvious examples include immunoglobulin molecules on the cell surface as a shared B cell characteristic, with some cells expressing a particular isotype (i.e., IgG, IgM), subclass (IgG1, IgG2), light chain (kappa or lambda), or characteristic binding site (idiotype). In addition, B cells bear HLA antigens, common stem cell antigens, and "activation" antigens as described above.

The previous paragraph describes the types of antigens that might be found on peripheral blood lymphocytes. These lymphocytes exist in "suspension" in blood, whereas other lymphocytes form part of the architecture of lymphoid organs—such as thymus, spleen, or lymph node. Cells in lymphoid organs may bear additional characteristic antigens that allow them to differentiate into particular lymphoid structures and participate in important cell–cell interactions. The nature of the lymphocyte surface molecules that govern this "differentiation" remain largely unknown (Weissman et al., 1978). However, it is likely that the cell–cell communication required for the differentiation of lymphoid organ architecture is dependent on particular cell surface antigens. Thus, human lymphoid cells express a wide variety of antigens and the resulting hydridomas may detect molecules characteristic of a cell lineage, of a specific organ, or of the state of activation. This wide range of antigens must be taken into account when interpreting the pattern of reactivity (or cross-reactivity) of a given monoclonal antibody.

Table 3
Types of Antigens on Lymphocytes

I. *T Cells from Peripheral Blood*
    A. Antigens characterizing all T cells
        (pan-T cell)
    B. Antigens characteristic of T cell subsets (including
        immature thymic cell markers and differentiation
        antigens on mature subsets)
    C. Antigens on activated T cells but not resting
        T cells (e.g., HLA-D and other activation antigens)
    D. HLA-A, -B, -C, and antigens common to other lymphoid or
        monocytic cells

II. *B Cells from Peripheral Blood*
    A. Antigens characterizing all B cells
    B. B-cell subset antigens (including pre-B cell and
        plasma cells)
    C. Activation antigens—not present on resting B cells,
        but that appear after stimulation

III. *Tissue-Specific Antigens*
    A. Antigens characteristic of a particular lymphoid organ,
        such as thymus, lymph node, spleen, or marrow
    B. Antigens characteristic of a particular subset of
        lymphocytes within a lymphoid organ
    C. Activation antigens—not found normally on resting
        cells within the lymphoid organ, but that appear after
        antigen stimulation

IV. *Leukemia or Autoimmune Disease*
    A. Antigens found on normal blood lymphocytes or in tissue
        lymphocytes (e.g., antigens normally present only on
        thymocytes appear on leukemic blasts in bone marrow)
    B. Antigens that represent altered forms of normal antigens
        (owing to altered transcription, translation, or post-
        translational modification)
    C. *De novo* antigens not normally found on normal cells,
        such as viral-specific or tumor-specific antigens

As outlined in Table 3, particular antigens may be detected on lymphocytes from patients with leukemia. These cells may be derived by expansion of a clone of "rare" cells that exists normally at a level too low to be
appreciated. An example of this situation was the finding of myelomas that
produced the previously undescribed class of IgD immunoglobulin (Rowe
and Fahey, 1965; Van Boxel et al., 1972). Antigens may also appear on
cells in disease conditions that are altered forms of "normal" antigens, re-

sulting from transcriptional, translational, or post-translational alteration (Watanabe and Hakomori, 1976; Taub et al., 1980; Nakahara et al., 1980).

Although there has been an intense search for leukemia specific markers, there have (as yet) been no generally agreed upon antigens that are unique to leukemia (reviewed by Bowman et al., 1980). Numerous antigens have been proposed as leukemia specific, but more extensive studies have subsequently demonstrated the presence of such markers on a minor population of normal adult or fetal cells (Mohanakumar and Roney, 1978; Mann et al., 1971; Billing and Terasaki, 1974). One example was the preparation of heteroantisera against the "common ALL antigen" that was present on many ALL blast cells but absent from normal mature lymphoid cells, or activated lymphocytes (Greaves et al., 1975). It has been detected, however, on a minor subpopulation of cells in fetal liver and on lymphoid cells in the bone marrow during lymphoid rebound after cessation of chemotherapy (Greaves and Janossy, 1978). Although the presence of this antigen is strongly associated with ALL, it appears to be a differentiation antigen whose normal expression is highly restricted.

Several authors have suggested that malignant blast cells in the various forms of leukemia seem to be "frozen" at a particular stage of lymphoid maturation. In support of this hypothesis, the phenotype of the "common form" of acute lymphoblastic leukemia corresponds to the phenotype of normal small non-T, non-B cells of lymphoid morphology detected in normal and regenerating infant marrow and that the phenotype of T-ALL corresponds approximately to that of cortical thymocytes or immediate precursors (Sachs, 1978; Salmon and Seligman, 1974; Greaves and Janossy, 1978; McMichael et al., 1979). However, Bradstock et al. (1980) noted that human ALL cells express a greater amount of HLA-A, -B, -C antigens on their cell membranes as compared to cortical thymocytes. These studies suggest that leukemia cells were not simply counterparts of normal thymocytes, but that they had aberrant expression of thymic antigen markers owing to "gene derepression." However, in lymphoid and nonlymphoid tumors, it remains difficult to rule out that a particular neoplasm has not resulted from a "rare" precursor cell that has now increased by clonal expansion.

2.2. Monoclonal Antibodies Reactive with PBL-T Cells

The preceding section describes the spectrum of possible antigens that might be detected. As expected, there will be substantial overlap between these groups: antigens found on peripheral blood cells will also be found on some thymocytes or leukemias. Detailed studies in future years will be required to outline the tissue distribution and molecular properties of the antigens detected by various monoclonal antibodies.

2.2.1. Comparison of Pan-T Cell Monoclonal Antibodies

Pan-T cell monoclonal antibodies have been defined as those that react with sheep rosette positive (SRBC+) PBL, but not with sheep rosette negative (SRBC−) PBL. An example of fluorescent staining of PBL with this type of antibody is shown in Fig. 1. Several groups have prepared such pan-T antibodies and a partial listing is presented in Table 4. It is important to note that these groups have used different cell types as an immunogen and that some of the antibodies show different reactivity with various target cells. The last pan-T antibody, OKT3, apparently recognizes a determinant on a different antigen, which has a distinct cell distribution (i.e., OKT1 and T101 both react with cell line CEM whereas OKT3 does not; Kung, 1979; Royston, 1980a). Further OKT3 probably precipitates an antigen of different molecular weight (C. Terhorst, personal communication). Perhaps the most provocative difference between OKT3 and the other pan-T antibodies is that OKT3 stimulates normal peripheral blood T cells to divide (Van Wauuve et al., 1980). In contrast, other pan-T antibodies that have been tested (OKT1, T101) are not mitogenic (Kung and Royston, unpublished observations).

Immunoprecipitation studies have been used to characterize the antigen detected by several of these different monoclonal antibodies. As shown in Fig. 2, ^{125}I-lactoperoxidase labeled membrane extract of PBL yielded a predominant 67,000-dalton band from four of the different antibodies tested. (Additional minor bands of lower molecular weight can also be detected using longer exposure of the autoradiographs.) The important point is that a similar antigen was recognized by each antibody. Sequential immunoprecipitation studies (lanes E,F) indicate that the antigenic determinants recognized by each of these antibodies are carried on the same molecule. Finally, in order to determine whether these independently generated antibodies detected identical antigenic determinants, "cross-blocking" experiments were performed, as shown in Fig. 3. Normal PBL were pre-incubated with increasing amounts of "unlabeled" monoclonal antibodies. Biotin-conjugated antibody L17F12 was added, followed by fluorescent avidin. The cells were analzyed by flow cytometry and the median fluorescent intensity was calculated. As expected, "unlabeled" L17F12 completely blocks the binding of biotin-L17F12, while a "control" antibody that was not reactive in indirect immunofluorescence with PBL (such as antibody OKT6) did not. Antibody SC1 was also able to inhibit binding while antibody OKT1 showed only a slight ability to block. These results demonstrate that some antibodies (e.g., OKT1) detect a different determinant on the 67K dalton antigen than detected by the other monoclonals (e.g., L17F12).

Since different research groups each use their own particular pan-T cell antibody, we now present a side-by-side comparison of cytofluorographs obtained by using each antibody in indirect immunofluorescent

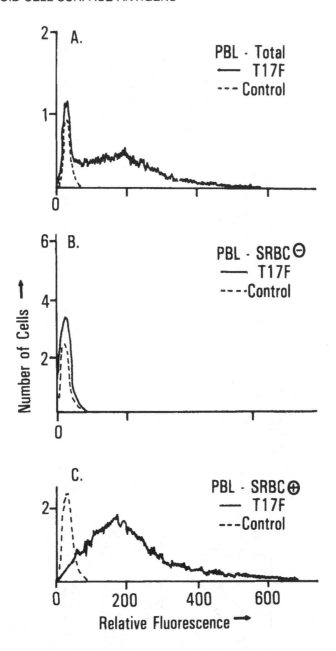

Fig. 1. Indirect immunofluorescence of PBL using a pan-T monoclonal antibody. Normal PBL were separated with Ficoll/Hypaque and stained with antibody T17F plus fluorescent rabbit anti-mouse Ig (frame A). Next, PBL were fractionated into SRBC − (frame B) and SRBC + (frame C) fractions, and each was stained with the same antibodies. For a control, a nonbinding myeloma protein of the same class and concentration as antibody T17F was employed.

Table 4
Monoclonal Antibodies with Pan-T Cell Reactivity

	Immunogen	Target antigen	H-chain isotype	Cytotoxicity	Protein A binding	Binding to E±PBL	Binding to T-ALL	Binding to T-CLL	Reference
17F12	T-ALL	67,000	IgG_{2a}	+	+	+	+	+	Engleman et al. (1980)
3F1	T-ALL	67,000	IgG_2	−	−	+	+	+	Levy and Fox (unpublished observation)
T101	T-cell	65,000	IgG_{2a}	+	+	+	+	+	Royston et al. (1980)
T17F	T-CLL	67,000	IgG_{2a}	+	+	+	+	+	Fox (unpublished observation)
OKR1	SRBC(+)	67,000[a]	IgG_1	+	+	+	−	+	Reinherz (1979)
OKT3	SRBC(+) PBL	20,000[a]	IgG_{2a}	+	+	+	−	+	Kung et al. (1979)
SK1	SRBC(+)	70,000		0	0	+	0	+	Wang et al. (1980)

[a]Terhorst, C., personal communication.

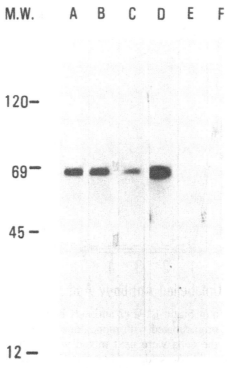

Fig. 2. Immunoprecipitation of ^{125}I-labeled membrane extract from normal peripheral blood lymphocytes (PBL). PBL were labeled with ^{125}I using lactoperoxidase and cell membranes were prepared using detergent extraction as previously described (Fox and Weissman, 1979). Nonspecifically precipitating material was removed by pretreatment with *Staph.* Cowan Strain I (SaCI). Then the immunoprecipitations were performed with specific monoclonal antibody + SaCI. In the case of antibodies of class IgG1, which do not bind directly to SaCI, a "bridging" antibody of goat anti-mouse Ig was also added (Levy et al., 1979): lane A, antibody 17F12 + SaCI (Engleman et al., 1980); lane B, antibody T101 + SaCI (Royston et al., 1980a) lane D, antibody T17F + SaCI; lane C, antibody OKT1 + goat anti-mouse Fab + SaCI. In order to determine whether these antibodies were detecting determinants on the same molecule, "immunodepletion" experiments were carried out by first reacting the ^{125}I-membrane extract with excess 17F12 + SaCI, then performing a sequential immunoprecipitation with another antibody. Lane E, membrane extract pretreated with 17F12 + SaCI, then sequentially with T101 + SaCI; lane F, membrane extract pretreated with 17F12 + SaCI, then sequentially with OKT1 + goat anti-mouse Ig + SaCI.

staining assays (Fig. 4). PBL T cells were prepared by formation of SRBC rosettes and stained with antibodies L17F12 (frame A, Fig. 4), T101 (frame B), T17F (frame C), 3 F1 (frame D), and OKT1 (frame E). When analyzed on a fluorescence-activated cell sorter, these cytofluorographs

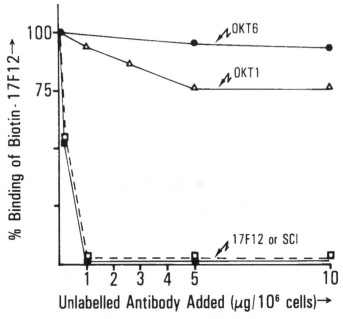

Fig. 3. Competition of biotin-L17F12 antibody binding to normal PBL T cells. Normal PBL were preincubated with monoclonal antibody, then the cells were washed twice and the cells were next mixed with biotin conjugated-L17F12. Finally, fluorescent avidin was added and cells were analyzed on a FACS I to calculate median fluorescence. Antibody OKT6 is nonreactive with PBL. Separate experiments using these PBL cells demonstrated that the dilutions of antibody OKT1 yielded maximal intensity of fluorescent staining (i.e., that failure of block did *not* owe to failure to saturate all antigenic sites).

had virtually identical patterns. In contrast, the staining pattern obtained with OKT3 was slightly different (frame F) with fewer dull staining cells. Each of these antibodies reacts with greater than 90% of thymocytes and peripheral blood T cells.

    After these studies were completed, an additional monoclonal antibody (clone 9.6), reactive with the sheep erythrocyte receptor on T cells, was reported (Kamoun, 1981). Since human T cells have been operationally defined on the basis of this receptor, antibody 9.6 can be conveniently used to quantitate precisely the number of T cells. Recent studies have compared the reactivity of antibodies OKT3, 9.6, and L17F12, indicating that the vast majority of normal PBL T cells express each antigen. However, in some cases, significant differences in reactivity were noted. For example, Tγ cells expressed antigens detected by antibodies 9.6 and L17F12, but reacted with antibody OKT3 to a lesser extent. Therefore, disease states in which rare T cell subsets are clonally expanded may be characterized by reactivity with only some pan-T cell antibodies.

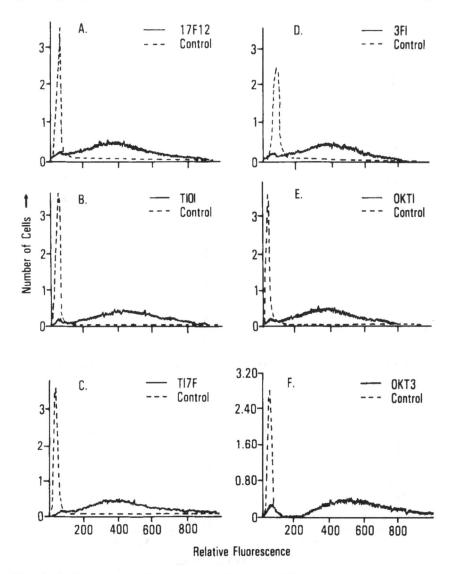

Fig. 4. Indirect immunofluorescence of sheep red blood cell (SRBC) rosette-positive PBL. Normal PBL were purified using Ficoll/Hypaque and "T" cells were prepared by 1 cycle of SRBC rosettes. Erythrocytes were lysed and the cells were stained in indirect immunofluorescence, then analyzed on FACS. In each frame, the "control" represents a monoclonal antibody that was of the same class and concentration as the antibody tested; however, the control antibody was negative in binding assays of PBL (e.g., MOPC-21 as an IgG_1 or GPC-7 as an IgG_{2a}). Antibodies used included: Frame A, antibody L17F12 (Engleman, 1980); frame B, antibody T101 (Royston, 1980); frame C, antibody T17F; and frame D, antibody 3F1 (Fox and Levy, additional "pan-T" antibodies derived separately from L17F12); frames E and F, antibodies OKT1 and OKT3 (Kung, 1979).

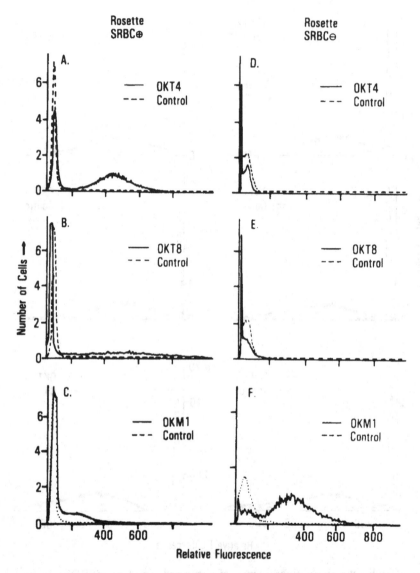

Fig. 5. Indirect immunofluorescence of normal peripheral blood lymphocytes (PBL) after separation into sheep red blood cell (SRBC) positive and negative rosette fractions using T lymphocyte subset antibodies. Normal PBL were prepared by Ficoll/Hypaque and subjected to two cycles of SRBC rosette fractionation. Each fraction was then stained with monoclonal antibody or control antibody (same class and concentration as the other antibodies, but negative in binding assays), then fluorescent sheep antimouse Ig was added as previously described (Levy et al., 1979). Cells were analyzed on FACS. Frames A through C show staining of SRBC rosette-positive cells, while frames D through K with SRBC rosette negative cells. Antibodies used included T subset antibodies OKT4 (Frames A and B) and OKT8 (frames C and D) [(Kung, 1979); frames E and F show staining with antibody OKM1 (Breard, 1980)].

2.2.2. T Cell Subset Antibodies

The next category of antigens are those that are present on T cell subsets. This topic has been recently reviewed by Kung et al. (1979) and Kung and Goldstein (1980). These investigators have demonstrated that "helper" T cells bear a particular antigen (recognized by antibody OKT4) and that "suppressor" T cells are recognized by antibody OKT5 or OKT8. For illustration, the indirect immunofluorescent staining patterns obtained with these antibodies are shown in Fig. 5, where only a subset of the PBL T cells are stained: about 60% with antibody OKT4 and about 35% with antibody OKT8. Studies using complement-mediated lysis and cell sorting have demonstrated that these antigens are present on different cell subsets (Reinherz et al., 1980a,b). A monoclonal antibody (OKM1) has been described recently that reacts with a subpopulation of T $^-$ lymphocytes as well as with some monocytes (Breard, 1980). In Fig. 5, frame C, the reactivity of antibody OKM1 with SRBC + lymphocytes is shown. T cell subsets defined by monoclonal antibodies OKT4 and OKT8 did not correspond to T cell subsets defined by receptors for immunoglobulin (Fc-γ, Fc-μ), Tγ + cells appear enriched for OKM-1 and OKT8 cells compared to T cells lacking Fc-γ receptor (Fox, 1981). Additional examples of monoclonal antibodies recognizing subsets of T lymphocytes are listed in Table 5. Further work will be necessary to determine if similar subsets are being detected by these antibodies.

2.2.3. Activation Antigens

An additional group of antigens are not present on PBL, but have been demonstrated after mitogen stimulation. In some cases, the newly appearing antigen (activation antigens) represents a molecule that previously

Table 5
Monoclonal Anti-Human Lymphoid Antibodies
Reactive with T Cell Subsets

Antibody	Reference
T Cell Subset	
OKT 4 (helper/inducer)	Reinherz et al. (1980b)
OKT 5, 8 (suppressor/cytotoxic)	Reinherz et al. (1980b)
3A1	Eisenbart et al. (1980)
Leu 2, 3	Ledbetter et al. (1981)
HuLyt-1	Hansen et al. (1980)
OKM 1	Reinherz et al. (1980d)
Thymocyte	
HTL	McMichael et al. (1979)
OKT 6	Kung and Goldstein (1980)
12E7	Levy et al. (1979)

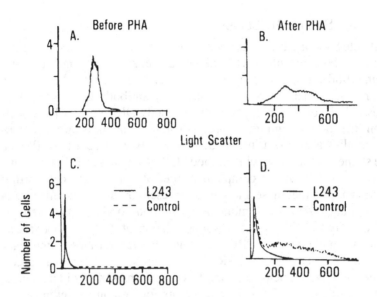

Fig. 6. Effect of mitogen phytohemaglutinin (PHA) on peripheral blood lymphocytes (PBL) T cells. PBL T cells were prepared by Ficoll/Hypaque and 2 cycles of
rosettes with SRBC. These cells were then incubated with PHA (5 µg/mL) for 60
h, at which time over 60% had undergone blast transformation. The increased size
of these blasts was confirmed by the shift in increased light scatter as shown in
frames A and B. (The arrow indicates the scatter of standard latex beads.) In frame
C the untreated T cells were stained with antibody L243, which detects an
HLA-DR like antigen (Lampson and Levy, 1980). Less than 5% of the cells
stained above the fluorescence noted with control antibody. However, after PHA
stimulation, as shown in frame D, over 70% of the cells were stained. Both large

was appreciated only on other cell types. For example, Ia-like antigens are
found on B cells and some monocytes, but not on resting T cells; but after
activation a high percent of T cells express Ia antigens. (Reviewed by
Winchester and Kunkel, 1980.) In other cases, the identity of the newly
appearing antigen (activation antigens) remains unclear. An example of
the latter type is detected by monoclonal antibody L22 that was derived
from mice immunized with the B cell line 8392 by Royston and coworkers
(in preparation); subsequent screening demonstrated that it detected antigens not present on resting T or B cells, but that can be induced after
mitogen stimulation.

An example of the induction antigen is shown in Fig. 6. In this experiment, PBL T cells have first been prepared by rosetting with SRBC and
then treated with phytohemagglutinin (PHA) for 60 h to induce blastogenesis. The increase in large cells (blasts) can be seen by the shift towards
increasing light scatter (frames A and B). Before treatment with the

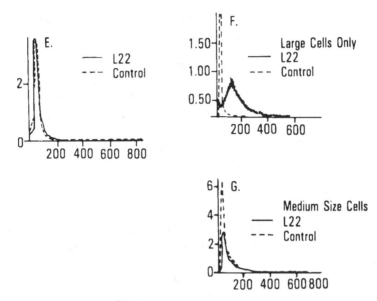

Relative Fluorescence

and medium sized cells were positive. Antibody L22 also was unreactive with T cells before PHA (frame E). Large cells were reactive after PHA (frame F), which shows the FACS analysis of fluorescence of the largest 30% of cells (based on light scatter). In contrast, medium sized cells, as shown in frame G, showed no significant increase in staining compared control antibody. Frames F and G demonstrate the ability of FACS to separately analyze the fluorescence of different cell size populations, using "size-gated fluorescence" (Loken and Herzenberg, 1975).

mitogen, fewer than 5% of the resting peripheral blood T cells are stained with monoclonal anti Ia (frame C). However, after blastogenesis, over 65% of the cells are Ia positive (frame D). These cells are greater than 85% T cells, based on their reactivity with the pan-T cell monoclonal L17F12 (data not shown). An additional type of activation antigen is shown in frames E, F, and G, where blastogenesis leads to expression of antigens reactive with monoclonal antibody L22. The L22 reactive antigen was found only on the "large" lymphoblasts (those exhibiting increased light scattering, as shown in frame F); it was not present on resting T cells (frame E) or on smaller size cells after PHA (frame G). It is unlikely that antibody L22 recognizes HLA-D molecules since B cells do not react with antibody L22 while Ia-negative T-cell lines (such as CEM) are reactive. Other examples of activation antigens are the new appearance of reactivity with monoclonal antibodies OKT9 and OKT10 after mitogen stimulation of PBL (Fox and Kung, unpublished observations).

2.3. Antigens Detected on Thymocytes
by Monoclonal Antibodies

As expected, thymocytes express antigens recognized by the pan-T and subset T monoclonal antibodies described above. In addition, some antigens appear to be expressed only on thymocytes. Examples are antibody HTL (McMichael et al., 1978) or antibody OKT6 (Kung and Goldstein, 1980), which may represent antigens characteristic of a particular stage of intrathymic differentiation. Another marker, such as the one detected by antibody OKT10, may represent a precursor stage since it is found on ~20% of bone marrow cells, >90% thymocytes, but less than 10% of PBL T cells (Reinherz et al., 1980a).

An additional antigen found on thymocytes is detected by antibody 12E7 (Levy et al., 1979). Cortical thymocytes stain very brightly with this antibody while medullary thymocytes and PBL show relatively dull immunofluorescence (Levy et al., 1979). This difference in fluorescence intensity reflects a difference in the quantity of cell surface antigen per cell (Loken and Herzenberg, 1975). Thus, the antigen density per cell is a helpful characteristic in enumerating lymphocyte subsets and may be an important correlate of lymphocyte differentiation (Ledbetter and Herzenberg, 1980).

2.4. Cell Surface Markers
on B Cells and Monocytes

Both normal and malignant B cells have been defined by their expression of cell surface immunoglobulin. Other markers of the B cell membrane, including receptors for the Fc portion of human immunoglobulin (Dickler and Kunkel, 1972), Ia-like antigens (Winchester and Kunkel, 1980) and receptors for complement components, are less useful because they are not restricted to cells of B lineage (Moretta et al., 1976) and are also found on normal and malignant monocytes (Huber, 1969). In addition, immunoglobulin bound to the cell membrane via Fc receptors may give spuriously positive results when enumerating B cells (Kumagi et al., 1975). Because of the overlap of many cell surface markers between B and non-B cells, monoclonal antibodies specific for B cells would be extremely valuable reagents. Recently, Nadler et al. (1981) reported a monoclonal antibody (anti B1) reactive with normal B cells that was not reactive with T cells, null cells, PMN, or monocytes. Abramson et al. (1981) also reported a monoclonal antibody (Ba-1) that was reactive with B cells and also with PMN. Of interest is that neither anti-B1 nor anti-Ba1 react with multiple myeloma- or mitogen-induced plasma cells (Abramson et al., 1981; Nadler, personal communication). The relationship of antigens detected by these monoclonal antibodies to those detected by heteroantiserum (Balch et al., 1978; Stashenko et al., 1980) remains to be determined.

Ault and Springer (1981) have reported a monoclonal antibody M 1/70 that detects an antigen present on all human monocytes and PMN. This antibody also reacted with a small population of null lymphocytes, but not with highly purified T cells. Breard and coworkers (1980) have also reported a monoclonal antibody (OKM1) reactive with monocytes, PMN, and null cells. However, this antibody also reacted with a small number of SRBC rosette-positive cells including T_γ cells (Reinherz, 1980d). Finally, LeBien and Kersey (1980) have reported a monoclonal antibody (TA-1) that reacts with all monocytes and the majority of PBL T cells, but not with granulocytes. Thus it appears that various monoclonals reactive with monocytes may also bind to cells of different lineage.

2.5. Monoclonal Antibodies Reactive with Leukemias and Lymphomas

As described earlier in this chapter, acute lymphoblastic leukemia (ALL) is generally considered to be a malignancy of lymphoid progenitor cells. Some cases are known to contain cytoplasmic immunoglobulin (pre-B phenotype), membrane immunoglobulin (B cell phenotype), or receptors for SRBC (T cell phenotype). An additional group (common ALL or cALLa phenotype) is felt to arise from terminal deoxynucleotidyl transferase (TdT) positive lymphocytes in normal bone marrow (Janossy et al., 1979). There has been an intense search for cell surface markers characteristic of leukemia cells, but to date there is no clear evidence for a leukemia-specific antigen. However, this search has led to recognition of antigens characteristic of progenitor cells and/or cells undergoing rapid replication. In addition, the reactivity (or lack of reactivity) of particular leukemia cases with monoclonal antibodies has led to some surprising results that may shed light on the lineage of these neoplasms. We summarize the reactivity of several monoclonal antibodies with various leukemias in Table 6. The references and description of reactivity of each antibody are described below. We have simplified the results for graphical purposes: if a significant percent of cases are reactive (but not necessarily all cases) they have been designated "+"; we have used an "R" to designate that only rare cases of leukemia are reactive or that a small percent of normal cells bear that antigen.

Reinherz et al., (1980a) used monoclonal antibodies to examine 26 cases of T-ALL. The vast majority (20/26) reacted with antibodies OKT9 and OKT10, but not with antibody OKT6 (found on thymic cortical cells) or antibody OKT3 (found on thymic medullary cells). However, it is likely that T-ALLs are of T cell lineage since they bear receptors for SRBC and also react with antibody L17F12 (Zipf et al., 1980) or T101 (Royston, 1980a). It has been postulated that T-ALL cells are derived from a normal thymocyte subpopulation that contains large blast cells ("prothymo-

Table 6
Reactivity with Monoclonal Antibodies

Antibody[a]	Thymus	PBL T	PBL B	PBL null	Mono-cytes	PMN	T-ALL	c-ALL	AML	AMML	B-CLL
OKT9	R	–	–	–	–	–	+	R[b]	–		–
OKT10	+	R[b]	–	R	–	–	+	+	+		–
OKT6	+	–	–	–	–	–	R	–	–	–	–
OKT3	+	+	–	–	–	–	R	–	–	–	–
L17F12	+	+	–	–	–	–	+	+	–	–	+
B1	–	–	+	–	–	–	–	+	–	–	+
Ba1	–	–	+	–	–	+	–	+	–	–	+
J-5	–	–	–	–	–	–	–	+	–	–	–
Ba2	–	–	–	–	–	–	R	+	–	–	+
OKM1	–	R	–	–	+	+	–	–	R	+	–
TA1	+	+	–	+	+	–	+	–	–	+	–

[a] References to each antibody are given in text.

[b] R refers to rare cases of staining for a particular ALL or only a few percent of normal cells.

cytes'') (Bradstock et al., 1980b). The presence of reactivity with antibody OKT9 and OKT10 may reflect a rapid rate of cell replication since these antigens can be induced by mitogens on normal PBL in vitro (Fox and Kung, unpublished observations). Thus the majority of T-ALL cases appear to arise from a precursor cell that is relatively rare in normal tissues and may represent a failure to achieve further lymphoid differentiation.

In order to study leukemias of B cell lineage, Nadler et al. (1981) developed antibody B1 and found it was reactive with all cases of B-CLL and B cell lymphoma. Of considerable interest is that approximately 50% of cases of ALL of non-T origin were also reactive with anti-B1. However, anti-B1 did not react with myelomas or B cells driven to plasma cells by mitogens. This suggests that anti-B1 detects a particular stage of B cell differentiation that characterizes certain ALL cases. In independent studies, Abramson et al. (1981) reported monoclonal antibody Ba-1 that appears to have a similar pattern of reactivities with ALL as noted for antibody B1. Further experiments will be required to determine if these antibodies are detecting similar antigens.

A surprising finding in the study of B-CLL was the expression of the 67,000 dalton antigen normally found on T cells (but not B cells) detected by antibody T101 (Royston, 1980a) or antibody SC1 (described earlier in this chapter). It is possible that B-CLL arises from a rare precursor of leukemic transformation.

Monoclonal antibodies that recognize antigens on lymphohematopoietic precursor cells also react with certain leukemia cells. For example, Janossy et al. (1979) reported that the antigen found on "common" ALL (the cALLa antigen on gp100) is also found on a small population of normal bone marrow lymphocytes that also contain the enzyme TdT. Recently, monoclonal antibody J-5 has been reported that also detects this antigen (Ritz et al., 1980). As another example, Kersey et al. (1981) recently reported monoclonal antibody Ba-2 that detects an antigen with molecular weight 24,000 daltons on normal bone marrow cells and in most cases of non-T, non-B ALL. Approximately 50% of B-CLL and 20% of T-ALL cases were also reactive with anti-Ba-2; also, some carcinomas and neuroblastomas were found to be reactive. These results suggest that different types of progenitor cells may express the Ba-2 antigen. A third example of an antigen found on precursor cells as well as ALL cells is the antigen recognized by antibody OKT10. This antibody reacts with the vast majority of T-ALL (Reinherz, 1980a) and AML cases (Reinherz and Schlossman, 1981a). It also reacts with greater than 90% of normal thymocytes and with TdT positive bone marrow cells, myeloblasts, and bone marrow B lymphocytes (Janossy et al., 1981). Antibody OKT10 reacts with a larger number of bone marrow mononuclear cells (16–20%) than does antibody Ba-2 (3–5%). Antibody Ba-2 may recognize a subset of precursor cells detected by antibody OKT10.

Monoclonal antibodies reactive with monocytes have also been found to react with certain leukemias. Antibody OKM1 (reactive with normal monocytes, null cells, PMN and a subset of T cells) was found to stain acute myelomonocytic (AMML) cells and to stain weakly only two out of eight cases of AML (Breard et al., 1980). Therefore, antibody OKM1 was able to stain normal mature PMN but not the majority of AML cases. As another example, antibody TA-1 (that detects all PBL T cells and monocytes but not PMN) was reactive with all cases (5/5) of AMML but no cases (0/12) of AML (LeBien and Kersey, 1981). The TA-1 antigen was not found on common ALL, pre B-ALL, or B-CLL. However, 6/11 cases of T-ALL were reactive. Thus, antibody TA-1 detects an antigen restricted to a particular stage of monocyte or T-cell differentiation. Both antibody OKM1 and TA-1 appear able to distinguish AMML from AML.

Recently, Nadler et al. (1981b) developed a monoclonal antibody (Ab 89) that was specific for a lymphoma-associated antigen on the tumor cells of a patient with poorly differentiated B cell lymphoma (D-PDL). This antibody was unreactive with this patient's normal PBL cells, but did react with lymphoma cells from other patients with B cell D-PDL. These studies suggest that there may be significant heterogeneity among B cell lymphomas.

Finally, Omary et al. (1980) have already reported an elegant series of experiments where they characterized an antigen found on rapidly dividing cells, such as normal PBL after mitogen stimulation. Antibody 3/25 apparently detects the same molecule as does antibody OKT9 and both antibodies react with the majority of ALL cells (Trowbridge and Omary, 1981). They demonstrated that the 100,000 dalton molecular weight glycoprotein identified by antibody 3/25 serves as the transferrin receptor on the cell membrane. Thus, the 3/25 antigen is the first cell surface molecule identified by a monoclonal antibody for which a biological function has been determined. Monoclonal antibodies to other cell surface antigens associated with precursor cells and leukemia may also represent receptors for polypeptide hormones or growth factors. Alternatively, these antigens may function as enzymes necessary for cell growth. Using heteroantiserum, Checkik et al. (1980), have demonstrated that human thymus/leukemia associated antigen (HThy-L) was identified to be a low molecular weight form of the enzyme adenosine deaminase. However, the HThy-L antigen could not be detected on the cell membrane and thus appears to be distinct from the antigens detected by the monoclonal antibodies described above.

2.6. Precautions in Interpreting the Reactivity of Monoclonal Antibodies

Although monoclonal antibodies are powerful tools for elucidation of lymphocyte subsets, potential pitfalls must carefully be avoided.

1. Monoclonal antibodies react only with a single antigenic determinant. Failure to react with antibody implies that the particular antigenic group is absent (or blocked by other determinants). For example, an antibody might recognize an oligosaccharide determinant on a membrane glycoprotein molecule. An identical protein backbone might also be present on different subsets of lymphocytes (or lymphoid tumors) with only minor differences in glycosylation, yet such cells would not react with the particular monoclonal antibody. Previous studies have demonstrated that cell membrane proteins undergo post translational modifications that are dictated by their state of differentiation (Barclay et al., 1976; Hoessli et al., 1980).

2. Cells may be characterized not only according to presence or absence of an antigen, but also by the relative amount of antigen on a particular cell type. For example, pan-T antibodies such as T101 also react with chronic lymphocytic leukemia cells (Royston et al., 1980a). However, CLL cells have less of the 67,000 dalton antigen than do T lymphoma or normal T cells. Thus, if only the ability to react with pan-T antibody is considered, then both CLL and T cells would be considered positive and might be grouped together. However, the difference in amount of antigen per cell is of obvious significance since CLL cells and T cells have many other clear differences.

3. Monoclonal antibodies may react with determinants that are only present in some individuals (i.e., alloantigens that are polymorphic). For example, the presence of reactivity with a given monoclonal antibody may enumerate a particular lymphocyte subset in the majority of individuals. However, in some other "normal" individuals, this antigenic marker may not be detectable although the lymphocyte subset is actually present. Therefore, the absence of reactivity with a monoclonal antibody may not necessarily imply a pathologic alteration of lymphocyte subsets.

4. Hybridomas grown as tissue culture supernatants express a single monoclonal antibody. However, hybridomas grown as "ascites" also contain other immunoglobulins in addition to the desired monoclonal antibody. Fortunately, the "titer" of the resulting ascites is sufficiently high that irrelevant antibodies *may* not be significant at the dilutions employed.

5. Monoclonal antibodies may exhibit a true cross-reactivity between distinct molecules and the extent of this cross-reactivity may vary with the experimental conditions employed (Mosman et al., 1980).

6. Cells that bear a particular antigen may not be susceptible to complement-mediated lysis. Ledbetter et al., (1980b) has demonstrated that all mouse T cells react with monoclonal Lyt-1, but only some T cells are lysed by anti Lyt-1 plus complement.

7. Many investigators use immunoprecipitation and gel electro-

phoresis to characterize the antigens identifiable by monoclonal anti-bodies. These reported molecular weights serve as an important parameter for comparison of the reactivity of various antibodies. Since many of the antigens are glycoproteins, their apparent molecular weights in SDS gels are higher than would be expected from other methods of molecular weight determination. For example, antibodies reactive with T cells (such as L17F12 or T101), have reported molecular weights ranging from 65,000 to 71,000 daltons (Royston et al., 1980a; Engleman et al., 1980; Wang et al., 1980). When immuno-precipitates are run side by side, a similar molecular weight antigen is precipitated by each antibody, as shown in Fig. 3.

3. Clinical Applications

3.1. Lymph Node Architecture:
Normal and Malignant

The previous discussion has dealt with the cell membrane antigens on lymphocytes in suspension, either as normal PBL or as leukemias. Another important question in clinical and research studies has been to determine characteristics of neoplastic lymphocytes as they assemble to form structures we term lymphomas. "Do lymphomas mimic the structure of the normal lymphoid system?" This leads to an important secondary question: "If lymphoma cells mimic normal lymphoid cells, does the histological appearance or expression of surface markers of a lymphoma provide a clue as to how it arose?" Figure 7 is a schematic representation of a normal human lymph node. It is simplified for clarity. The structure is oval, with afferent lymphatics, through which lymphoid cells enter, and efferent lymphatics, through which cells leave. The node is conventionally divided into two regions: cortex and medulla. The cortex contains most of the lymphocytes. The medulla is the region of confluence of the sinusoids. Within the cortex there are three subregions: primary follicles, secondary follicles, and the diffuse cortex. These are easily recognized histologically and are domains for different types of lymphocytes (Weissman et al., 1978). Primary follicles are round aggregates of cells, most of which are small B lymphocytes. A few T cells as well as a few macrophages and dendritic reticular cells are also present. These cells have been defined by immunofluorescent techniques using antibodies to cell surface immuno-globulin to detect B cells. Phagocytosis has been used as a marker for macrophages, and antigen fixation as a marker for dendritic reticular cells. Under conditions of antigenic stimulation, primary follicles become sec-

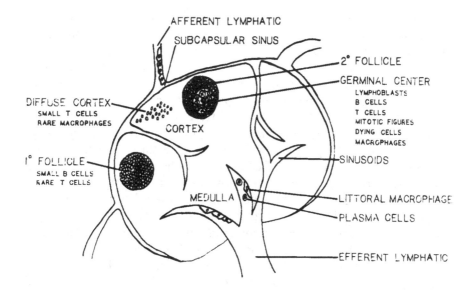

Fig. 7. Schematic representation of a normal lymph node.

ondary follicles: a rim of B cells surrounds lymphoblasts, mitotic figures, dying cells, macrophages, and reticular cells. By immunofluorescence, both B and T cells are always detected in this center area, which is usually called a "germinal center." Today it is common to assert that "follicular lymphomas" arise in germinal centers, or mimic germinal centers.

In non-Hodgkin's lymphoma, two major alterations in lymph node morphology may be seen: "nodular" (or follicular) and "diffuse" (Rappaport, 1966). Nodular lymphomas replace the entire architecture of the lymph node with nodules of cells reminiscent of normal secondary follicles. Immunofluorescence studies have shown that these nodules are composed of B cells that express monoclonal surface immunoglobulin (Jaffe et al., 1974). In the lymph nodes of an individual lymphoma patient, all the nodules react with antibody to kappa chains only or to lambda chains only. (Normal follicles have both kappa- and lambda-bearing cells.) Between the follicles of a lymphoma one does not usually see T cells as one would in a normal lymph node. Instead one sees either a heterogeneous population of B cells with kappa- and lambda-bearing cells, or one sees a monoclonal proliferation of B cells bearing the same light chain as that seen in the follicles. A comparison of the structure of normal lymph nodes and "follicular" lymphomas shows considerable differences among the cell populations in all regions of the node. Diffuse lymphomas are easy to recognize. All of the normal architecture of the lymph node is replaced by a sheet of lymphoid cells. In humans, most diffuse lymphomas are also composed of B cells bearing monoclonal surface immunoglobulin (Aisenberg and Long, 1975). Because spread of B cells from follicles to the cortex may be seen in follicular lymphomas, some investigators have concluded that many diffuse lymphomas have evolved from follicular lymphomas. This may be true in some cases, particularly since both patterns may occasionally be seen in one patient. It is almost certainly not true for some types of lymphoma, such as diffuse well-differentiated lymphocytic lymphoma and chronic lymphocytic leukemia. These entities always diffusely replace lymph nodes with histologically unremarkable lymphocytes (hence the term "well-differentiated"). The lymphocytes are also B cells that display monoclonal immunoglobulin on their surfaces.

Hodgkin's disease is distinguishable from non-Hodgkin's lymphomas by histological criteria. When one studies surface markers on cells in involved lymph nodes, the differences between Hodgkin's disease and non-Hodgkin's lymphoma are considerable. Hodgkin's disease lymphocytes are a mixture of T cells, B cells, and macrophages. There is no evidence of a monoclonal proliferation unless one considers the Reed Sternberg cell or other atypical "histiocytes" *the* malignant cells. Reed Sternberg cells often bear surface Ig that can be demonstrated by fluorescent antibodies, but the Ig is not monoclonal. These cells probably adsorb Ig on surface Fc receptors and are thought to be malignant monocytes (Mann et al., 1979). The demonstration that Hodgkin's disease is characterized by a proliferating mixture of cell types, but still behaves in a malignant fashion leads to two quite different possibilities. The generally accepted interpretation is that the Reed Sternberg cell or other atypical histiocytes are malignant and that the rest of the cells in the involved lymph node are reactive. But, one should also consider that some tumors are not necessarily monoclonal proliferations. Self-stimulatory mixtures of cells may also escape normal control mechanism and proliferate endlessly, or at least long enough to kill the host.

This brief review of lymphoid architecture should point out some problems in the common interpretation of data derived from lymph nodes stained with fluorescent antibodies. Many investigators accept that "all nodular lymphomas regardless of cytologic subtype, arise from follicular (or germinal center) B lymphocytes" (Jaffe et al., 1974). But there is a difference between primary and secondary follicles. B lymphocytes of primary follicles probably arise in the bone marrow and migrate to primary follicles, where they await antigenic stimulation; they are probably short-lived. Germinal center B lymphocytes differentiate to form plasma cells, and presumably memory cells. Whether the memory cells return to primary follicles, recirculate, or remain *in situ* is not known. We do know that malignant B cells do recirculate and form follicle-like structures (Warnke and Levy, 1978). The rate of cell division varies greatly from patient to patient. If we suppose that malignant B cells are more like primary follicle B lymphocytes, one might guess that transformation took place in the bone marrow and the transformed cells migrated to lymph nodes. If we suppose that the malignant B cells are more like germinal center B cells, we would guess that malignant cells were transformed in lymph nodes and recirculated to other nodes. We need to resolve all these questions. Hopefully, a systematic study of markers on the surface of normal and malignant cells will be helpful.

3.2. Clinical Applications of Monoclonal Antibody Technology

Following the description of markers on the surface of lymphocytes many investigators have sought to establish correlations between surface markers and disease states that are believed to be related to lymphocyte abnormalities. In the case of lymphocytic lymphoma and leukemia, surface marker analysis has demonstrated that the great majority of these patients have a monoclonal proliferation of lymphocytes. These studies, including the prognostic implications, have been extensively reviewed (Greaves et al., 1980; Reinherz et al., 1979b, 1979d,1980a; Sallen et al., 1980; Nadler et al., 1980). The value of such tests for aiding the diagnosis or therapy of leukemia is only beginning to be appreciated. The advent of monoclonal antibody technology affords the chance for standardized reagents to become available to the multiple centers that study these problems.

Initially, this new technology will be used to investigate the biologic mechanisms in health and disease. With the widespread availability of monoclonal antibodies, they will be increasingly used to help make diagnostic decisions and to monitor patients' progress. Therefore, it is important that initial studies be sufficiently complete to avoid potentially misleading results. Ransohof and Feinstein (1978) have found many published articles describing diagnostic tests that were useful when the tests compared patients with advanced disease to normal subjects. However, in clinical practice, the problem is often to distinquish minimal disease from normal states or from other diseases in the differential diagnosis. For this reason, many tests that appear useful in the laboratory have proved disappointing in clinical practice. Therefore, the value of monoclonal antibodies must be proven in carefully controlled studies before they are used for widespread clinical diagnosis.

4. Summary

Initial studies have demonstrated that lymphocyte subsets can be defined with rosetting techniques and heteroantisera. These studies were limited by technical difficulties in performing the assays as well as by availability and specificity of standardized antibody reagents. It now appears that the limitations associated with heteroantisera can be overcome by using monoclonal antibodies. Since these reagents will be increasingly used in clinical research, we have reviewed the basic aspects of their preparation and use. Next, we have outlined the types of antigens that might be detected on lymphoid cells and listed examples of some reported monoclonal antibodies. Finally, we have given side-by-side comparisons of monoclonal antibodies that have been prepared by different groups of investigators and reported to have pan-T cell activity. Next, we have reviewed monoclonal antibodies reactive with B cells, monocytes, and various types of leukemia. Finally, we have discussed normal lymph node structure and the alterations that lead to the diagnosis of lymphoma.

The use of monoclonal antibodies does appear to be a promising technique that may help describe how normal cells differentiate and how cells transform. However, realization of the full potential use of monoclonal antibodies in clinical medicine will depend on continued exchange and comparison of these reagents among different investigators.

Acknowledgments

We would like to thank Nilima Sabharwal and Ted Benson for their expert technical assistance. We are grateful to Drs. S. Fong, L. Thompson, J. Huddlestone, C. Tsoukas, and J. Vaughan for their suggestions regarding these experiments and proofreading this manuscript. We thank Shari Brewster and Anna Milne for their secretarial assistance.

References

Abramson, C., J. Kersey, and T. LeBien (1981), *J. Immunol.* **126,** 83.
Ades, E., R. Zwernor, R. Acton, and C. Balch (1980), *J. Exptl. Med.* **151,** 400.
Aisenberg, A., and J. Long (1975), *Am. J. Med.* **58,** 300.
Anderson, J., and R. Metzgar (1978), *J. Immunol.* **120,** 262.
Ault, K., and T. Springer (1981), *J. Immunol.* **126,** 359.
Balch, C., P. Dourgert, L. Volger, E. Ades, and S. Ferrone (1978), *J. Immunol.* **121,** 232.
Balch, H., E. Ades, M. Loken, and S. Shore (1980), *J. Immunol.* **124,** 1845.
Barclay, A., M. Letarte-Muirhead, A. Williams, and R. Foulker (1976), *Nature* **263,** 563.
Bentwich, Z., S. Douglas, E. Skutelsky, and H. Kunkel (1973), *J. Exptl. Med.* **137,** 1532.
Billing, R., and P. Terasaki (1974), *J. Natl. Cancer Inst.* **53,** 1635.
Borella, L., and L. Sen (1973), *J. Immunol.* **111,** 1257.
Bowman, P., S. Melvin, and A. Mauer (1980), *Adv. Int. Med.* **25,** 391.

Bradstock, K., G. Janossy, M. Bollum, and C. Milstein (1980a), *Nature* **284** (in press).

Bradstock, K., G. Janossy, G. Pizzolo, V. Hoffmand, A. McMichael, J. Pilch, C. Milstein, P. Beverly, and F. Bollum (1980b), *J. Natl. Cancer Inst.* **65**, 33.

Breard, J., E. Reinherz, P. Kung, G. Goldstein, and S. Schlossman (1980), *J. Immunol.* **124**, 1943.

Broder, S., and T. Waldmann (1978), *New Engl. J. Med.* **299**, 1281.

Brooks, H., I. Beckman, and H. Zola (1980), *Clin. Exptl. Immunol.* **39**, 477.

Brouet, J., and M. Seligmann (1978), *Cancer* **42**, 817.

Brown, G., M. Greaves, T. Lister, and N. Rapson (1974), *Lancet* **2**, 753.

Cantor, H., F. Shen, and E. Boyse (1976), *J. Exptl. Med.* **143**, 1391.

Checkik, B., M. Percy, and E. Gelfand (1978), *J. Natl. Cancer Inst.* **60**, 69.

Checkik, B., J. Rao, M. Greaves, and V. Hoffbrand (1980), *Leukemia Res.* **4**, 343.

Claman, H., and E. Chaperon (1969), *Transpl. Rev.* **1**, 92.

Cooper, M. (1979), *J. Exptl. Med.* **150**, 792.

Cordier, G., C. Samarut, J. Brochier, and J. P. Revillard (1976), *Scand. J. Immunol.* **5**, 233.

Dickler, H., and H. Kunkel (1972), *J. Exptl. Med.* **136**, 191.

Eisenbarth, G., J. Haynes, A. Schroer, and A. Fauci (1980), *J. Immunol.* **124**, 1237.

Engleman, E., R. Fox, R. Warnke, and R. Levy (1981), *Proc. Natl. Acad. Sci.* (in press).

Evans, R., J. Breard, H. Lazarus, S. Schlossman, and L. Chess (1977), *J. Exptl. Med.* **145**, 221.

Evans, R., T. Faldetta, R. Humphrey, D. Pratt, E. Yunis, and S. Schlossman (1978), *J. Exptl. Med.* **148**, 1440.

Ferrarini, M., T. Hoffman, S. Fu, R. Winchester, and H. Kunkel (1977), *J. Immunol.* **199**, 1525.

Fox, R., and I. Weissman (1979), *J. Immunol.* **122**, 1697.

Friedman, H., J. Brochier, and J. Revillard (1976), *Immunol.* **31**, 759.

Gonzales, A., and H. Spiegelberg (1977), *J. Clin. Inv.* **59**, 616.

Greaves, M., G. Brown, N. Rapson, and T. Lister (1975), *Clin. Immunol. Immunopath.* **4**, 67.

Greaves, M., and G. Janossy (1978), *Biochem. Biophys. Acta* **516**, 193.

Greaves, M., W. Verbi, L. Vogler, M. Cooper, and R. Ellis (1980), *Leukemia Res.* **3**, 353.

Hanaumi, K., T. Abo, and K. Kumagi (1976), *Nature* **259**, 124.

Hansen, J., P. Martin, and R. Nowinski (1980), *Immunogenetics* **10**, 247.

Haynes, B., J. Schooley, C. Grouse, R. Payling, R. Dolin, and A. Fauci (1979), *J. Immunol.* **122**, 699.

Hayward, A., L. Layward, P. Lydyard, L. Moretta, M. Dagg, and A. Lawton (1978), *J. Immunol.* **121**, 1.

Hoessli, D., C. Bron, and R. Pink (1980), *Nature* **283**, 576.

Jaffee, E., E. Shevach, M. Frank, C. Breard, and I. Green (1974), *New Engl. J. Med.* **290**, 813.

Janossy, G., F. Bollum, A. McMichael, N. Rapson, and M. Greaves (1979), *J. Immunol.* **123**, 1525.

Janossy, G., N. Tidman, E. Papageorgiou, P. Kung, and G. Goldstein (1981), *J. Immunol.* **126,** 1608.

Jondal, M., G. Holm, and H. Wigzell (1972), *J. Exptl. Med.* **136,** 207.

Kamoun, P., Martin, P., Hansen, J., Brown, M., Siadek, A. and Nowinski, R. (1981), *J. Exp. Med.* **153,** 207

Katz, D. (1977), *Lymphoid Differentiation, Recognition and Regulation.* Academic Press, New York, pp. 1–119.

Katz, D., and B. Benacerraf (1972), *Adv. Immunol.* **15,** 1.

Kersey, J., T. LeBien, C. Abramson, R. Newman, R. Sutherland, and M. Greaves (1981), *J. Exptl. Med.* (in press).

Ko, H., S. Fu, R. Winchester, D. Ya, and H. Kunkel (1979), *J. Exptl. Med.* **150,** 246.

Köhler, G., and C. Milstein (1975), *Nature* **256,** 495.

Kumagi, K., T. Abo, T. Sekizawa, and M. Sasaki (1975), *J. Immunol.* **115,** 982.

Kung, P., G. Goldstein, E. Reinherz, and S. Schlossman (1979), *Science* **206,** 347.

Kung, P., and G. Goldstein (1980), *Vox Sanguinis* **39,** 121.

Huber, H., S. Douglas, and H. Fudenberg (1969), *Immunology* **17,** 7.

Lampson, L., and R. Levy (1980), *J. Immunol.* **125,** 293.

Le Bien, T., and J. Kersey (1980), *J. Immunol.* **125,** 2208.

Ledbetter, J., R. Evans, and L. Herzenberg (1981), *J. Exptl. Med.* **153,** 310.

Ledbetter, J., J. Goding, T. Tsu, and L. Herzenberg (1979), *Immunogenetics* **8,** 347.

Ledbetter, J. and L. Herzenberg (1980), *Immunol. Rev.* **47,** 63.

Levy, R., J. Dilley, R. Fox, and P. Warnke (1979), *Proc. Natl. Acad. Sci.* **76,** 6552.

Limatibul, S., A. Shore, H. Dosch, and E. Gelfund (1978), *Clin. Exptl. Immunol.* **33,** 503.

Loken, M., and L. Herzenberg (1975), *Ann. NY Acad. Sci.* **254,** 163.

Lum, L., M. Keren, W. Strober, and R. Bloese (1979), *J. Immuno.* **122,** 65.

Mackler, B., E. Richie, and T. Swate (1980), *Clin. Immunol. Immunolpath.* **15,** 238.

Mann, D., G. Rogentine, R. Halterman, and B. Leventhal (1971), *Science* **1974,** 1136.

Mann, R., E. Jaffe, and C. Breard (1979), *Amer. J. Pathol.* **94,** 105.

McMichael, A., J. Pilch, G. Golfre, D. Mason, and C. Milstein (1979), *Eur. J. Immunol.* **9,** 205.

Merrill, J., G. Biberfeld, G. Kolmodin, S. Landin, and E. Norrby (1980), *J. Immunol.* **124,** 2758.

Mingari, M., L. Moretta, A. Moretta M. Ferrarini, and J. Preud'homme (1978), *J. Immunol.* **121,** 767.

Minowada, J., T. Ohnuma, and G. Moore (1972), *J. Natl. Cancer Inst.* **49,** 891.

Mohanakumar, T., and R. Roney (1978), *Clin. Haem.* **7,** 363.

Moretta, L., M. Ferranini, C. Mingari, A. Moretta, and S. Webb (1976), *J. Immunol.* **117,** 2171.

Moretta, L., S. Webb, P. Grossi, P. Lydyard, and M. Cooper (1977), *J. Exptl. Med.* **146,** 184.

Moriya, N., T. Nagaoki, N. Okuda, and N. Taniguchi (1979), *J. Immunol.* **123,** 1795.

Nadler, L., E. Reinherz, H. Weinstein, C. Orsi, and S. Schlossman (1980a), *Blood* **55,** 806.

Nadler, L., J. Ritz, R. Handy, J. Pesando, and S. Schlossman (1981), *J. Clin. Invest.* **67,** 134.

Nadler, L., P. Stashenko, R. Hardy, and S. Schlossman (1980b), *J. Immunol.* **125,** 570.

Nakahara, K., T. Ohashi, T. Oda, T. Hirano, M. Kasai, K. Okumura, and T. Tada (1980), *New Engl. J. Med.* **302,** 675.

Niaudet, P., and M. Greaves (1980), *J. Immunol.* **124,** 1203.

Niaudet, P., M. Greaves, and D. Horwitz (1979), *Scand. J. Immunol.* **9,** 387.

Noorloos, A., H. Pegels, R. Oors, J. Wilberbusch, T. Vroom, R. Goudsint, W. Zeijlemaker, A. Bornee, and C. Melief (1980), *N. Engl. J. Med.* **320,** 933.

Omary, M., I. Trowbridge, and J. Minowada (1980), *Nature* **286,** 888.

Owen, R., G. Bernier, and M. Farger (1976), *Immunochemistry* **13,** 129.

Ozer, H., A. J. Strelkauskas, R. T. Callery, and S. F. Schlossman (1979), *Eur. J. Immunol.* **9,** 112.

Pellegrino, M., S. Ferrone, M. Dierich, and R. Reisfeld (1975), *Clin. Immuno. Immunopath.* **3,** 324.

Pesando, J., J. Ritz, H. Levine, C. Terhorst, H. Lazarus, and S. Schlossman (1980), *J. Immunol.* **124,** 2794.

Pichler, W., and S. Broder (1978), *J. Immunol.* **121,** 887.

Pratt, D., S. Schlossman, and J. Strominger (1980), *J. Immunol.* **124,** 1449.

Preud'homme, J., M. Klein, S. Labaume, and M. Seligman (1977), *Eur. J. Immunol.* **1,** 840.

Ransohof, D., and A. Feinstein (1978), *N. Engl. J. Med.* **299,** 926.

Rappaport, H. (1966), in *Atlas of Tumor Pathology,* sect. III, fasc. 8, Armed Forces Institute of Pathology, Washington, D.C.

Reinherz, E., P. Kung, G. Goldstein, and S. Schlossman (1979a), *J. Immunol.* **123,** 1312.

Reinherz, E., P. Kung, G. Goldstein, and S. Schlossman (1979f), *Proc. Natl. Acad. Sci.* **76,** 4061.

Reinherz, E., P. Kung, G. Goldstein, and S. Schlossman (1979g), *J. Immunol.* **123,** 2894.

Reinherz, E., P. Kung, G. Goldstein, and S. Schlossman (1980b), *J. Immunol.* **124,** 1301.

Reinherz, E., P. Kung, G. Goldstein, R. Levy, and S. Schlossman (1980a), *Proc. Natl. Acad. Sci.* **77,** 1588.

Reinherz, E., P. Kung, J. Resando, J. Ritz, G. Goldstein, and S. Schlossman (1979c), *J. Exptl. Med.* **150,** 1472.

Reinherz, E., L. Moretta, M. Roper, J. Breard, M. Mingari, M. Cooper, and S. Schlossman (1980d), *J. Exptl. Med.* **151,** 969.

Reinherz, E., L. Nadler, D. Rosenthal, W. Moloney, and S. Schlossman (1979d), *Blood,* **53,** 1066.

Reinherz, E., L. Nadler, S. Sallon, and S. Schlossman (1979b), *J. Clin. Invest.* **64,** 392.

Reinherz, E., R. Parkman, J. Rappaport, F. Rosen, and S. Schlossman (1979e), *N. Engl. J. Med.* **300,** 1061.

Reinherz, E., and S. Schlossman (1980c), *Cell* **19,** 821.

Reinherz, E., and S. Schlossman (1980e), *Cancer Treatment Reports.*

Ritz, J., J. Pesando, J. Notis-McConarty, H. Lazarus, and S. Schlossman (1980), *Nature* **283,** 583.

Rowe, D., and J. Fahey (1965), *J. Exptl. Med.* **121,** 171.

Royston, I., J. Majda, S. Baird, G. Yamamoto, B. Meserve, C. Ivor, and J. Griffiths (1980a), *J. Immunol.* **125,** 725.

Royston, I., J. Majda, G. Yamamoto, and S. Baird (1980b), *Proc. 28th Colloquium,* Pergamon Press, London, 1980.

Sachs, L. (1978), *Nature* **274,** 535.

Sallan, S., J. Ritz, J. Pesando, R. Geller, C. O'Brien, S. Hitchcock, F. Coral, and S. Schlossman (1980), *Blood* **55,** 395.

Salmon, S., and M. Seligman (1974), *Lancet* **2,** 1230.

Schuster, D., B. Bongiovani, D. Pierson, D. Wond, and A. Levinson (1980), *J. Immunol.* **124,** 1662.

Seligman, M., J. Preud'homme, and J. Brovet (1973), Transplant. Rev. **16,** 83.

Sell, S. (1980), *Cancer Markers,* Humana, Clifton, N.J.

Shore, S. L., F. M. Melewicz, and D. S. Gordon (1977), *J. Immunol.* **118,** 558.

Taub, R., M. Baker, and K. Madyastha (1980), 55, 294.

Touraine, J. (1978), in *Human Lymphocyte Differentiation: Its application to cancer,* Serrou, B., and C. Rosenfeld, eds., Elsevier/North-Holland, NY, p. 93.

Trowbridge, I., and M. Omary (1981), *Proc. Nat. Acad. Sci.* (in press).

Unanue, E., H. Grey, E. Rabellino, P. Campbell, and J. Schmidtke (1971), *J. Exptl. Med.* **133,** 1188.

Van Boxel, J., W. Paul, W. Terry, and I. Green (1972), *J. Immunol.* **109,** 648.

Van Wauwe, J., J. DeMey, and J. Goossens (1980), *J. Immunol.* **124,** 2708.

Wang, C., R. Good, P. Ammirati, G. Dymbort, and R. Evans (1980), *J. Exptl. Med.* **151,** 1539.

Warnke, R., and R. Levy (1978), *N. Engl. J. Med.* **298,** 481.

Watanabe, K., and S. Hakomori (1976), *J. Exptl. Med.* **144,** 644.

Weiner, M., C. Bianoc, and V. Nussenzweig (1973), *Blood* **42,** 939.

Weissman, I., A. Warnke, E. Butcher, R. Rouse, and R. Levy (1978), *Human Path.* **9,** 325.

West, W. H., R. B. Boozer, and R. B. Herberman (1978), *J. Immunol.* **120,** 90.

Winchester, R., and H. Kunkel (1980), *Adv. Immunol.* **28,** 221.

Wybran, J., M. Carr, and H. Fudenberg (1973), *Clin. Immunol. Immunopath.* **1,** 408.

Wybran, J., and H. Fudenberg (1973), *Clin. Immunol. Immunopath.* **52,** 1026.

Zipf, T., R. Fox, J. Dilley, and R. Levy (1981), *Cancer Res. Treat. Rpts.*

3

An Immunochemical Approach to the Isolation of Human Melanoma-Associated Antigens

D. R. Galloway and R. A. Reisfeld

Department of Molecular Immunology, Scripps Clinic and Research Foundation, La Jolla, California

1. Introduction

"One of the principal hopes of the control of cancer lies fundamentally in a knowledge of the chemical nature of the malignant cell, and in successful development of chemotherapeutic approaches which must depend upon this knowledge." So wrote Dr. Jesse P. Greenstein in his book, *The Biochemistry of Cancer* in 1947 (Greenstein, 1947). The enormous complexity of this task is apparent when one considers that thirty-three years later many attempts are still in progress to characterize neoplastic cells biochemically. Although the general literature on cancer research and the publication of this volume *per se* indicate that a great deal of progress has been made, the search for relevant tumor markers continues.

A major emphasis in cancer research has been placed upon the study of relevant cell surface proteins and glycoproteins since there is ample experimental evidence to support the idea that malignant cells differ in their expression of such cell surface markers (Lewis, 1974; Ferrone and Pellegrino, 1977; Gold and Goldenberg, 1980). The appearance of new antigens or the alteration of existing macromolecules on the cell surface of neoplastic cells has important implications in terms of the detection and possible control of cancer. In recent years several new techniques have been developed that have resulted in a more precise study of the molecular nature of cell surfaces. As a result, a better detailed description of the neoplastic cell surface has gradually emerged.

Another development in the area of cell surface research is the discovery of antigen "shedding," that is, the release of such macromolecules as proteins, glycoproteins, lipoproteins, glycolipids, and glycosaminoglycans, either alone or in combination with other cell membrane constituents from the surface of viable cells. This phenomenon has been observed in a number of systems and has been the subject of a recent review (Black, 1980). The concept of shed antigens has important implications in terms of tumor versus host interactions by suggesting a mechanism for tumor escape from the imm   e surveillance of the host. Whether or not this is the basis for tumor survival or metastasis remains to be proven, but an increasing amount of evidence indicates that tumor-associated antigens are spontaneously released from the surface (Grimm et al., 1976; Bystryn, 1977; Stuhlmiller and Seigler, 1977; McCabe et al., 1978b, 1979; Gupta et al., 1979; Morgan et al., 1981). Consequently, when studying a particular tumor antigen, it has become important to establish its cell surface association and whether or not it is spontaneously released into the surrounding medium. Malignant melanoma was chosen as a model system for our studies since, of the various human tumors investigated thus far, it seems to be one of those most influenced by immunological factors that may be partially responsible for this tumor's unusual behavior (Lewis, 1974; Clark et al., 1977; Ferrone and Pellegrino, 1977). Therefore, it is important to characterize thoroughly the molecular profile of the antigenic mosaic on melanoma cells and to delineate the role of antibodies directed against these antigens during the clinical course of the disease. The ready availability of a number of well-characterized long-term human culture lines that definitely shed melanoma-associated antigens (MAA) aids this task since it provides the opportunity for comparative studies as well as a consistent source for the eventual purification and molecular characterization of these tumor cell markers.

The goal of our studies has been the development of immunochemical approaches for the isolation and molecular characterization of MAA and we thus concentrated our previous efforts on the production and serological characterization of functionally specific antimelanoma xenoantisera (McCabe et al., 1978a, 1979; Galloway et al., 1981a). In this paper we describe the utilization of this immunochemical approach in applying specific xenoantisera for the identification and purification of two glycoprotein antigens. We have concentrated our efforts to isolate and identify by immunochemical means the shed MAA in serum-free spent culture medium of cultered human melanoma cells, a readily available source of soluble antigens that precludes the use of cumbersome extraction procedures.

2. Methods

2.1. Intrinsic Labeling

In order to investigate the nature of cellular antigens shed from tumor cell surfaces, cultured human tumor cells were intrinsically radiolabeled by culturing the cells in the presence of labeled essential amino acids for 72 h. Typically, 2×10^7 cells were grown, either adherent or nonadherent in RPMI 1640 medium supplemented with 10% fetal calf serum, 1% glutamine, 0.01% gentamycin, and containing ^{3}H-valine (1 mCi, 50 mCi/mmol). In order to ensure selective incorporation of the radiolabel, the usual concentration of unlabeled valine (0.1 mg/mL) was reduced to one-quarter (0.025 mg/mL). Various radiolabeled amino acids were successfully used, including ^{3}H-valine, ^{3}H-phenylalanine, ^{3}H-leucine, ^{3}H-arginine, ^{3}H-lysine, and ^{35}S-methionine. The 72-h labeling period allowed intrinsically radiolabeled proteins released from the cell surface to accumulate in the spent culture medium. Following the incorporation of radiolabel, the spent medium was collected, centrifuged to remove cells, and then dialyzed against several changes of phosphate buffered saline pH 7.2 (PBS) containing 0.02% sodium azide, and the spent medium was finally stored in frozen aliquots. In the few cases where antigens were extracted from melanoma cells, radiolabeled cells were washed with PBS and cell surface macromolecules extracted with either 0.5% NP-40 in PBS (Stuhlmiller and Seigler, 1977), $3M$ KCl (Reisfeld et al., 1971), or $4M$ urea (Kishi et al., 1980).

2.2. SDS Polyacrylamide Gel Electrophoresis (SDS-PAGE)

Intrinsically labeled antigen preparations from spent culture medium or cell extracts were analyzed directly using discontinuous SDS-polyacrylamide gel electrophoresis (SDS-PAGE) according to the method of Laemmli (1970) and described by Weber and Osborn (1969). All analytical SDS-PAGE were performed using a slab gel format employing gels of 1.5-mm thickness and varying percentages of acrylamide, including gradient gels from 4 to 12% acrylamide concentration. Following electrophoresis, the gels were placed overnight in a fixative solution of 10% acetic acid and 20% methanol. The protein patterns were revealed by staining the gels in Coomassie Blue R-250 or by autoradiographic analysis following the incorporation of a fluor into the gels as described by Laskey and Mills (1975). All gels were dried onto Whatman 3mm filter paper using a Hoeffer slab gel dryer prior to autoradiography.

2.3. Indirect Immunoprecipitation

SDS-PAGE analysis of immunoprecipitates obtained by reacting specific antimelanoma xenoantisera with the labeled antigen preparations provided a sensitive method for identifying antigens being recognized by the antimelanoma antibody populations. The antimelanoma xenoantiserum #6522 used in these studies was prepared from rabbits injected repeatedly with intact cultured human melanoma cells (M21) and has been previously described in detail (McCabe et al., 1978a,b, Galloway et al., 1981b). This procedure was carried out essentially as described by Kessler (1975) using either protein A-bearing *Staphylococcus aureus* Cowan I (SACI) or protein A covalently coupled to Sepharose 4B (Pharmacia). The latter reagent resulted in less nonspecific binding of labeled protein and was therefore the reagent of choice. Immunoadsorbents were prepared just prior to use of reacting the xenoantisera with a 10% suspension of the protein A support at a ratio of 10:1. This experimental approach is outlined in Fig. 1.

3. Identification of MAA in Spent Culture Medium

Using the techniques outlined (Fig. 1) the known serological specificity of antimelanoma xenoantisera was compared with the molecular profiles obtained upon SDS-PAGE analysis of spent media antigens reacting with these antisera by immunoprecipitation. Figure 2 is an example of this type of analysis. Comparisons of immunoprecipitation patterns of spent media from several melanoma cell lines obtained with a specific antimelanoma xenoantiserum (#6522) resulted in the highly reproducible identification of two antigens (Fig. 2). One of these antigens has an approximate molecular weight of 240,000 daltons (240K), has only been found in association with cultured human melanoma cells, and thus far appears to be melanoma-specific. The other antigen has an approximate molecular weight of 94,000 daltons (94K) and has been found in association with both melanoma and carcinoma cells.

An interesting observation in these studies has been the frequent presence of fibronectin in the spent culture media (Fig. 2). The identification of this protein was achieved through the use of a specific antifibronectin xenoantiserum made to human fibronectin (Fig. 3). This highly immunogenic molecule is not only present in spent culture medium of all melanoma cell lines tested, but is also found in the spent media of many human

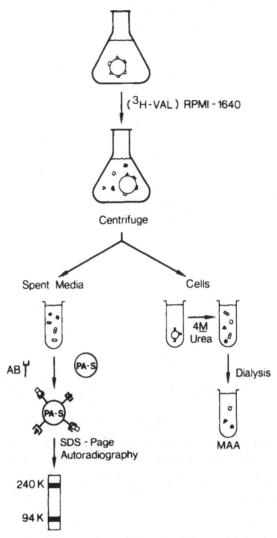

(^{3}H-VAL) RPMI-1640

Centrifuge

Spent Media

Cells

AB

PA-S

4M Urea

Dialysis

PA-S

SDS - Page
Autoradiography

MAA

240 K

94 K

Fig. 1. Schematic representation of the approaches used for the molecular characterization of human melanoma-associated antigens isolated from spent medium of cultured melanoma cells.

carcinoma lines (Fig. 2). In addition, antisera made to tumor cells frequently contain antifibronectin antibodies, as revealed by SDS-PAGE profiles of numerous immunoprecipitates. Consequently, an important consideration in the purification of MAA or the production of specific xenoantiserum to MAA was the removal of fibronectin from antigen preparations, especially since this molecule not only adheres to many other macromolecules, but also has proved to be highly immunogenic. The re-

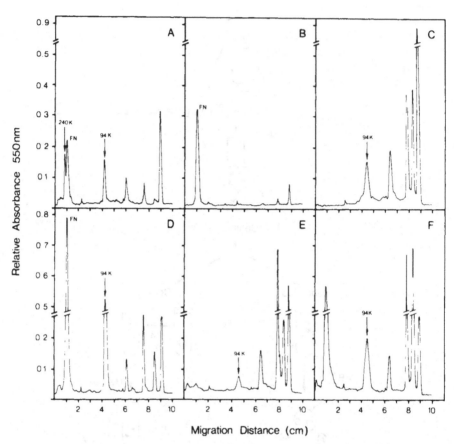

Fig. 2. SDS-PAGE molecular profiles of indirect immunoprecipitates obtained by reacting intrinsically labeled (^{3}H-valine) spent culture medium from various tumor lines with anti-MAA xenoantiserum #6522. A: M14 melanoma; B: HAM SK fibroblast; C: HT-29 carcinoma; D: T-24 carcinoma; E: D-98 carcinoma; F: MANO carcinoma.

moval of fibronectin was readily achieved by affinity chromatography using gelatin convalently coupled to Sepharose 4B, as described by Engvall and Ruoslahti (1977). Figure 3 demonstrates the effect of the removal of fibronectin from the spent culture medium and clearly shows the distinction between the 240K antigen and fibronectin.

The 240K and 94K antigens are specifically bound by antimelanoma xenoantiserum #6522. Intrinsically labeled (^{3}H-valine) spent media from cultured human melanoma cells (M21), first depleted with antilymphocyte xenoantiserum (coupled to Protein A-bearing SACI) in order to remove any proteins that might bind nonspecifically to antimelanoma immunoadsorbents, and subsequently analyzed by indirect immunoprecipitation using serum #6522, still showed the presence of the 240K and 94K MAA

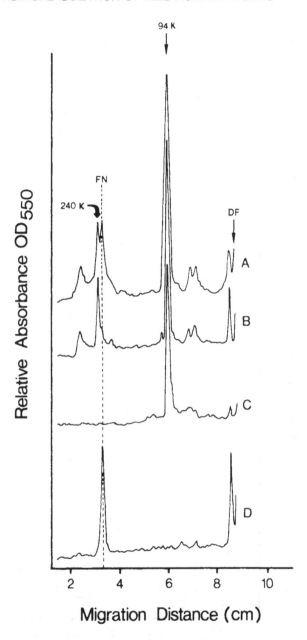

Fig. 3. SDS-PAGE profiles on 5% acrylamide gels of indirect immuno-precipitates obtained by reacting spent culture medium depleted of fibronectin from intrinsically labeled (^{3}H-valine) 21 SCRF cells with anti-MAA xeno-antisera. A, Anti-MAA xenoantiserum #6522 vs nondepleted spent medium (M21); B, anti-MAA xenoantiserum #6522 vs FN-depleted spent culture medium; C, anti-94K xenoantiserum #9446 vs FN-depleted spent medium; D, Xenoantiserum to human fibronectin vs M21 spent culture medium.

76 D. R. GALLOWAY AND R. A. REISFELD

(Fig. 3). Furthermore, the 240K and 94K antigens detected by antimelanoma xenoantiserum #6522 are not present in spent culture medium or cell extracts from several lymphoblastoid cell lines (MOLT 4, RPMI 1788, WIL-2, RAJI, Victor) or fibroblast cells. However, absorption of serum #6522 with cultured melanoma cells (M14 or M21) removed antibodies to the 240K and 94K proteins while #6522 absorbed with cultured carcinoma cells (T24) lost antibodies to 94K, but still retained the ability to precipitate the 240K antigen (Fig. 4). The radioimmunometric antibody

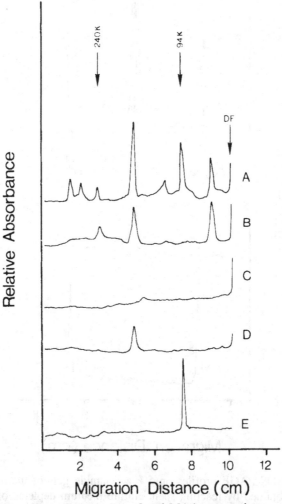

Fig. 4. The effect of absorption of anti-MAA xenoantiserum #6522 using whole cultured melanoma cells or carcinoma cells. SDS-PAGE analysis of 3H-valine-labeled spent culture media (FN-depleted) immunoprecipitated with serum #6522. A, Directly; or following depletion of serum #6522 using B, T-24 carcinoma cells; C, M14 melanoma cells; D, M12 melanoma cells; E, 94K antigen immunoprecipitated by monoclonal antibody (Galloway et al., 1980).

Table 1
Summary of Distribution of MAA

Cell type	Cell line	94K	240K
Melanoma	BW V	+	+
Melanoma	Carr I	+	+
Melanoma	M10	+	+
Melanoma	M14	+	+
Melanoma	M21	+	+
Melanoma	M51	+	+
Carcinoma	HeLa (D-98)	+	−
Carcinoma	HT-29	+	−
Carcinoma	Mano	+	−
Carcinoma	T-24	+	−
B-lymphoblast	Victor	−	−
B-lymphoblast	WI-L2	−	−
Fibroblast	IMR-90	−	−
Fibroblast	HAM SK	−	−

binding assay described by McCabe et al. (1978b; 1979) has shown that specific antisera directed to each of these proteins detect their presence on the cell surface and offers further proof of the specificity of these reagents (McCabe 1978a; 1978b; Galloway 1981a; 1981b). Finally, the production of a monoclonal antibody specific for the spent media 94K protein has revealed an absolute association of this glycoprotein antigen with melanoma and carcinoma cells by immune precipitation (Ferrone et al., 1980; Imai and Ferrone, 1980) and by immunofluorescence studies that show no crossreactivity with normal tissues or nevi (P. G. Natali, personal communication).

The distribution of these MAA among cultured human cell lines is given in Table 1. These results were obtained by analyzing intrinsically labeled culture medium from each of these cell lines using melanoma antiserum #6522 or by using xenoantiserum to each of these cell lines to precipitate intrinsically labeled spent media proteins from cultured human melanoma cells (M21).

4. Characterization of Melanoma-Associated Antigens

4.1. Molecular Characterization

The molecular characterization of the 240K and 94K antigens has thus far been accomplished primarily through immunochemical methods until larger amounts of these antigens become available to study. The molecular weights assigned to these proteins are determined by SDS-PAGE analysis in the presence of standard protein markers. The subunit composition of these MAA was analyzed by SDS-PAGE under reducing and nonreducing conditions (Fig. 5), which suggested that the 240K antigen is part of a larger molecular weight complex, since it failed to enter a 5% gel under nonreducing conditions (Fig. 5a,b) whereas the 94K antigen apparently exists as a single chain structure with intrachain disulfide bridges since this protein migrates slightly faster under nonreducing conditions (Fig. 5b).

The 240K and 94K antigens reveal no crossreactivity with antisera to CEA, BCG, β_2-microglobulin, HLA-A, B, DR, or plasma fibronectin, which indicates structural distinction from any of these proteins. The 240K

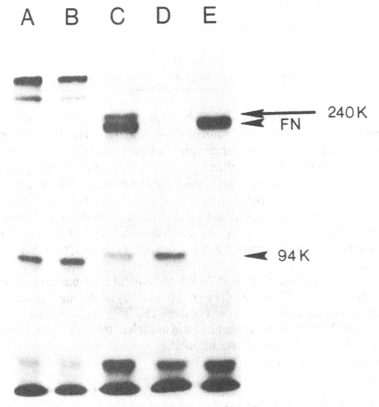

Fig. 5. Radiofluorograph showing the SDS-PAGE profiles of spent media proteins from intrinsically labeled (^{3}H-valine) human melanoma cells (M14), as revealed by indirect immunoprecipitation with anti-MAA xenoantiserum #7051 (A) or #6522 (B) under nonreducing or reducing (C) conditions. Lane D shows the position of the 94K antigen (serum #9446), while lane E reveals the position of human fibronectin using antihuman fibronectin antisera reacted against labeled spent culture media from M14 cells.

antigen shows no apparent relationship to fibronectin since it is not removed by gelatin-sepharose chromatography, does not react with antifibronectin antisera, and elicits the production of a specific xenoantisera that does not bind fibronectin.

The glycoprotein nature of the 240K and 94K antigens was determined by reacting intrinsically radiolabeled spent culture medium from M14 cells with lectins covalently coupled to Sepharose 4B. SDS-PAGE analysis revealed that the 240K antigen bound to *Lens culinaris* (lentil) lectin whereas the 94K antigen was bound by the *ricinus communis* (ricin) lectin (data not shown).

4.2. Cell Surface Location

Three lines of evidence indicate that these proteins are expressed on the cell surface. In the first place, xenoantisera specific for each antigen bind directly to the cell surface, as determined by a radioimmunometric binding assay (Galloway, 1981a; 1981b), as shown in Fig. 6. Futhermore, adsorption studies using whole cells indicate that cultured melanoma cells remove antibodies to the 240K and 94K antigens, whereas carcinoma cells only remove antibodies directed to 94K (Fig. 4). Finally, since it was reported that buffered urea solution can be used to extract cell surface proteins from cultured mouse cells (Kishi et al., 1980), we used a modification of this technique to extract cultured human melanoma cells with $4M$ urea in PBS (Galloway, 1981b), which resulted in the removal of the 240K and 94K antigens from these cells. However, similar extracts from cultured carcinoma cells (T24) did not yield any detectable 240K antigen.

5. Preparation of Specific Antimelanoma Xenoantisera to 240K and 94K Antigens

Initial studies dealing with the identification of MAA made use of xenoantisera prepared against intact cultured human melanoma cells (M21) (McCabe et al., 1978a, 1978b; Galloway et al., 1981a; 1981b). The procedure used to produce a specific xenoantiserum against each of the 240K and 94K antigens described in this report is outlined schematically in Fig. 7. The key elements in the production of specific antisera from partially purified melanoma extracts were (1) the removal of HLA-A, -B, -C, and -DR antigens by KBr flotation ($d = 1.23$ g/mL); (2) the removal of fibronectin from the antigen preparations and (3) utilization of the specific lectin affinities of each of the specific glycoprotein antigens. Specifically, histocompatibility antigens that are highly immunogenic, and thus interfere in the production of antimelanoma antibodies, are quantitatively removed by flotation on KBr as described previously (McCabe et al.,

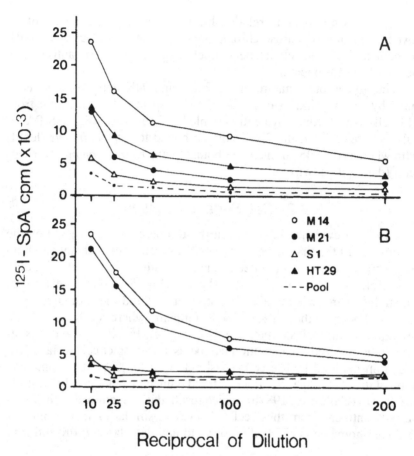

Fig. 6. Specificity of two xenoantisera to cell surface MAA following absorption with human erythrocytes and pooled cultured lymphoblasts as determined with a radioimmunometric ^{125}I-SpA antibody-binding assay. Twofold serial dilutions of the xenoantiserum (50 μL) were reacted against 5 × 10^5 M21 (●), M14 (○), HT-29 (▲), SI (△), and pooled lymphoblastoid (---) cells: A, specificity of anti-94K xenoantiserum #9446; B, specificity of anti-240K xenoantiserum #8995.

1978a). Lectins were utilized to produce anti-240K xenoantiserum (#8995) in rabbits by injecting the antigen bound to a lentil lectin Sepharose matrix. The source of the 240K antigen was a 3M KCl extract from melanoma cells partially purified over a CM-cellulose ion exchange column or a 4M urea extract depleted of fibronectin. Both of these antigen extracts were subsequently coupled to *lens culinaris* lectin bound to Sepharose 4B and injected biweekly into White New Zealand rabbits. A specific xenoantiserum against 94K·antigen (#9446) was produced by injecting rabbits with partially purified antigen specifically bound to ricin

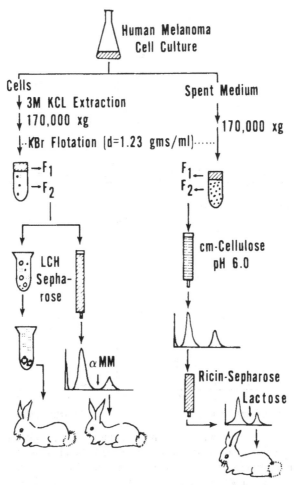

Fig. 7. Purification scheme for human melanoma-associated antigens to be used as immunogens for the production of specific xenoantisera directed against 94K and 240K antigens.

lectin coupled to Sepharose 4B. The 94K antigen was contained in serum-free spent culture medium that had been depleted of histocompatibility antigens by KBr flotation of medium from M14 cells and of 240K antigen by passage over CM-cellulose.

Other polyclonal xenoantisera to the 94K antigen have been produced in the same fashion, but were made more specific by the removal of fibronectin from the antigen preparation prior to lectin binding. Figure 8 shows the specificity of the anti-MAA xenoantisera prepared as described. Antifibronectin antiserum was produced by the injection of purified plasma fibronectin into rabbits.

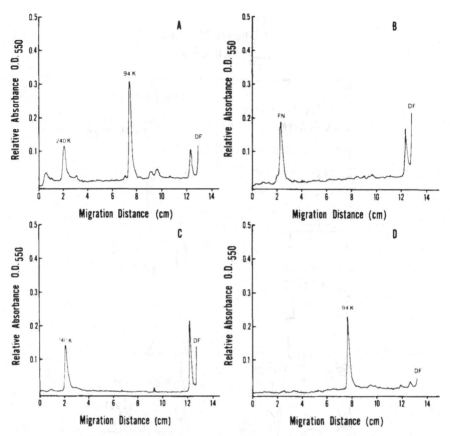

Fig. 8. SDS-PAGE analysis of indirect immunoprecipitates using specific anti-MAA xenoantisera reacted against intrinsically labeled spent culture media. A, FN-depleted spent media vs xenoantiserum #6522; B, α -FN xenoantisera; C, α -240K xenoantisera #8995; D, α -94K xenoantiserum#9446.

6. Purification of 240K and 94K MAA from Spent Culture Medium

The primary source of MAA for purification purposes has been the spent culture medium from a human melanoma cell line (M14) specially adapted to grow in a serum-free medium supplemented with vitamins and free fatty acids (Grimm et al., 1976; Gupta et al., 1979). The advantages of using this antigen source are (1) the absence of serum proteins, simplifying the purification of MAA; (2) the availability of already soluble antigens, thus avoiding the use of extraction procedures; (3) economy, since media can be harvested repeatedly from a given batch of cultured cells; and (4) simulation of in vivo shedding of tumor-associated antigens into the circulation, thereby providing a relevant working model to develop immuno-diagnostic and prognostic approaches. We have developed an approach to purify MAA from spent media of cultured melanoma cells by using intrinsically radiolabeled macromolecules and specific anti-MAA xenoantisera. The strategy used for the purification of MAA from spent culture media is outlined in Fig. 9. Following harvesting of the spent media and high speed ($\sim$170,000g, 1 h) centrifugation to remove particulate matter, the preparation is dialyzed vs PBS and then passed over a gelatin–Sepharose column in order to remove fibronectin, which selectively binds to the gelatin. The fibronectin-free media is then equilibrated against 0.01M phosphate

MAA Purification Scheme

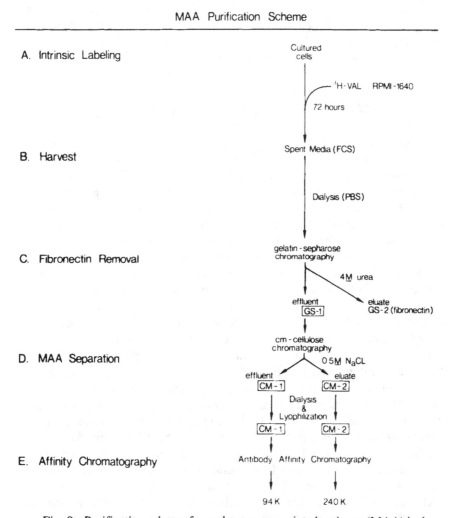

A. Intrinsic Labeling

Cultured cells

³H - VAL RPMI -1640

72 hours

B. Harvest

Spent Media (FCS)

Dialysis (PBS)

C. Fibronectin Removal

gelatin - sepharose chromatography

4M urea

effluent
GS-1

eluate
GS-2 (fibronectin)

cm - cellulose chromatography

D. MAA Separation

0 5M NaCL

effluent
CM-1

eluate
CM-2

Dialysis
&
Lyophilization

CM-1

CM-2

E. Affinity Chromatography

Antibody Affinity Chromatography

94 K

240 K

Fig. 9. Purification scheme for melanoma-associated antigens (MAA) isolated from spent media of intrinsically labeled cultured melanoma cells.

buffer, pH 5.7, and fractionated by CM-cellulose chromatography into material binding to the column, designated CM-2, and material passing through the column, the CM-1 fraction. The CM-2 fraction is obtained by column elution using buffered 0.5M NaCl. This procedure effectively separates the 240K (CM-2) antigen from the 94K (CM-1) protein. The final step in this purification scheme was based upon the ability of immunoadsorbents containing specific antibody to 240K (#8995) and 94K (#9446) antigens to concentrate and selectively purify each of these macromolecules. The results achieved with this type of purification scheme are illustrated in Fig. 10. Direct SDS-PAGE analysis of crude spent culture medium from M14 melanoma cells reveals the complex assortment of shed proteins (Fig. 10a). Following the depletion of fibronectin and subsequent fractionation over CM-cellulose, the 240K and 94K antigens are effectively separated (Fig. 10b, c). The two fractions containing these MAA are concentrated and then passed over small affinity columns consisting of either anti-240K or anti-94K xenoantisera coupled to protein A-Sepharose. When these immunoadsorbents are eluted at low pH (0.01M phosphoric acid, pH 3.0) and the eluates analyzed directly on SDS-PAGE, the results shown in Figs. 10d and 10e are obtained. These data clearly indicate the feasibility of MAA purification from spent culture media. This is further illustrated by the purification of 94K antigen from spent media of T-24 bladder carcinoma cells. Figure 11 indicates the efficiency in purifying the 94K antigen to a high degree following fibronectin removal, CM-cellulose fractionation, and indirect immunoprecipitation with specific anti-94K xenoantiserum #9446.

The ability to grow human melanoma cells (M14) in serum-free media provides a unique opportunity to obtain large amounts of soluble MAA from spent medium for purification purposes without the use of extraction procedures. At the time of this writing our primary efforts at large-scale purification have been concerned with the 94K antigen since this glycoprotein appears to be present in larger quantities than the 240K protein, and is found in greater amounts on human carcinoma cells than on melanoma cells. Typically, large scale purification of the 94K antigen from serum-free spent culture media begins with the collection of large amounts of spent medium followed by 100-fold concentration using an Amicon concentrator. The concentrated spent media is then dialyzed extensively against PBS plus 0.02% sodium azide and then fibronectin is removed by gelatin–Sepharose affinity chromatography. The fibronectin-free spent medium is then fractionated by CM-cellulose chromatography, after which the fractions are concentrated by ammonium sulfate fractionation at 0.8 saturation. The dialyzed and concentrated fractions are then ready for lectin affinity chromatography, which serves to concentrate and further purify the MAA for a final purification step using specific antibody affinity chromatography. Specifically, in the case of the 94K antigen, the CM-1

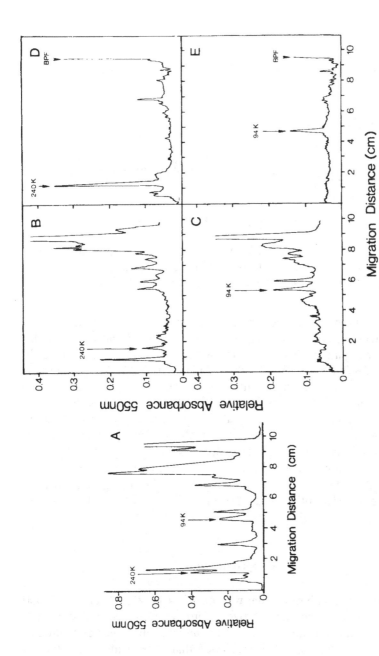

Fig. 10. 5% SDS-PAGE analysis of ³H-valine-labeled spent culture media from M14 melanoma cells. A, Unfractionated spent media; B, CM-cellulose eluate (CM-2) fraction; C, CM-cellulose effluent (CM-1) fraction; D, antibody affinity column eluate of CM-2 fraction; E, antibody affinity column eluate of CM-1 fraction.

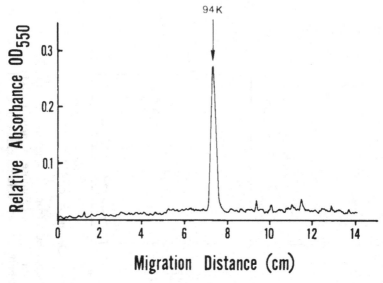

Fig. 11. 5% SDS-PAGE profile of ^{3}H-valine-labeled highly purified 94K antigen isolated from spent media of cultured bladder carcinoma cells and immunoprecipitated with specific anti-94K xenoantiserum (#9446).

fraction containing this antigen is placed over a small column of *Ricinus communis* lectin covalently coupled to Sepharose 4B, at a rate of 0.9 mL/h. Following an extensive washing with lectin column buffer (0.01M Tris·HCl, pH 8.0; 0.01M MgCl$_2$; 0.01M CaCl$_2$; 0.025M NaN$_3$), the proteins binding to the column are eluted in this same buffer containing 2% D-galactose. From 100 mg of CM-1 purified protein applied to a small (2 mL) ricin–Sepharose column, estimated yields are about 5 mg of eluted protein, of which 0.2–0.8 mg appears to be the 94K glycoprotein. The actual yield based upon cell numbers is difficult to estimate since the spent culture media are repeatedly collected from the same cultures over a period of time. Final purification using antibody affinity chromatography is anticipated, since the 94K antigen eluted from the ricin column still reacts with antibody.

7. Summary

Two glycoproteins with molecular weights of 240,000 (240K) and 94,000 (94K) were isolated and characterized from among macromolecules expressed and shed from cultured human melanoma cells. The key feature of the immunochemical approach developed that proved most effective to isolate these two melanoma-associated antigens from spent culture medium of intrinsically radiolabeled melanoma cells was the use of antibody affinity chromatography together with cation-exchange and lectin affinity chromatography. The two antigens could be separated by CM-cellulose ion exchange chromatography since the 240K molecule was bound at pH 5.7 and low salt concentration whereas the 94K molecule eluted under these conditions. A marked difference in their affinity for lectins led to further purification since the 240K molecule bound to lentil lectin and the 94K molecule to ricin lectin. This particular property of the two melanoma-associated antigens, together with the removal of highly immunogenic fibronectin molecules by gelatin–Sepharose chromatography made it feasible to produce highly specific xenoantisera to the 240K and 94K antigens as the lectin-bound, fibronectin-depleted spent culture media proved to be highly effective immunogens. The highly specific xenoantisera produced in this manner were effective in assessing the molecular profile of the two melanoma associated antigens when used for their indirect immunoprecipitation and subsequent analysis by SDS-PAGE. The 94K molecule appears to be a single polypeptide chain whereas the 240K molecule is part of a larger complex, possibly linked by interchain disulfide bridges. Results from radioimmunometric antibody-binding assays indicated that both antigens are expressed on the surface of cultured melanoma cells from which they are readily shed in the spent culture medium. The 240K antigen has thus far only been detected on cultured melanoma cells, whereas the 94K antigen was also found expressed on a variety of carcinoma cells as well as on fetal melanocytes. Human fibroblasts and lymphoblastoid cell lines fail to express both antigens. It is anticipated that the availability of the two highly purified and well-characterized tumor markers and specific xenoantibody directed against them will contribute to a better understanding of the biochemical nature of the neoplastic cell and make it feasible to critically assess their usefulness as cancer markers.

References

Black, P. H. (1980), *Adv. Cancer Res.* **32,** 75.

Bystryn, J. C. (1977), *J. Natl. Cancer Inst.* **59,** 325.

Clark, W. H., M. S. Mastrangelo, A. M. Ainsworth, O. Berd, R. E. Bellet, and E. A. Bernardino (1977), *Adv. Cancer Res.* **24,** 267.

Engvall, E., and E. Ruoslahti (1977), *Int. J. Cancer* **20,** 1.

Ferrone, S., and M. A. Pellegrino (1977), in *Handbook of Cancer Immunology* (Walters, H., ed.), Garland STPM Press, New York, pp. 155–173.

Ferrone, S., K. Imai, R. P. McCabe, G. A. Molinaro, D. R. Galloway, and R. A. Reisfeld (1980), in *Serologic Analysis of Human Tumor Antigens* (Rosenberg, S. A., ed.), Academic Press, New York.

Galloway, D. R., K. Imai, S. Ferrone, and R. A. Reisfeld (1981a), *Fed. Proc.* **40,** 59.

Galloway, D. R., R. P. McCabe, M. A. Pellegrino, S. Ferrone, and R. A. Reisfeld (1981b), *J. Immunol.* **126,** 62.

Gold, D. V., and D. M. Goldenberg (1980), in *Cancer Markers* (Sell, S. A., ed.), Humana, Clifton, New Jersey, pp. 329–364.

Greenstein, J. P. (1947), in *Biochemistry of Cancer*, Academic Press, New York, pp. 1–389.

Grimm, E. A., H. K. Silver, and J. A. Roth (1976), *Int. J. Cancer* **17,** 559.

Gupta, R. V., R. F. Irie, D. O. Chee, D. H. Kern, and D. L. Morton (1979), *J. Natl. Cancer Inst.* **63,** 347.

Kessler, S. (1975), *J. Immunol.* **115,** 1617.

Kishi, M., S. Nakajo, T. Shibayama, K. Nakaya, and Y. Nakamura (1980), *J. Biochem. (Japan)* **87,** 135.

Laemmli, U. K. (1970), *Nature* **227,** 680.

Laskey, R. A., and A. D. Mills (1975), *Eur. J. Biochem.* **47,** 335.

Lewis, M. G. (1974) *Curr. Topics Microbiol. Immunol.* 63, 49

Morgan, A. C., Galloway, D. R., Imai, K., and Reisfeld, R. A. (1981), *J. Imminol.* **126,** 365.

McCabe, R. P., S. Ferrone, M. A. Pellegrino, D. H. Kern, E. C. Holmes, and R. A. Reisfeld (1978a), *J. Natl. Cancer Inst.* **60,** 773.

McCabe, R. P., V. Quaranta, L. Frugis, S. Ferrone, and R. A. Reisfeld (1978b), *J. Natl. Cancer Inst.* **62, 455.**

McCabe, R. P., D. R. Galloway, S. Ferrone, and R. A. Reisfeld (1979), in *Current Trends in Tumor Immunology* (Reisfeld, R. A., S. Ferrone, L. Gorino, and R. B. Heberman, eds.), Garland STPM Press, New York, pp. 269–286.

Reisfeld, R. A., M.A. Pellegrino, and B. D. Kahan (1971), *Science* **172,** 1134.

Stuhlmiller, G. M., and H. F. Seigler (1977), *J. Natl. Cancer Inst.* **58,** 215.

Weber, S., and Osborne, J. (1969), *J. Biol. Chem.* **244,**4406.

4

Skin Tumor Markers

Jean-Claude Bystryn

*Department of Dermatology, New York University School of
Medicine, New York, New York*

1. Introduction

Skin cancers are the most common malignant tumors of man, constituting
approximately one-third of all human cancers. The most common malignant tumors of skin are basal-cell carcinomas, and the next most common
are squamous-cell carcinomas. The rarest, but most serious, is malignant
melanoma. There are approximately 8000–10,000 new cases of melanoma
per year in the United States, and this cancer accounts for 1% of all human
cancers. A variety of other malignancies arise from specialized cells present in skin or its appendages, but these are very rare and will not be considered.

Both basal- and squamous-cell carcinomas arise from keratinocytes,
though the exact cell of origin has not been determined. Presently, it is believed that basal-cell carcinomas arise from pluripotential cells that reside
in the basal layer of the epidermis or its appendages and differentiate toward basal cells, whereas squamous-cell carcinomas differentiate to cells
that have a tendency to form prickles and keratin. Melanomas arise from
melanocytes, pigment making cells of neural origin, which are interspaced
among the cells of the basal layer.

Because skin cancers are visible, thorough inspection of the skin and
the education of patients to bring suspicious lesions to the attention of physicians may be more practical measures at this time than the use of cancer
markers for early diagnosis or screening. The unequivocal identification of

89

unique cancer markers, however, would be of value in the differential diagnosis of skin tumors that mimic malignant lesions, such as keratoacanthomas or Spitz nevi; as aids in evaluating prognosis, monitoring the results of treatment, and for the early detection of recurrent disease; in differentiating between normal and malignant epidermal cells in culture; and in studies designed to understand better the process of malignant transformation.

2. Melanoma

2.1. Immunological Markers

A great deal of effort has been expended and an astounding variety of tests developed to study immunological markers associated with melanoma. Unfortunately, there is at present still no immunodiagnostic test that has definitely been shown to be of use in the clinical evaluation of patients with this cancer. The reasons for this are many and include the following: No standardized reagents (tumor antigens, antisera, cell lines) to assay melanoma-associated antigens (MAA) are available, though the recent development of monoclonal antibodies to some MAA may partially rectify this problem in the near future. Melanoma cells may not express MAA, or may not express MAA recognized by the assay used. Melanoma cells may express normal tissue antigens or fetal antigens of restricted distribution that may be mistaken for MAA. The MAA expressed by the cells may shift from time to time or from cell to cell within the same tumor. The expression of MAA may be cell cycle-related or shift when the cells are placed in tissue culture. Furthermore, some individuals may not develop immune reactions to MAA. Lastly, most immunodiagnostic tests have not been properly evaluated in terms of reproducibility, specificity, and sensitivity, and adequate controls have often not been used in the preliminary evaluation of the test leading to over optimistic initial reports that do no stand up to more critical reanalysis.

The immunological markers associated with melanoma and other cancers can be divided into two categories, according to whether they are products of the tumor, such as tumor antigens, or immunological reactants induced by these products, such as humoral or cell-mediated immune reactions to tumor antigens or circulating or tissue-fixed immune complexes. Only the former will be discussed in detail. However, the results obtained with a variety of assays of specific humoral or cell-mediated immunity to melanoma have recently been reviewed (Reisfeld, 1979). None has been found to be useful as yet for screening, early detection, or staging of melanoma.

2.1.1. Melanoma-Associated Antigens (MAA)

Most animal and human tumors carry antigens that differ quantitatively and/or qualitatively from those in normal adult cells. These antigens are thought to play a major, though complex, role in host resistance to cancer. Their existence has generated an intense search to determine whether their detection in tumor tissue or body fluids can yield clinically useful information. To date it has not, despite numerous optimistic reports to the contrary.

A number of antigens are associated with human melanoma and can be demonstrated serologically or by assays of cellular immunity (Morton et al., 1968; Lewis et al., 1969; Nairn et al., 1972; Gray et al., 1971; Shiku et al., 1976; Hellström et al., 1971a; Heppner et al., 1973). The antigens differ in their anatomical location (cell-surface, cytoplasmic, melanosomal, and nuclear) and distribution (individual specific, shared by some, or present on all melanomas). MAA can be classified into three categories according to whether they are: (a) individual melanoma-specific antigens unique for each tumor; (b) common melanoma-specific antigens shared with some, but not all, melanomas. There appears to be a family of such antigens that have only partially overlapping expression on individual tumors (Hellström and Hellström, 1973; McCoy et al., 1975; Seiberg et al., 1977); or (c) antigens present on other cells as well. Whether any MAA are qualitatively rather than quantitatively different from antigens in normal cells is still not completely clear. Tumor cells may express a wide variety of antigens, and melanoma specifically has been reported to carry histocompatibility (Pellegrino et al., 1977), viral (Parsons et al., 1974), fetal (Avis and Lewis, 1973; Fritze et al., 1976), blood group (Bloom et al., 1973), and tissue-specific (Fritze et al., 1976) antigens, neoantigens that arise in tissue culture or are derived from fetal calf serum components (Irie et al., 1974), and other potentially antigenic unique macromolecules, i.e., nerve growth factor binding sites (Fabricant et al., 1977). Consequently, specificity for melanoma is difficult to establish without extensive absorption and direct tests that unfortunately are only rarely performed. The presence of "natural" antibodies (Hersey et al., 1975; Kodera and Bean, 1975), and sensitized lymphoid cells (DeVries and Rumpke, 1976; Hellström et al., 1973) to melanoma in normal and black individuals, and of various autoantibodies to normal tissue in patients with melanoma (Bystryn et al., 1973; Whitehouse, 1973), complicates the task of establishing specificity.

A number of investigators have partially purified MAA. Jehn et al. (1970) fractionated the fluid in a cystic melanoma by starch gel electrophoresis. An antigenic fraction, identified by lymphocyte stimulation, was found to have the mobility of a beta-globulin and a molecular weight of 40,000. Carrel and Theilkaes (1973) obtained soluble MAA by saline extraction of homogenized tumor tissues and from the urine of patients with this tumor. The MAA were partially purified by chromatography on Sephadex G-10, G-100, and G-75, followed by Pevikon electrophoresis and electrofocusing. The MAA were found to be common to all melanoma and to have a mw of 40,000–60,000. Hollinshead et al. (1974) solubilized MAA by sonication of membrane fractions and partially purified these by Sephadex G-200 chromatography and electrophoresis on stacked acrylamide gels. Two groups of antigens were found. One appeared to be specific for melanoma. This was a glycoprotein with a mw of 38,500 (Hollinshead, 1975). Similar antigens were extracted from melanoma by a group in the USSR (Hollinshead et al., 1975). The other antigens appeared to be fetal, were expressed on other tumors, and had a mw of 9950. Roth et al. (1976) solubilized MAA by $3M$ KCl extractions of fresh tumor tissue and partially purified these by G-200 chromatography and acrylamide gel electrophoresis. Antigenic activity, assayed by delayed cutaneous hypersensitivity, was present in multiple fractions. The most active fraction (Sephadex peak fraction II, acrylamide gel region 2) appeared to be similar to Hollinshead's specific MAA. In further studies, soluble MAA were obtained from spent culture media and found to be large molecules excluded from Sephadex G-200, which eluted at an ionic strength of $0.1M$ NaCl on anion exchange chromatography (Grimm et al., 1976). MAA could be separated from HLA antigens by density gradient ultracentrifugation (Reisfeld et al., 1977). MAA could not be identified in extract of metastatic tumors, suggesting loss of antigen owing to immunoselection or to the presence of inhibitors or blocking factors. Thompson et al. (1976) solubilized MAA by limited papain digestion of membrane fractions of fresh melanoma tissue, in a manner similar to that described for the preparation of histocompatibility antigens. MAA, assayed by leukocyte adherence inhibition, were eluted in the heavy molecular weight fractions (70,000–150,000 daltons) on Sephadex G-150 and were bound by β_2-microglobulin affinity columns. MAA, when reduced and analyzed on acrylamide gels, consisted of three molecular species (11,000; 25,000; 40,000). These structural units are similar to those of HLA antigens, which are also rich in β_2-microglobulins, suggesting that some MAA may be altered histocompatibility antigens. Carey et al. (1979) have partially characterized a class 1 melanoma antigen that was uniquely expressed on a single line of melanoma cells. Following limited papain digestion, the antigen was found to be glycoprotein with a mw of 20,000–50,000. No β_2-microglobulin was associated with this antigen.

Following the demonstration that MAA were rapidly released into culture medium by viable melanoma cells (Bystryn, 1977), Smalley and Bystryn (1978) partially purified an MAA that was expressed on the surface of these cells. The MAA was a glycoprotein with a mw of 120,000–130,000. It was expressed by many, but not all, melanomas examined.

Lastly, Reisfeld et al. (1980) purified two distinct MAA, MGP-1 and MGP-2, from spent melanoma medium. MGP-1 was a glycoprotein with a mw of 240,000 that was found only on melanoma cells, whereas MGP-2 was another glycoprotein with a mw of 94,000 that was also expressed by fetal cells and unrelated cancers. A similar antigen has been described by Hellström et al. (1980) using monoclonal antibodies. (See Chapter 3.)

It appears from these studies that there is a striking variety of MAA. It is not clear how many of these are expressed concurrently on melanoma cells. The results of the above studies cannot readily be compared since different antisera, cells, and procedures were used for antigen purification. Furthermore, in many instances the limited specificity studies performed do not permit a complete evaluation of the specificity of the isolated antigens.

In any event, despite extensive efforts and considerable progress in identifying MAA, no clinical application of this information has been developed to date.

2.1.2. Soluble MAA

The detection of MAA in a tumor has limited clinical applications as a cancer marker, since in most instances the diagnosis of melanoma can be made readily by histological criteria. However, soluble MAA may be present in various body fluids of patients with melanoma, particularly those with disseminated disease. Consequently, it has been suggested that assay of urine or serum for MAA may permit the early detection of recurrent disease, aid in the evaluation of prognosis, and in monitoring therapy.

Viza and Phillips (1975) found antigens in the sera of most patients with melanoma that were not present in patients with leukemia or normal controls. Antibodies to this antigen cross-reacted with embryonic extracts, suggesting that the antigen was an oncofetal antigen. Several patients with circulating antigen, but free of tumor at the time of assay, eventually developed recurrent melanoma, suggesting that the assay could predict recurrence in patients who appeared to be clinically free of disease. In addition, a number of investigators have demonstrated that the serum of melanoma patients contain factors that can block immune reactions to melanoma cells (Hellström et al., 1971b). Although initially believed to be tumor-specific antibodies, it is now believed that in the majority of cases the blocking factors are soluble tumor antigens or immune complexes containing tumor antigens (Hellström et al., 1969; Murray et al., 1978). The presence of soluble tumor antigens in serum can readily be explained by the observation that viable melanoma cells can release in 24 h several times the amount of some of the MAA expressed on their surface (Bystryn and Smalley, 1979). A number of studies have suggested that there is an association between the presence and levels of blocking factors and the extent and prognosis of melanoma (Hellström and Hellström, 1973;

Holliday et al., 1975; Hersey et al., 1978). MAA have also been reported in the urine of patients with melanoma (Jehn et al., 1970), and urinary levels of antigen have been reported to correlate with the extent of disease (Bennet and Cooke, 1978).

Unfortunately, the same difficulties that limit the clinical usefulness of assays of MAA in tissue apply to assays of soluble MAA in body fluids. To date these approaches have not found clinical applications.

2.1.3. Other Antigens

In addition to melanoma-associated antigens, a number of other antigens have been suggested as potentially useful markers of melanoma because their expression is limited to a few tissues. Although of no use for the diagnosis of melanoma, change in the levels of these antigens could be of use as markers of disease recurrence or progression.

2.1.3.1. Oncofetal Antigens. A variety of proteins normally present in biological fluids of the fetus are also present in certain forms of cancers. Two of these, carcinoembryonic antigens and alphafetoprotein, may also be expressed by melanoma cells (Morgan et al., 1977; Waldman and McIntire, 1979). The detection of these proteins is of no value for diagnosis since they are elevated in a wide range of malignancies as well as in some nonmalignant diseases. However, fluctuations in their levels could prove of use in monitoring the course of melanoma. As yet, too few studies have been done to determine whether this will prove to be the case.

2.1.3.2. DR (Ia-like) Antigens. This is a group of histocompatibility antigens involved in cell–cell interactions. They consist of two glycoprotein chains of mw of 34,000 and 29,000 held by noncovalent bonds. The DR antigens are analogous to the Ia antigens of mice, and like these antigens have a restricted tissue distribution, being expressed predominantly on cells involved in immune functions. These antigens have been found on a small proportion of melanoma cells. They are expressed only minimally by neuroblastoma or other solid tumors (Howe et al., 1980) and are not expressed by normal human melanocytes or by normal human epidermal cells (Winchester et al., 1978; Wilson et al., 1979).

2.1.3.3. Nerve Growth Factor Receptors. Specific receptors for nerve growth factor have been found on the surface of human melanoma cells (Fabricant et al., 1977). Four of six melanomas examined had levels of NGF receptors that were 20–100 times greater than those expressed on the surface of a variety of normal tissues and unrelated malignancies.

2.1.3.4. Steroid Hormone Receptors. Human melanoma cells may express receptors for a number of steroid hormones including estrogens, androgens, progesterone, and glucocorticoids. However, the value of these receptors as markers of melanoma is rather limited, since they are expressed by only a minority of melanomas (20–45%) and are expressed more frequently on unrelated tumors (Neifeld and Lippman, 1980).

2.2. Biochemical Markers

Because melanocytes and melanoma cells have a unique capacity to produce melanin, a good deal of effort has been expended to determine whether melanogens, intermediates or derivatives formed during the synthesis and catabolism of melanin, can serve as biochemical markers of the extent or course of melanoma. Unfortunately, as in the case of immunological markers, the results to date have not yielded information that can be applied clinically.

One of the difficulties in using melanogens as markers of melanoma is that an extremely wide variety of melanogens is produced. There are over 40 phenolic melanogens such as p-hydroxyphenylacetic acid, salicyluric acid, homovanilic acid, salicylic acid, and so on, as well as a wide variety of catecholic compounds such as dopa, dopamine, norepinephrine, etc. Because of this variety, and because the melanogen that best correlates with melanoma is still not known, procedures that measure levels of individual melanogens are not as suitable as chromatographic procedures that permit the analysis of a wide spectrum of different melanogens.

2.2.1. Urinary Melanogens

Most investigators who have studied melanogens agree that increased levels of these compounds are present in the urine of patients with melanoma, and that there is a correlation between the extent of the tumor and the levels of melanogens. There is disagreement about which melanogen is most often excreted in large amounts. Some investigators have found it to be dopa, which is present in elevated levels in approximately 65% of patients with disseminated melanoma (for review, see Duchon and Matous, 1973). Others have found the principal melanogens in the urine of patients with disseminated melanoma to be different products whose identities have not yet been established (Banda et al., 1976).

Another melanogen that has attracted specific attention is 5-cysteindopa, an amino acid that is present only in melanocytes; in contradiction to dopa and other melanogens that are also found in other tissues such as brain, nerves, or adrenal glands. This amino acid is excreted in small amounts in the urine of normal individuals, and is present in increased amounts in the urine of patients with metastatic melanoma. It appears to be a more sensitive indicator of melanoma than dopa, since it will be elevated in patients with melanoma and normal urine levels of dopa (Agrup et al., 1977). Increased excretion of the amino acid may be observed before metastasis becomes clinically evident. However, its value as a marker of melanoma progression is limited by the pronounced increases in urinary excretion of 5-cysteindopa that occur in the summer in normal individuals as a result of stimulation of the pigmentary system by UV light.

It appears that the profile of melanogens excreted in the urine is unique for each patient (Banda et al., 1976) and that the level of a particular melanogen in the urine may vary from patient to patient (Banda et al., 1977). Furthermore, each method of analyzing melanogens selectively detects different classes of melanogens. For these reasons, and because it is not yet evident that melanogen levels are increased at a stage prior to clinically evident disease, their determination has not yet found any clinical application (Blois and Banda 1976).

2.2.2. Serum Tyrosinase

Melanocytes contain a unique enzyme, tyrosinase, that is involved in the synthesis of melanin. A number of investigators have attempted to determine whether increased levels of this enzyme occur in persons with melanoma. The results are not consistent. Most studies indicate that the enzyme is elevated in persons with melanoma. However, some investigators have found that this occurs only in persons with melanoma (Nishioka et al., 1979), while others have found tyrosinase to be elevated as well in persons suffering from a variety of other cancers including carcinomas of the breast, rectum, mouth, and cervix, in hepatomas, and in Hodgkin's disease (Chen et al., 1979). Although increased levels of tyrosinase in breast cancer may result from estrogen-induced melanogenesis, the high levels in other malignant diseases are not explicable at the present. Assays of serum tyrosinase are complicated by the presence of multiple forms of this enzyme and by the presence of inhibitors of tyrosinase activity in the serum. Attempts have been made to increase the sensitivity and specificity of this test by electrophoretic classification of the different tyrosinases or by removing low molecular weight inhibitors by dialysis of serum (Nishioka et al., 1979), but the full value of these modifications remains to be evaluated. Whether tyrosinase levels become elevated prior to clinically evident disease also remains to be determined.

2.2.3. Sialic Acid and Sialyltransferase

Malignant transformation is associated with increased serum levels of sialic acid, a component of cell membrane glycoproteins. It has been reported that serum levels of sialic acid are elevated in patients with melanoma (Silver et al., 1978; Kessel and Allen, 1975) and that the levels correlate with tumor burden and recurrence rate (Silver et al., 1979). Serum levels of sialyltransferase, the enzyme that adds sialic acid to membrane-bound and soluble glycoproteins may also be elevated in patients with melanoma (Kessel and Allen, 1975; Henderson and Kessel, 1977). However, both parameters may be equally elevated in patients suffering from a variety of cancers other than melanoma as well as in patients with nonmalignant skin diseases (Herrman and Gielen, 1979) so that they are not markers of melanoma. Because the highest levels of sialic acid and sialyltransferase are found in patients with widely disseminated disease, it has been suggested that these parameters might be of use to follow disease progression. However, more recent studies have shown that a high proportion of patients with observable melanoma do not have demonstrable serum sialic acid elevations (Silver et al., 1978) and have failed to reveal a distinct correlation between clinical progression of disease and significant alterations in serum levels of sialyltransferase (Silver et al., 1979), so that the value of these parameters as markers of disease progression or of metastatic involvement is in question.

2.2.4. Other Enzymes

Acceleration of the glycolytic pathway is a common biochemical alteration in many tumors. The activity of most enzymes involved in the main metabolic pathways, particularly the enzymes involved in the glycolytic pathways, are increased in human melanoma and to a lesser degree in benign nevi. By contrast, the activity of alanine transaminase is reduced by about 50% in melanoma (Cerimele et al., 1976). No clinical application of these findings has yet been described.

2.2.5. Melanosomal Proteins

Over 25 different proteins can be resolved by polyacrylamide gel electrophoresis of triton A extracts of human melanosomes. Approximately half of these proteins are found only in melanosomes obtained from melanoma, whereas conversely several of these proteins are present in normal melanosomes, but not in those of melanoma patients (Klinger et al., 1977). No clinical application of this finding has yet been described, though the presence of melanoma-specific melanosomal proteins suggests that their use as markers of disease progression should be examined.

3. Basal- and Squamous-Cell Carcinoma

These two tumors will be considered together because relatively little is known about markers associated with either cancer in humans, and because in many instances the markers that have been described are similar in both instances.

3.1. Immunological Markers

There is ample evidence in animal systems that carcinomas of keratinocytes express distinct tumor specific antigens. In general it appears that skin tumors induced by chemical or physical agents express antigens that are unique for each individual tumor, whereas virally induced tumors express common antigens (Old et al., 1968; Sjögren and Bansal, 1971). Unfortunately, the same has not been shown for carcinomas of keratinocytes in man. There are observations that individuals with such tumors can develop humoral or cell-mediated immune reactions to tumor tissue (Hellström et al., 1971a; Ibrahim et al., 1979; Tong et al., 1978) suggesting the tumors do express new antigens. However, little has been done to identify the antigens in question. What is known at present is that carcinomas of keratinocytes may express oncofetal antigens and may lose a number of tissue-specific antigens expressed by epidermal cells.

3.1.1. Tissue-Specific Antigens of Epidermal Cells

The most striking and reproducible immunological change associated with malignant transformation of keratinocytes is the loss of tissue-specific antigens normally expressed by these cells. At least four distinct types of tissue-specific antigens of keratinocytes are lost in basal- and squamous-cell carcinomas. Two of these are antigens on the surface of the cells, and the other two are cytoplasmic antigens. The cell-surface antigens that are lost are basement zone antigens that are expressed in the lamina lucida of the epidermis and produced by basal cells, and intercellular antigens that are present in the intercellular substance that separates suprabasal keratinocytes from each other (DeMoragas et al., 1970a; DeMoragas et al., 1970b; Muller and Flannery, 1973; Bystryn and Frances, 1979). The cytoplasmic antigens that are lost are BCL antigens present only in cells of the basal layer and U-CYT antigens that are expressed only in suprabasal keratinocytes (Bystryn et al., 1978). Figure 1 illustrates the loss of BCL antigens in a basal-cell carcinoma and the retention of this antigen in adjacent normal epidermis. Little is known about the biochemical nature of these antigens. However, their distribution in different tissues has been studied thoroughly, and it is clear that they are expresssed only in stratified squamous epithelium. All these antigens are lost or greatly decreased in expression in basal- and squamous-cell carcinomas. They are all retained by benign skin tumors such as seborrheic keratosis and keratoacanthomas that histologically resemble basal- or squamous-cell carcinomas, respectively. It is of interest that the antigens that are lost are expressed in subpopulations of keratinocytes that are stratified in distinct layers of the epidermis. Thus, these antigens appear to be differentiation antigens whose expression is linked to the terminal differentiation of epidermal cells as they migrate upward through the epidermis. By contrast, another type of tissue-specific antigen of keratinocytes, the G-CYT antigens, which are expressed in all epidermal cells, are retained in malignant carcinomas of the skin (Bystryn and Frances, 1979). Thus, it is only the antigens that express specialized differentiated properties of subpopulations of epidermal cells that are lost during malignant transformation.

The study of these antigens may find clinical application in distinguishing between squamous-cell carcinomas and keratoacanthomas, tumors of the skin that clinically and histologically are difficult to differentiate from the other. In addition, the detection of these antigens may be of

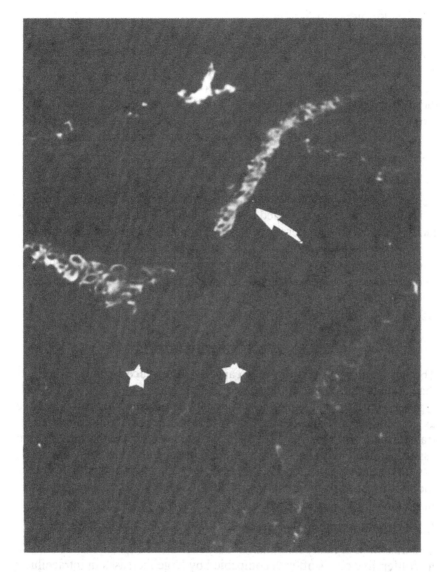

Fig. 1. Immunofluorescence photomicrograph of basal-cell carcinoma reacted with antibodies to BCL antigens. These antigens are expressed in the cytoplasm of basal cells in normal tissue (↑), but are lacking in tumor tissue (*). (Original magnification × 312.)

use in differentiating between normal and transformed cells in vitro, where the morphological criteria normally used to make this decision are difficult to apply. Loss of these antigens, being a clear marker of malignant transformation, may help in studying this process.

3.1.2. Oncofetal Antigens

Alphafetoprotein (Soltani et al., 1976) and carcinoembryonic antigens (Wang et al., 1979) have been reported in a few patients with squamous-cell carcinomas. Though only few studies of oncofetal antigens in basal- and squamous-cell carcinomas have been done, these findings suggest that these two tumors can be added to the large list of other tumors in which these antigens are expressed. There is no information as to the potential significance of measuring serum levels of these markers as guides to the presence and extent of metastatic disease.

3.1.3. Other Antigens

β_2-microglobulin appears to be present on the surface of all human nucleated cells that have been studied to date. It can be demonstrated on the surface of normal human keratinocytes by immunofluorescence techniques. This molecule is completely absent or greatly decreased in amount in basal-cell carcinomas (Tjerlund and Forsum, 1977). Interestingly, the antigen appears to be retained by squamous-cell carcinomas (Nilsson et al., 1974) as well as by benign growth of the skin. Again no clinical application of this finding has been described.

3.2. Biochemical Markers

Though keratinocytes do have a capacity to produce keratin, a product that, though not unique to these cells, is present in only a few other cell types, no biochemical marker associated with this metabolic pathway have as yet been studied in skin cancer. The biochemical markers of malignant transformation of keratinocytes that have been studied are markers that are associated with malignant transformation in general. Thus, they are not of use for diagnosis or screening. Although they may turn out to be useful for monitoring disease progression, no studies have yet been done to determine their clinical usefulness.

3.2.1. Ornithine Decarboxylase

The transition of many mammalian tissues from a nonproliferative state to a proliferative one is often accompanied by large increases in intracellular levels of polyamines and of polyamine decarboxylases. In particular, the levels of ornithine decarboxylase are increased in basal-cell carcinomas and in melanomas (Scalabrino et al., 1980; Helson et al., 1977). This elevation is not unique to basal-cell carcinomas since similar increases occur in benign proliferative disease of the skin such as psoriasis, as well as unrelated malignancies (Janne et al., 1978).

3.2.2. Glutathione and Glutathione Reductase

Glutathione plays an important role in maintaining the high glycolytic activity that is one of the most important biochemical alterations associated with carcinogenesis. Tissue levels of this enzyme are elevated in basal-

and squamous-cell carcinomas of the skin (Engin, 1976) and the levels correlate with mitotic activity. Glutathione reductase catalyzes the reduction of glutathione. Its levels are elevated in basal-cell carcinomas and in benign seborrheic keratosis, and appear to be normal in squamous-cell carcinomas (DeBersaques, 1979).

3.2.3. Transglutaminase

These are soluble crosslinking enzymes recently identified as markers for mature differentiation of several cell types. In epidermis, the enzyme is found in normal keratinizing cells of the epidermis and hair follicle. The enzyme is absent in basal-cell carcinomas (Buxman and Wuepper, 1978).

3.2.4. Acid Hydrolases

Acid hydrolases are often elevated in many skin diseases. Two of these in particular, arylsulfatases A and B, increase dramatically in hyperproliferative disorders such as psoriasis. It has recently been reported that in basal-cell carcinomas, the levels of the B form of this enzyme increase to a much greater extent than that of the A form, suggesting that the ratio of these two enzymes may provide a marker of malignant transformation (Orfanos et al., 1979).

3.2.5. Sulfhydryl Groups

By histochemical staining it has been found that sulfhydryl groups are more abundant in the cytoplasm and nuclei of human squamous-cell carcinomas than in normal epidermal cells of the same patient (Ogawa and Taneda, 1979).

4. Conclusion

No immunological or biochemical marker of skin cancer has yet been recognized as clinically useful. However, the distinct antigens and biochemical pathways associated with epidermal cells and melanocytes provide a rationale for believing that markers will eventually be found that will prove of value for monitoring the progression of skin cancers.

Acknowledgment

This work was supported in part by funds provided by NIH Research Grant CA 13844-08.

References

Agrup, G., P. Agrup, and T. Anderson (1977), *Acta Dermatovenerol.* **57**, 113.
Avis, P., and M. G. Lewis (1973), *J. Natl. Cancer Inst.* **51**, 1063.
Baldwin, R. W., D. Glaves, and M. V. Pimm (1971), *Prog. Immunol.* **1**, 907.

Banda, P. W., A. E. Sherry, and M. S. Blois (1976), *Pigment Cell* **2**, 254.

Banda, P. W., A. E. Sherry, and M. S. Blois (1977), *Clin. Chem.* **23**, 1397.

Bennet, C., and K. B. Cooke (1978), *Aust. J. Dermatol.* **19**, 19.

Blois, M. S., and P. W. Banda (1976), *Cancer Res.* **36**, 3317.

Bloom, E. T., J. L. Fahey, I. A. Peterson, G. Geering, M. Bernhard, and G. Trempe (1973), *Int. J. Cancer* **12**, 21.

Bystryn, J-C. (1977), *J. Natl. Cancer Inst.* **59**, 325.

Bystryn, J-C., and C. Frances (1979), *Transplantation* **27**, 392.

Bystryn, J-C., and J. Smalley (1979), *Pigment Cell* **5**, 155.

Bystryn, J-C., E. Abel, and S. Weidman (1973), *Arch. Dermatol.* **108**, 241.

Bystryn, J-C., M. Nash, and P. Robins (1978), *J. Invest. Derm.* **71**, 110.

Buxman, M. M., and K. D. Wuepper (1978), *J. Histochem. Cytochem.* **26**, 340.

Carey, T. E., K. O. Lloyd, T. Takahashi, L. R. Travassors, and L. J. Old (1979), *Proc. Natl. Acad. Sci. USA* **76**, 2898.

Carrel, S., and L. Theilkaes (1973), *Nature* **242**, 609.

Cerimele, D., M. Torsellini, and F. Serri (1976), *Pigment Cell* **2**, 290.

Chen, Y. M., B. T. Lim, and W. Chavin (1979), *Cancer Res.* **39**, 3485.

DeBersaques, J. (1979), *Arch. Dermatol. Res.* **265**, 139.

DeMoragas, J. M., R. K. Winkelmann, and R. E. Jordon (1970a), *Cancer* **25**, 1399.

DeMoragas, J. M., R. K. Winkelmann, and R. E. Jordon (1970b), *Cancer* **25**, 1404.

Devries, J. E., and P. Rumpke (1976), *Int. J. Cancer* **17**, 182.

Duchon, J., and B. Matous (1973), *Pigment Cell* **1**, 317.

Engin, A. (1976), *Arch. Dermatol. Res.* **257**, 53.

Fabricant, R. N., J. E. DeLargo, and G. J. Todaro (1977), *Proc. Natl. Acad. Sci. USA* **74**, 565.

Fritze, D., K. H. Kern, C. R. Drogemuller, and Y. H. Pilch (1976), *Cancer Res.* **36**, 458.

Gray, B. K., J. T. Mehigan, and D. L. Morton (1971), *Cancer Res.* **12**, 79.

Grimm, E. A., H. K. Silver, J. A. Roth, D. O. Chee, R. K. Gupta, and D. L. Morton (1976), *Int. J. Cancer* **17**, 559.

Hellström, I., J. P. Brown, R. Woodbury, M-Y. Yeh, K. Nishiyama, and K. E. Hellström (1980), *Proc. Amer. Assoc. Cancer Res.* **21**, 221.

Hellström, I., K. E. Hellström, C. A. Evans, G. H. Heppner, G. E. Pierce, and J. P. S. Yang (1969), *Proc. Natl. Acad. Sci USA* **62**, 362.

Hellström, I., K. E. Hellström, H. O. Sjögren, and G. A. Warner (1973), *Int. J. Cancer* **11**, 116.

Hellström, K. E., and I. Hellström (1973), *Fed. Proc.* **32**, 156.

Hellström, K. E., I. Hellström, and H. O. Sjögren (1971a), *Int. J. Cancer* **7**, 1.

Hellström, I., H. O. Sjögren, G. Warner, and K. E. Hellström (1971b), *Int. J. Cancer* **7**, 226.

Helson, I., C. Helson, and A. Majeranowski (1977), *Proc. Amer. Assoc. Cancer Res.* **18**, 166.

Henderson, M., and D. Kessel (1977), *Cancer* **39**, 1129.

Heppner, G. H., L. Stolbach, M. Byrne, F. J. Cummings, E. McDonough, and P. Calabresi (1973), *Int. J. Cancer* **11**, 245.

Herrman, W. P., and W. Gielen (1979), *Arch. Dermatol. Res.* **265**, 321.

Hersey, P., J. Edwards, A. Edwards, E. Adams, R. Kearney, and G. W. Milton (1975), *Int. J. Cancer* **16**, 164.

Hersey, P., E. Murray, and S. Ruygrok (1978), *Aust. N. Z. J. Surg.* **48**, 346.

Holliday, W. J., A. E., Maluish, J. H. Little, and N. C. Davis (1975), *Int. J. Cancer* **16**, 645.

Hollinshead, A. C. (1975), *Cancer* **36**, 1282.

Hollinshead, A. C., and V. V. Gorodilova (1975), *Science* **190**, 391.

Hollinshead, A. C., R. B. Herberman, W. J. Jaffurs, L. K. Alpert, J. P. Minto, and J. E. Harris (1974), *Cancer* **34**, 1235.

Howe, A., R. C. Seeger, and G. A. Molinaro (1980), *Clin. Res.* **28**, 104A.

Ibrahim, A., R. A. Robinson, and L. Marr (1979), *J. Natl. Cancer Inst.* **63**, 319.

Irie, R. F., K. Irie, and D. L. Morton (1974), *J. Natl. Cancer Inst.* **52**, 1051.

Janne, J., H. Poso, and A. Raina (1978), *Biochim. Biophys. Acta* **473**, 241.

Jehn, U. W., L. Nathanson, R. S. Schwartz, and M. Skinner (1970), *New Engl. J. Med.* **283**, 329.

Kessel, D., and J. Allen (1975), *Cancer Res.* **35**, 670.

Klinger, W. G., P. M. Montague, and P. B. Chretien (1977), *Arch. Dermatol.* **113**, 19.

Kodera, Y., and M. A. Bean (1975), *Int. J. Cancer* **16**, 579.

Lewis, M. G., R. L. Ikonopisov, R. C. Nairn, T. M. Phillips, G. Hamilton Fairley, D. C. Bodenham, and P. Alexander (1969), *Brit. Med. J.* **3**, 547.

McCoy, J. L., L. F. Jerome, J. H. Dean, E. Perlin, R. K. Oldham, D. H. Char, M. H. Cohen, E. L. Felix, and R. B. Herberman (1975), *J. Natl. Cancer Inst.* **55**, 19.

Morgan, G., W. H. McCarthy, and P. Hersey (1977), *Brit. J. Cancer* **36**, 446.

Morton, D. L., R. A. Malmgren, E. C. Holmes, and A. S. Ketcham (1968), *Surgery* **64**, 233.

Muller, H. K., and G. R. Flannery (1973), *Cancer Res.* **33**, 2181.

Murray, E. S. Ruygrok, and G. W. Milton (1978), *Int. J. Cancer* **21**, 578.

Nairn, R. C., A. P. Nind, E. P. Guli, and D. J. Davies (1972), *Med. J. Aust.* **1**, 397.

Neifeld, J. P., and M. E. Lippman (1980), *J. Invest. Derm.* **74**, 379.

Nilsson, K., P. E. Ervin, and K. I. Welsh (1974), Transplantation Rev., **21**, 53.

Nishioka, N., M. M. Romsdahl, and M. J. McMurtrey (1979), *Pigment Cell* **5**, 300.

Ogawa, H., and A. Taneda (1979), *Arch. Dermatol. Res.* **264**, 77.

Old, L. J., E. A. Boyse, G. Geering, and H. F. Oettgen (1968), *Cancer Res.* **28**, 1288.

Orfanos, C. E., H. Roeltzema, P. D. Mier, and Jose S. M. A. van den Hurk (1979), *Br. J. Dermatol.* **100**, 591.

Parsons, P. G., P. Goss, and J. H. Pope (1974), *Int. J. Cancer* **13**, 606.

Pellegrino, M. A., S. Ferrone, R. A. Reisfeld, R. F. Irie, and S. H. Golub (1977), *Cancer* **40**, 36.

Reisfeld, R. A. (1979), *Dev. Cancer Res.* **1**, 571.

Reisfeld, R. A., D. Galloway, and K. Imai (1978), *Fed. Proc.* **39**, 351.

Reisfeld, R. A., R. P. McCabe, and S. Ferrone (1977), *Proc. Amer. Assoc. Cancer Res.* **18**, 205.

Roth, J. A., H. K. Slocum, M. A. Pellegrino, E. Carmack Holmes, R. A. Reisfeld (1976), *Cancer Res.* **36,** 2360.

Scalabrino, G., P. Pigatto, M. E. Ferioli, D. Modena, M. Puerari, and A. Caru (1980), *J. Invest. Derm.* **74,** 122.

Seiberg, E., C. Sorg, R. Happle, and E. Macher (1977), *Int. J. Cancer* **19,** 172.

Shiku, H., T. Takahashi, H. F. Oettgen, and L. J. Old (1976), *J. Exptl. Med.* **144,** 873.

Silver, H. K., K. A. Karim, E. L. Archibald, and F. A. Salinas (1979), *Cancer Res.* **39,** 5036.

Silver, H. K., D. M. Range, and D. L. Morton (1978), *Cancer* **41,** 1497.

Sjögren, H. O., and S. C. Bansal (1971), *Prog. Immunol.* **1,** 921.

Smalley, J., and J-C. Bystryn (1978), *Fed. Proc.* **37,** 1595.

Sohn, N., H. Gang, S. L. Gumport, M. Goldstein, and L. M. Deppisch (1969), *Cancer* **24,** 897.

Soltani, K., S. Yachnin, and F. Brickman (1976), *J. Invest. Dermatol.* **70,** 204.

Thompson, D. M. P., P. Gold, S. O. Freedman, and J. Shuster (1976), *Cancer Res.* **36,** 3518.

Tjerlund, U. M., and U. Forsum (1977), *Acta Dermatovenerol.* **57,** 503.

Tong, A. W., W. Kraybill, and D. R. Burger (1979), *Fed. Proc.* **38,** 1218.

Viza, D., and J. Phillips (1975), *Int. J. Cancer* **13,** 312.

Waldman, T. A., and K. R. McIntire (1979), *Immunodiagnosis of Cancer*, part 1, R. Herberman and K. McIntire, eds., Dekker, New York.

Wang, N., S. Huang, and P. Gold (1979), *Cancer* **44,** 937.

Whitehouse, J. M. A. (1973), *Brit. J. Cancer* **28,** 170.

Wilson, B. S., F. Indiveri, M. A. Pellegrino, and S. Ferrone (1979), *J. Exptl. Med.* **149,** 658.

Winchester, R. J., C-Y Yang, A. Gibofsky, H. G. Kunkel, K. O. Lloyd, and L. J. Old (1978), *Proc. Natl. Acad. Sci. USA* **75,** 6235.

5

Gastrointestinal Cancer Markers

Hans O. Sjögren[1] and Britta Wahren[2]

*[1]The Wallenberg Laboratory, University of Lund, Lund,
and [2]Radiumhemmet, Karolinska Hospital, Stockholm, Sweden*

1. Introduction

A neoplastic transformation is usually associated with alterations in cell differentiation (Matsushima et al., 1968; Potter, 1969). Several of the markers characteristic of cancer cells are associated with such alterations in differentiation. Molecules that normally occur at certain stages of embryonal development can be demonstrated by immunological techniques. Several of these molecules are also produced normally in small quantities in adult tissues. Some are not immunogenic in the host of origin, but can be detected by antisera produced in other animal species; others are immunogenic in the host of origin and induce demonstrable immune responses. The appearance of altered nuclear nonhistone proteins detectable by xenogeneic antisera may reflect alterations in the transcriptional restrictions of cell DNA associated with transformation from the normal to the neoplastic phenotype. The altered cell differentiation may also result in the disappearance of molecules that are present in the untransformed cells. Finally, entirely new or altered macromolecules, which are not present in either embryonic or normal adult cells, may appear and elicit immune responses.

The various markers of gastrointestinal tract cancer will be reviewed, with emphasis on those that are detectable by immunological techniques (Table 1). Cancer markers are of interest for various reasons and the requirements differ accordingly. When used for cancer detection and cancer diagnosis with respect to the tissue of origin, the markers must have good specificity and sensitivity. As a basis for monitoring tumor therapy, the marker should correlate quantitatively to the tumor mass. Cancer markers may also be used as a basis for immunotherapy and possibly immuno-prevention; a prerequisite here is that the marker is or can be made immunogenic in the host of origin. The usefulness of markers will be dis-cussed in the respective sections.

2. Enzymes and Hormones in Gastrointestinal Tumor Disease

Isoenzymes have been described that, when specific for certain tissues, may be very useful for tumor monitoring by determination of serum con-centrations. The glycolytic enzyme aldolase A that normally occurs mainly in muscle and fetal liver may be increased in gastric cancer tissue when compared to normal gastric mucosa. The pattern of increased con-centration of subunits of aldolase A resembles that seen in fetal gastric tis-sue (Saito and Hokkaido, 1975). Aldolases B and C, on the other hand, are decreased in gastric carcinoma tissue (for a review, see Balinsky, 1980).

Many enzymes may be elevated in serum with disseminated disease, especially when the liver is involved (Schwartz, 1976; Beck et al., 1979). The most common metastatic site of gastrointestinal cancer is the liver. Enzymes that signify liver damage (such as alanine and aspartate trans-minases, γ-glutamyltransferase, lactate dehydrogenase, and alkaline phosphatase) are then often raised in the peripheral blood.

Ectopic hormone production by tumor tissue is not uncommon (Griffing and Vaitukaitis, 1980). Human chorionic gonadotropin (HCG) is the hormone most frequently associated with stomach, small intestinal, and colon cancer. It is measured in tissue or serum using a radioimmuno-assay with heterologous sera to the β-chain of HCG. An increased serum HCG can be seen in 12–25% of these cancers. HCG may also be found in the urine (Papapetrou et al., 1980). With gastrointestinal tumors, the HCG levels are usually very low, at least compared to levels found in preg-nancy. Also growth hormone-like substances have occasionally been dem-onstrated in tissue extracts of gastric cancer.

3. Tissue Antigens of Human Gastrointestinal Cancers Defined by Xenogeneic Antisera

The tissue antigens may be divided into those that normally occur in the re-spective organs and are also detectable in tumors of the same organ, those that are significantly increased in tumor compared to normal tissue, and

Table 1
Cancer Markers of Human Gastrointestinal Cancers

Marker	Cancer localization	Examples
Isoenzyme alteration	Stomach	Aldolase
Enzymes in altered quantity	Liver metastases of, e.g., gastrointestinal cancer	Lactic dehydrogenase, alkaline phosphatase
Ectopic hormone synthesis	Stomach	Human chorionic gonadotropin
Tumor and/or organ-associated antigens in man, defined by xenogeneic antisera	Colon, stomach	Carcinoembryonic antigen, other colon- and gastric-derived antigens
Normal antigens deleted from tissue of origin	Colon	ABH blood group substances
Tumor and organ associated antigens immunogenic in the host of origin	Colon, rectum	Tissue-type specific antigens Antigens detectable by demonstration of humoral antibodies Antigens detectable by demonstration of cell-mediated immune reactivity

others, such as blood group isoantigens, which may be deleted in tumor disease and accordingly constitute a third group that may be of histopathological and clinical significance (Table 1). The borderlines between these groups are not very distinct and since relatively insensitive methods have sometimes been used for antigen characterization, it has not always been possible to arrive at a definitive classification (see also Goldenberg, 1976).

3.1. Carcinoembryonic Antigen (CEA)

The first substance of gastrointestinal origin to be characterized by heteroantisera was the carcinoembryonic antigen. Two methods were employed to demonstrate the distinctive antigenicity of CEA, which occurs in adenocarcinomas of the gastrointestinal tract (Gold and Freedman, 1965a). In the first, newborn rabbits were made tolerant to human normal gut tissue by immunization with adenocarcinoma of colon (Gold and Freedman, 1965b); the rabbits then developed antibodies, reacting mainly with tissue extracts of colorectal adenocarcinomas. The second method involved immunizing adult animals with human colon adenocarcinomas, and then absorbing the resulting antisera with normal gut tissue, blood cells, and serum proteins. This yielded antisera with a similar specificity.

Antisera for analytic or diagnostic purposes have generally been produced in rabbits, goats, and sheep. The antigen defined by such sera is a glucoprotein of molecular weight around 180,000.

A more homogeneous species of CEA, called CEA-S, has been isolated by Plow and Edgington (1975). Clinical studies have shown that antisera to CEA-S can also be used in assays to detect gastrointestinal cancers (Edgington et al., 1975). The efficiency of detection seems to be similar to that with the conventional CEA assay (Brooks et al., 1979; Reynoso, personal communication).

3.1.1. Tissue CEA

CEA appears early during human fetal life. From the third month of gestation there are high amounts in the entodermal germ layer, mainly the fetal gut (Gadler et al., 1980; Lindgren, 1980). Adult normal tissues have a comparatively low content of CEA. The normal gut contains 1–10% of the amount found in adenocarcinoma (Martin and Martin, 1972).

The CEA isolated from tumors of the gastrointestinal tract is indistinguishable from the CEA obtained from fetal and adult normal bowel tissue. Primary or metastatic adenocarcinomas of the stomach, pancreas, colon, and rectum usually contain large amounts of CEA. Highly differentiated colonic cancers have been demonstrated to contain more CEA per unit weight than those that are less well differentiated (Denk et al., 1972). Since serum CEA levels are nonetheless high with undifferentiated colon carcinomas, these tumor cells are thought to synthesize and release CEA at a high rate, though more differentiated tumor cells retain CEA intracellularly.

Metabolic blocking experiments performed in vitro show that CEA is accumulated in nondividing cells with a high protein synthesis (G_o cells). The release occurs mainly in the lag phase (Drewinko and Yang, 1980). CEA accordingly seems to be characteristic of cells of a certain differentiation that can also maintain protein synthesis.

The histopathological localization of CEA to the tumor cell surface is well established (Gold et al., 1968; Denk et al., 1972). Localization studies have also been performed on sections obtained for ordinary histopathology. Immunoperoxidase or immunofluorescence staining (Isaacson and Le Vann, 1976; Goldenberg et al., 1976b; Pihl et al., 1980) can be used to study formalin-fixed and paraffin-embedded specimens. In this way, CEA can be detected in stomach, colon, and rectum tumors, as well as in some nongastrointestinal carcinomas. The fixation procedure decreases the total CEA content compared to that of fresh tissue. To obtain true CEA values in cells, radioimmunoassay can be combined with microspectrophotometry of cytologically prepared cells (Wahren et al., 1977).

3.1.2. Serum CEA

3.1.2.1. Primary Disease. Determination of CEA in serum samples is usually performed with radioimmunoassay techniques. Making allowance for the statistical variations in the CEA assays, one can draw a nomogram to show which values represent statistically significant changes (Martin et al., 1977). Increased concentrations of CEA compared to normal, i.e., over 2.5 μg/L, are found in the blood of patients with gastrointestinal malignancies (Hansen et al., 1974; Zamcheck, 1978; Gold et al., 1973). The frequency of raised values and the content of CEA are higher in more advanced local disease. Most patients (77–95%) with metastases to other organs or with liver involvement have elevated CEA values. Very few patients with metastases have been found to have persistently low levels. The content of CEA in serum is also influenced by other factors, such as tumor cell differentiation and the state of the liver (Wahren, 1976; Zamcheck, 1978).

3.1.2.2. Evaluation of Prognosis. Several authors have shown that a raised preoperative CEA value (usually above 5 μg/L) confers a poorer prognosis than a low one (Dhar et al., 1972; Lo Gerfo and Herter, 1975; Wanebo et al., 1978; Chu et al., 1976). The combination of Dukes' classification and CEA determination gives the most sensitive prognosis for colorectal cancer. There is also a correlation between higher preoperative CEA values and a shorter time to recurrence. CEA plasma levels have been shown (Rieger and Wahren, 1975) to be high or rising mainly in primary cases known to have a poor prognosis, i.e., with serosal break through initially, with primary regional lymph-node involvement, or with distant metastasis to liver or other organs. Lo Gerfo and Herter (1975) have shown that the probability for recurrence is increased 1.8 times with a high CEA value preoperatively. Herrera et al. (1976) found that few patients with a low preoperative CEA level recur within 18 months, although those with elevated levels recur early.

3.1.2.3. Monitoring of Patients. It is in the followup of patients operated for colorectal carcinomas that CEA determinations have played their largest part (Fuks et al., 1980). Rising CEA levels predict tumor recurrence or metastasis, often several months before clinical detection (Mach et al., 1974). A study designed to evaluate the accuracy of CEA determination in indicating recurrence after curative surgery showed the test sensitivity for tumor recurrence to be 97% (Wood et al., 1980).

It is obviously important to distinguish local recurrence from distant metastases. Since rising serial CEA values often provide evidence of recurrence in asymptomatic patients, patients with two successively increasing CEA values have been explored operatively. Second-look operations (Martin et al., 1977; Martin et al., 1979) performed on 32 patients who fulfilled these criteria showed previously unknown and resectable disease in 41%; exploration was negative in 3 patients (9%), and the remainder had metastatic disease. This material has now been extended to include over 100 patients. According to these authors, two successive elevated CEA levels motivate a laparotomy in the post-operative followup of patients with colorectal carcinoma. Still, transient rises may occur without a detectable recurrence (Rittgers et al., 1978). A possible way to distinguish CEA elevations signifying recurrence from those that do not was suggested by Steele et al. (1978), who found that seven out of eight patients with increased CEA and tumor recurrence had a concurrent rise in circulating immune complexes; in seven patients without recurrence, the level of immune complexes was inversely related to the CEA level.

Slopes formed by sequentially increasing CEA determinations have been used to evaluate the type of recurrence. Gentle slopes (<0.6 μg/L rise of CEA in 10 days) tended to accompany local recurrence (Staab et al., 1978), while a steeper slope indicated general spread of the tumor. Especially patients with slow rises were shown to benefit from second-look surgery (Staab et al., 1978; Steele et al., 1980). Steele et al. (1980) showed that of 15 recurrences first detected at second-look operations, only two were apparently cured, while six other patients benefited from therapy. All but one of these patients had slowly increasing CEA values (less than 2.1 μg/L/30 days). In another investigation (Wood et al., 1980) a slow rise to less than 75 μg/L during 12 months was usually related to local recurrences and a relatively good prognosis; a fast rise up to more than 100 μg/L of CEA during 6 months was associated with metastatic disease.

The lead time between a CEA rise and clinically detectable tumor has shown to average 3–4 months, but may vary from zero up to more than 2 years. However, the rises may be transient and CEA determinations are no substitute for ordinary clinical assessment (Loewenstein and Zamcheck, 1978; Rittgers et al., 1978). Not all authors have found CEA reliable for the early detection of recurrent colorectal cancer (Moertel et al., 1978).

CEA levels over 25 μg/L suggest liver involvement. Serum assays of CEA were made from patients with advanced colorectal carcinoma receiving chemotherapy (Al-Sarraf et al., 1979; Mayer et al., 1978). With tumor remission, CEA decreased in 89% of the patients; with stable or progressing disease, CEA generally rose, although some decreases were noted (Al-Sarraf et al., 1979).

Blood CEA is also elevated with disseminated tumors from lung, breast and genital cancer (Laurence et al., 1972; Hansen et al., 1974). In long-standing infections that resist therapy, a substance is released that is immunologically cross-reactive with CEA. Thus even normal, i.e., not just malignant, cells may augment their CEA secretion if adequately stimulated. This supports the idea that the capacity to synthesize CEA is retained in all cells, but achieves maximal expression under certain circumstances only. CEA may therefore sometimes be elevated in benign gastrointestinal disease (Loewenstein and Zamcheck, 1978). Such elevated values may be seen in benign hepatic disease, such as cirrhosis or hepatitis, or with biliary obstruction, colitis, and pancreatitis. The levels usually do not exceed 10 μg/L of serum. Such benign conditions must therefore be taken into account in interpreting mildly elevated serum CEA.

3.1.2.4. Serum CEA in Cancer of Esophagus and Stomach.

Only a few reports have appeared on tumor markers in cancer of esophagus and stomach (Alexander et al., 1978; Wahren et al., 1979). The staging of esophageal cancer is difficult, especially with respect to local spread and node involvement. A CEA level above 2.5 μg CEA/L in 35/59 (59%) of patients has been demonstrated with localized esophagus cancer (Wahren et al., 1979). In metastatic disease this figure was 78%. High CEA levels preceded the clinical detection of metastases even when liver enzymes were normal. In primary or metastatic disease of the esophagus, the CEA levels may thus be raised, but usually they are below those associated with advanced colorectal cancer.

In advanced gastric carcinomas, 30–50% of the patients have elevated CEA levels. Prognostic information can be obtained from CEA determinations in patients with initially raised levels (Ellis et al., 1978).

3.1.2.5. Serum CEA with Polyps.

CEA can be demonstrated in polyps of the colon (Burtin et al., 1972; Alm and Wahren, 1975). Assays of tissue CEA content in histologically verified adenomas show values similar to those of overt carcinomas. Patients with hereditary adenomatosis were studied for elevation of blood CEA (Alm and Wahren, 1975). This disease is inherited as an autosomal dominant disorder and invariably leads to malignant transformation of the polyps unless the patient undergoes colectomy. Raised serum CEA was found in approximately 25% of this high-risk population, irrespective of the presence of adenomatous tissue. The non-affected first-degree relatives had about the same frequency of elevated serum CEA as the affected individuals. The raised serum values were between 5 and 20 μg CEA/L. Patients with unselected types of colorectal polyps have also presented a raised frequency of increased CEA values (Doos et al., 1975). Thus, in a population of persons known to be running a very high risk of cancer, an increased proportion of subjects had moderately raised serum CEA. A screening of blood CEA, however, to detect malignant gut cell transformation in this type of population does not seem meaningful. The adenomas are not invasive and therefore the tissue CEA does not reach the blood in a sufficiently high proportion of patients.

3.1.3. Fecal CEA

Measuring CEA in feces does not seem feasible for the diagnosis of colorectal cancer, since levels are high both in healthy persons and in cancer patients (Hirsch-Marie et al., 1973; Elias et al., 1974). In a closer study, Fujimoto et al. (1979) showed that feces from patients with primary colorectal cancer usually had a higher CEA content than the feces of healthy persons. The CEA level was not closely related to tumor size. Resection of the tumor was followed by a decreased fecal CEA content.

3.1.4. Radiolocalization of Tumors Using Anti-CEA Antibody

Recently, the demonstration of CEA in tumors has been used as a new approach to clinical diagnosis. By labelling anti-CEA antibodies with an isotope, the antibody can be traced after injection and CEA-producing tumors can be localized in vivo. Model experiments have been performed in animals (Mach et al., 1974). The method seems to be suitable for localization of tumors in patients. Goldenberg et al., (1978) and Kim et al. (1980) have shown a positive localization rate of 80–90% in known tumors with ^{131}I-labeled goat anti-CEA antibodies. In addition, tumor deposits that were not previously known could be found and were confirmed histopathologically by later biopsy or autopsy. Tumors of varying histopathology, which do not always have CEA secretion, have been localized. The limiting size with scintigraphy is 2 cm in diameter, which can possibly be improved by using emission tomography. Lower success rates have been obtained by other groups (Dykes et al., 1980; Mach et al., 1980). At present, the best method available for non-invasive tumor screening is computer-assisted tomography. If radiolocalization with anti-CEA or other types of antibodies proves to identify additional tumors, this method should become very important clinically. It might be used after primary surgery to determine whether adjuvant therapy should be given. The potential to treat micrometastases of disseminated disease is also apparent with this technique.

3.2. Colon Cancer Antigens Defined by Monoclonal Antibodies

A new technique for the detection and analysis of antigens is based on monoclonal antibodies. Colon cancer associated antigen(s) defined in this way has recently been reported (Herlyn et al., 1979). Cell lines derived from colon or rectal carcinomas were used to immunize mice, the mouse spleen cells were fused with mouse myeloma cells, and immunoglobulins produced by the hybrid cells were assayed for activity to the same colorectal cell lines or to primary colon tumor cells. Two clones produced antibodies that reacted with colorectal cell lines and freshly explanted colon carcinomas, but not with fibroblasts, normal cells of colonic mucosa, or melanoma cells, which were the control cells. Outgrowth of the colon cancer cell lines to tumors in nude mice was delayed after injection of the monoclonal anticolon cancer antibodies (Herlyn et al., 1980). Several further clones of antibody-producing cells have now been described with specificity for colorectal carcinoma. Most have no reactivity with CEA. By studying mutual blocking or enhancing of the antibody activity on target tumor cells, it was possible to describe antigenic determinants associated with molecules of 32, 36, and 39 K, respectively (Koprowski et al., 1979). It is not yet clear whether any of these molecules is immunogenic in the original tumor host.

3.3. Other Colon-Derived Antigens

3.3.1. Colon Mucoprotein Antigens (CMA)

Colon mucoprotein antigens extractable with phenol–water are present in normal and malignant colon tissue (Gold and Miller, 1974; 1975). The antigens were described to have molecular weights around 1.5×10^7 daltons. These high molecular weight substances were analyzed with rabbit antisera. They are not related to CEA or blood group substances. One type of CMA isolated from colon carcinomas seems to differ from that of normal colon mucosa, and there are also differences between CMA of individual tumors, at least quantitatively. The CMA that appears to be unique for tumors is called TCMA (Gold and Miller, 1978). The concentration of TCMA was diminished on colon tumor cells that were brought to differentiate in vitro, in contrast to CEA, which increases in more differentiated cells (Denk et al., 1972; Hager et al., 1980). CMA characteristic of normal colon mucosa also increased in concentration in differentiated tumor cells. Normal CMA may be an organ-specific antigen, though the tumor specificity of TCMA needs confirmation (Gold and Goldenberg, 1980).

3.3.2. Zinc Glycinate Marker (ZGM)

An α_2-mobile antigen from zinc glycinate-treated extracts of colon cancer has been described (Pusztaszeri et al., 1976). This antigen has a high molecular weight of 2×10^6 daltons and is not identical to CEA, nonspecific crossreacting antigen, or blood group antigens. Antibodies to ZGM were produced in rabbits made tolerant to normal human tissues and CEA. Antibodies that reacted with colon carcinomas and not with normal tissue were produced (Saravis et al., 1978). The antiserum, however, does not react with all colon carcinomas. Immunofluorescence localization studies showed ZGM in the cytoplasm, luminal border, and/or extracellularly in 26 out of 29 colon cancers, but weaker reactions also occurred in benign colon mucosa of the same patients (Doos et al., 1978). The localization pattern of ZGM was similar to CEA, i.e., on luminal borders of malignant glands. Also gastric cancer and associated normal tissues showed some ZGM immunofluorescence. In later publications (Saravis et al., 1979)

ZGM was demonstrated in all of 90 colon tumors, but also in the great majority of gastric, breast, lung, and prostatic cancers. This means that ZGM is not organ or tumor specific, although present in larger amounts in cancerous than in normal tissue. So far serum contents of ZGM have not been investigated.

3.3.3. Colon-Specific Antigens (CSA)

Organ-type specific antigens have been described in colon tissue and adenocarcinomas (Goldenberg et al., 1976a). Sera of hamsters immunized with phenol–alcohol extracts of whole colon adenocarcinoma cells were absorbed with normal human tissue, blood cells, and hamster tissue. Colon-specific antigens are associated with several glycoproteins of varying molecular weight, ranging from 46,000 upwards. The antigens are increased in both fetal and adult human colon compared to other organs. CSA with high molecular weights of 170,000–900,000 by immunodiffusion appear to be specific for the gastrointestinal tract. One of them, CSAp, with a molecular weight of 70,000–110,000, was described to be characteristic for tumors of the gastrointestinal tissues. CSAp is thermolabile and is isolated from the tumor by water extraction (Pant et al., 1978). Primary human colon carcinomas, fetal colon, and ovarian cystadenocarcinomas have high CSAp contents, but small concentrations also occur in normal adult colon. CSAp is present in higher concentrations in colon tumors and polyps than in normal adult or fetal intestinal tissues. There were no cross-reactions with CEA, alphafetoprotein, or ferritin.

3.3.4. Membrane Tissue Antigen (MTA)

This antigen has also been purified from primary and metastatic colonic carcinomas (von Kleist et al., 1974). It is one of the three perchloric acid-soluble substances easily demonstrated in colon carcinoma, i.e., CEA, nonspecific crossreacting antigen and MTA. MTA is a glucoprotein with α-mobility and a molecular weight between 23,000–44,000. Using rabbit antisera, MTA was shown to be located in the cytoplasm and cell membrane of colonic tumors. Immunodiffusion demonstrated that MTA also occurs in extracts of adult colon mucosa, renal and lung tissue, as well as in fetal intestine. MTA thus appears to be present both in normal and in malignant gastrointestinal specimens, as well as in other tissues. The amount found in colonic tumors, however, was higher than in normal colon. The claims for autoantigenicity of MTA (von Kleist et al., 1974) remain to be confirmed.

3.3.5. Nonspecific Crossreacting Antigens (NCA)

NCA (von Kleist et al., 1972; Mach and Pusztaszeri, 1972) is a glycoprotein with a molecular weight around 115,000 (Hammarström et al., 1978) that shares antigenic determinants with CEA. NCA is present in normal gut cells, but also in myeloid cells, lung and spleen tissue. It has been purified from liver metastases of colonic cancer and from normal lung and spleen. NCA serum levels in gastrointestinal disease have been measured and are often slightly raised in malignant as well as nonmalignant diseases. There is no specific elevation of NCA in the serum of patients with gastrointestinal tumors, apart from some cases of colon carcinoma with metastatic growth in the liver (von Kleist et al., 1977).

A second normal colon antigen (NCA-2) with a larger molecular weight than NCA has been described (Burtin et al., 1973). Semiquantitative determinations of NCA-2 with sheep or rabbit antisera were performed by immunodiffusion of fecal extracts (Hirsch-Marie et al., 1973). NCA-2 was detected in the feces of 73% of patients with gastrointestinal cancer, and in the same frequency in persons with noncancerous diseases. NCA-2 is therefore not cancer-related, but a normal component of the feces. NCA-2 is not yet well characterized, but may be similar to other fecal antigens (Matsuoka et al., 1973).

3.4. Gastric-Derived Antigens

3.4.1. Fetal Sulfoglycoprotein (FSA)

An antigen called fetal sulfoglycoprotein antigen (FSA) has been described in fetal stomach, in gastric cancer cells, and in gastric juice of patients with gastric cancer (Häkkinen, 1966; Häkkinen et al., 1968a; 1968b). Rabbit antisera were produced to the mucoproteins of gastric cancer juice. Immunofluorescence demonstrated FSA in gastric cancer cells, but also outside the tumor in superficial cells (Häkkinen et al., 1968a). FSA is antigenically related to CEA.

Population screenings performed in Finland for this antigen revealed thirty previously unknown gastric cancers (Häkkinen, 1974; 1979). FSA determinations of gastric juice by immunodiffusion have also been evaluated in patients with advanced gastric carcinomas (Parvinen et al., 1979). Partial remission or stable disease was followed by a temporary decrease of FSA in the gastric juice. In progressive disease, FSA was usually present.

FSA has not been sought for extensively in other tissues than gastrointestinal. Its relation to CEA and other gastric antigens will hopefully be clarified soon. Although this antigen is expressed not only in gastric cancers, but also sometimes in benign diseases such as gastritis, screening approaches may be worthwhile in high-risk populations.

3.4.2. CEA-like Antigen (CELIA)

A CEA-like antigen has been partially characterized (Vuento et al., 1976a; 1976b). CELIA was isolated from gastric juice of healthy persons. The purification was performed with anti-CEA affinity chromatography, and the material reactive in a radioimmunoassay for CEA was collected. Although the purification was made so as to obtain CEA-like material, the resulting substance differed somewhat from CEA. In gel filtration CELIA was slightly retarded compared to CEA. Immunodiffusion experiments indicated a minor difference between the antigenic determinants. Also, absorption of anti-CEA sera with CELIA reduced anti-CELIA activity but had only a minor effect on anti-CEA activity.

CEA-like activity in gastric juice did not differ between subjects with gastric cancer, ulcers, or healthy persons. Since other organs have not been studied, it is unclear whether CELIA is specifically related to gastric tissue. CELIA seems to differ from FSA because the latter is mainly found in a fraction of acid glycoproteins of cancerous but not normal gastric juice. Serum levels of CELIA have not been reported, but it should be noted that serum CEA often reaches high levels in advanced gastric cancer (Ellis et al., 1978).

3.4.3. Sulfoglycopeptide Antigen (SGA)

Bara et al. (1978) have described a sulfoglycopeptide that is detected after papain digestion of gastric carcinoma tissue. The antigen is a mucoprotein, rich in threonine and proline. Rabbit antisera were produced and used for immune histology. About 50% of colon carcinomas and some gastric cancers contained this antigen. Like CEA, SGA concentrations are higher in well-differentiated than in poorly differentiated carcinomas. No staining for SGA was seen in normal adult gastric mucosa. Normal colon, however, does contain a similar substance.

3.4.4. Gastric Cancer Antigen (GCA)

Rabbit antisera produced against gastric cancer juice detected an antigen called GCA (Deutsch et al., 1973). On electrophoresis, the antigen was found in the β-region. After absorption of this antiserum with gastric juice from noncancerous patients or with normal human plasma, immunodiffusion showed a reaction with 22/24 cancer secretions, but none of 28 normal or gastritis secretions. Since the technique is relatively insensitive, this may reflect a quantitative rather than a qualitative difference. The relation, if any, of GCA to FSA has not been studied.

3.5. Alphafetoprotein (AFP) in Esophageal and Gastric Cancer

AFP elevations are most common with primary hepatic and gonadal tumors. Serum AFP was increased in 4% of patients considered to have a localized esophageal carcinoma (Wahren et al., 1979) and in 15% of gastric cancer patients (McIntire et al., 1975). These frequencies are too low to be of any practical value. In patients who do have elevated serum AFP, tumor progression is usually accompanied by a rise in AFP.

3.6. Deleted Antigens

One of the earliest findings in gastrointestinal tumor immunology was deleted blood group antigens. Such antigens as ABH are defined by human sera and/or by lectins.

In the adult, ABH blood group activity can be detected in the upper gastrointestinal tract, but not lower than the transverse colon. In gastrointestinal tumors, a change to less or no blood group antigens of the water-soluble ABH types was seen in the parts of the gastrointestinal tract that normally express them (Davidsohn et al., 1966; Davidsohn, 1972). This was true both for gastric tumors and for tumors of the colon's proximal parts. Instead I-antigen, which is one of the precursor substances, was found in increased amounts in gastric cancer extracts (Picard et al., 1978). The loss of mature ABH antigens have been suggested to represent the functional dedifferentiation of cancer cells. In contrast, studies of the blood group antigen content of carcinomas located in the distal colon showed that around 50% of these tumors expressed blood group antigens (Abdelfattah-Gad and Denk, 1980).

In both gastric and colon tumor tissue, it has been noted that CEA may be present when the blood group isoantigens are absent (Denk et al., 1974). When morphologic differentiation and loss of tumorigenicity were induced by a polar solvent in a colon carcinoma cell line (Hager et al., 1980), blood group antigen H was decreased, while CEA increased.

Burtin et al. (1971) have described the loss of a normally occurring colonic membrane antigen in adenocarcinoma cells of the colon. The antigen was prepared from adult or fetal colon mucosa. It is present on the cell surface of normal mucosa. This α-mobile antigen was diminished in colon tumor cells compared with normal colon mucosa, as judged by immunofluorescence with rabbit antisera.

3.7. Conclusions

As a marker for gastrointestinal tumors, CEA at present seems to be the most useful substance. A high preoperative serum CEA indicates a poorer prognosis than a low one, both regarding survival time and the risk of developing recurrence. Such information can be used when considering more intensive modes of treatment for patients with elevated CEA. In monitoring patients after primary operation, frequent CEA determinations are the best non-invasive means to detect recurrence before clinical symptoms occur. CEA-containing tumors have been located by injecting isotope-labeled anti-CEA antibodies. Successful results have not been obtained in screening of asymptomatic persons since CEA elevations occur with some benign conditions. Therefore, an elevated CEA alone can not be used to establish the primary diagnosis of colorectal cancer.

Several colon- and gastric-derived substances other than CEA have been described. Closer study has revealed that most of them, like CEA, are also found in small quantities in nonmalignant tissues of the gastrointestinal tract. These antigens, as well as the phenomenon of normal antigen deletion, can be used to study regulatory mechanisms of benign and malignant cells. Antigen occurrence and quantification might help in histopathological classification of tumors. It is not yet clear whether any of these substances will offer advantages that CEA does not already give in the clinical diagnosis, followup, and possibly the treatment of patients with gastrointestinal tumors.

4. Tissue Antigens of Human Large Bowel Cancers Immunogenic in the Host of Origin

4.1. Antigens Defined by Demonstration of Cell-Mediated Reactivity in Vitro

The antigens discussed in the previous section are defined by xenogeneic antisera. They do not seem to be immunogenic in the host of origin. Other reports deal with antigens associated with large bowel cancer, which are indeed immunogenic in the patient in whom the tumor originates. The use of various assays for cell-mediated immunity has provided indications of reactivity in the majority of colon cancer patients against antigens common for colorectal cancer cells and not usually detectable in neoplastic or normal cells of other tissue origin. Lymphocyte cytotoxicity and colony inhibition tests have given evidence of selective effects on target tumor cells of recent origin (Hellström and Hellström, 1970; Hellström et al., 1971; Nairn et al., 1971; Baldwin et al., 1973a; Steele et al., 1975). A major problem in lymphocyte cytotoxicity tests has been to distinguish selective antitumor effects from spontaneous cytotoxicity of particular lymphocyte subpopulations (NK cells). The effects of the latter cells are not selective for tumor cells, but are recorded also on various normal cells, although the sensitivity varies. The NK effector cells have now been better defined and procedures for their enrichment or depletion have been established (Herberman and Holden, 1978; Timonen et al., 1979; Malmström et al., 1980a,b). This provides means for a more detailed reinvestigation of selective, lytic antitumor effects of lymphocytes from individual patients.

Lymphocytotoxicity was often stronger towards autochthonous than allogeneic colon carcinoma cells. Selective reactivity to tumor cells was also demonstrated more often on short-term tissue cultures than on established cell lines (Hellström et al., 1971; Nairn et al., 1971). Hellström et al. (1971) and Nind et al. (1971) demonstrated that sera of patients with growing colon cancer inhibited the lymphocyte cytotoxicity to autochthonous tumor cells. A similar inhibition of the lymphocyte effect was achieved by preincubation of the lymphocytes with papain-solubilized colon cancer preparations, but not with preparations from normal colon cells (Baldwin et al., 1973b). It is still not sufficiently clear whether the cytotoxicity owes to T cells or results from antibodies produced or carried by some of the lymphocytes used in the tests.

The lymphocytes of colon cancer patients were also cytotoxic to embryonal gut cells, as opposed to kidney cells of the same embryo (Hellström et al., 1970). These results thus indicated the existence of oncofetal antigens which were immunogenic in the host of origin. Koldovsky and Weinstein (1972) found lymphocytes of colorectal carcinoma patients cytotoxic to both embryonic and adult intestinal cells, indicating immunity to bowel specific antigens. However, the role of NK in these reactions has not been clarified. A similar organ-specific reactivity has been demonstrated in patients with the benign disease chronic ulcerative colitis (Perlmann and Broberger, 1963).

Also, assays that do not involve cytolytic effects have been used to demonstrate immunogenicity of colorectal carcinomas. When sensitized lymphocytes are exposed to antigen, they release lymphokines. Some lymphokines give rise to an inhibition of leukocyte migration (LMI), which can be measured. With this method, a positive reaction to colon carcinoma extracts, but not to normal mucosal extracts, has been demonstrated in a majority of patients with colon carcinoma (68–89%) (Bull et al., 1973; Guillou and Giles, 1973; McIllmurray et al., 1974). No reactivity was seen in patients free of tumor for more than 6 months (Bull et al., 1973). There was no obvious correlation to clinical stage in most studies. Elias and Elias (1975), however, reported nonreactivity in 14 of 15 patients with widespread disease, although 18 of 20 patients with resectable tumors were reactive. A correlation has been reported between reactivity in leukocyte migration inhibition tests and delayed hypersensitivity skin tests toward a $3M$ KCl extract of a colon carcinoma patient's own tumor (Mavligit et al., 1972). Hollinshead et al. (1970; 1972) have described most patients with colorectal carcinomas to be reactive in delayed hypersensitivity skin tests with antigen isolated from soluble fractions of intestinal cancer and of fetal gut cell membranes from the first and second trimester. These antigens were demonstrated to be distinct from CEA.

Lymphocytes of most patients with colon carcinomas, but not of patients with other neoplasms, showed a blastogenic response on exposure to $3M$ KCl extracts of colon carcinomas (Mavligit et al., 1973) or to irradiated cells of their own tumor. However, in general, there is still uncertainty about the significance of the lymphoblastogenic response to allogeneic cells or extracts as an indicator of presensitization to the antigen in question (Dean et al., 1975; Vanky et al., 1974).

The leukocyte adherence inhibition test (LAI) has also been utilized as an assay for patient immunity to one's own tumor. The leukocyte adherence to glass surfaces decreases when the cells are exposed to crude antigens against which the donor was sensitized (Halliday et al., 1974). In 36 of 38 colorectal carcinoma patients, a reaction with colon cancer extracts was seen in LAI. Similarly, Powell et al. (1975) found that leukocytes of 95% of cancer patients, comprising 9 different types of cancer, responded to the appropriate 3M KCl tumor extract. Halliday et al. (1977) also reported that 46 out of 47 colorectal carcinoma patients had serum factors that blocked the LAI response. They recommended the LAI assay as an immunodiagnostic test for cancer.

The LAI assay has also been used in studies of the β_2- microglobulin associated colon cancer antigens of Thomson et al. (1978; 1980). This antigen is a lipoprotein isolated by gel filtration from papain preparations of cell membranes. As a final purification step, a horse antihuman β_2-microglobulin immunosorbent was used. The isolated material with LAI activity was shown to consist of molecules of 12k, 25k, 40k, 50k, and 60k. These antigens show organ specificity. Depending on age, leukocytes of 60–100% of patients with colon cancer reacted with the antigen. The stage A patients had 100% reactivity. Leukocytes of patients with other tumors of gastrointestinal origin were reactive in less than 3%. No comparison has been made with fractions isolated in a similar way from normal colon. Since the antigen was coisolated with the β_2-microglobulin fraction, its relationship to normal histocompatibility antigens has to be clarified further before the tumor-specificity can be judged. The antigen is present in serum of patients with metastatic gastrointestinal cancer, but clinical evaluations have not yet been performed (Thomson et al., 1980).

Results obtained with LAI and leukocyte migration inhibition assays have been compared with those obtained with macrophage electrophoretic mobility (MEM) analysis (Field and Caspary, 1970). The latter technique measures the reduction in surface charge of leukocytes after exposure to cell extracts of tumor or control tissues. In all three tests, preparations by 3M KCl extraction of liver, lung, heart, kidney, and spleen of 3–5-month-old human fetuses were reported to affect lymphocytes of many tumor patients (69–80%), including those with gastrointestinal tract cancers (Pasternak et al., 1978). Healthy controls or patients with nonneoplastic diseases reacted much less frequently, 10% in MEM, 15–20% in LAI, and 25–30% in LMI. MEM tests on extracts of colon and stomach cancers affected lymphocytes of patients with the appropriate cancer type in a high proportion as measured by the MEM assay (Müller et al., 1978). Colon cancer extracts gave positive reactions in 95% of 82 colon cancer patients and in 25% of 59 stomach cancer patients, while only 6 out of 80 patients with other malignancies and 3 out of 77 without malignancy gave positive reactions. Extracts of normal colon mucosa gave positive results in only 2 out of 27 colon cancer patients. Analogous results were reported for stomach cancer patients, 94% of 96 stomach cancer patients and 17% of 70 colon cancer patients being positive, while control patients without malignancy or with other types of cancer were positive in 3 and 5%, respectively. Normal stomach mucosa yielded positive results with only 17% of stomach cancer patients and 6% of controls.

These results indicate that the MEM technique reflects sensitization to organ related antigens with quantitative differences between neoplastic and nonneoplastic tissue. Another possibility is the existence of antigens distinctive of the cancer cells. No attempt to purify the active tissue components has been reported. This is also true for most of the results with LAI and leukocyte migration inhibition.

4.2. Antigens Defined by Humoral Antibodies in Patient Serum

Serum antibodies from colorectal carcinoma patients have been tested for complement dependent cytotoxicity and antibody-dependent cellular cytotoxicity against allogeneic colon carcinoma cell lines (Baldwin et al., 1973a; Schultz et al., 1975; Hahn et al., 1978). Complement-dependent cytotoxicity was demonstrated in varying frequencies (14–75%) against established cell lines from colon and rectum carcinomas. Sera from healthy persons were found to be negative. Sera of 9 out of 14 patients were reactive against one or both of two colon carcinoma cell lines in the antibody dependent cellular cytotoxicity assay. The antigens involved in these reactions have not been defined. It has not been established that the antigens are truly organ related, although the data indicate that they might be. Reactivity to the patient's own tumor cells has not been demonstrated, nor has it been ruled out that the detected reactivity might be directed against blood group antigens or the HLA system. Bloom et al. (1973) showed that patients whose sera reacted against several tumor cells had antibodies to blood group A or A-like substances. It has also been demonstrated that a number of bowel and gastric cancers express the heterogenic Forssman glycolipid antigen, which is an A-like antigen (Hakamori et al., 1977). Sequential studies in individual patients have not yet been performed.

4.3. Conclusions

There is good support for the conclusion that patients with bowel carcinoma are often sensitized to antigens related to the large bowel. Strict tumor specificity has not yet been proven. However, there are indications of at least a quantitative difference in antigen content between cancer and normal tissues. Several of the assays have potential as standard assays when the antigens have been characterized and the specificity and sensitivity have been confirmed in larger materials.

The immunity reflected by these tests might be of importance in tumor rejection and thus in immunotherapy. This, too, remains to be established by, for example, sequential studies in the course of successful and unsuccessful immunotherapy and by analysis of reactivity both to the patients' malignant and nonmalignant cells.

5. Tissue Antigens of Rat Bowel Cancer

5.1. Antigens Defined by Xenogeneic Antisera

Rabbit antisera to rat colon carcinoma reacted with several rat colon carcinomas also after extensive absorption with various normal rat cells (Martin et al., 1975). These studies were performed by the immunofluorescence technique. These sera also recognized a membrane antigen in the rat fetal gut, but not in adult bowel cells, indicating that the common tumor-associated antigens were probably of oncofetal nature (Table 2).

5.2. Nonhistone Nuclear Protein Antigens

It has been demonstrated that histone and nonhistone nuclear proteins are involved in the restriction of DNA transcription. Such proteins might therefore differ in neoplastic cells as compared to normal. Chiu et al. (1980) produced antisera in rabbits against dehistonized chromatin isolated from rat transplantable colon carcinoma. Similar antisera were produced against analogous material from normal gut epithelium. The antisera to tumor material showed specificity for tumor chromatin and very little cross-reactivity with chromatin from normal colon (Wasserman and Levine, 1961). Using this serum, the appearance of the nonhistone nuclear antigen was studied in the course of 1,2-dimethylhydrazine (DMH) induced carcinogenesis in rats. Chromatin from the large bowel of rats

Table 2
Markers of Bowel Cancers in the Rat

Marker	Cancer localization	Examples
Antigens in animals defined by xenogeneic antisera	Colon	Oncofetal antigen, nonhistone nuclear antigen
Tumor-associated antigens immunogenic in the host of origin	Colon and small intestine	Unique antigens; tissue-associated embryonic antigens

treated with DMH for 6 weeks or more reacted with the antiserum against the tumor chromatin. At this time point there was no marked histological manifestation of the neoplastic transformation. No tumor specificity could be demonstrated against nonhistone proteins free of DNA. It was further shown that the antiserum demonstrated only nuclear antigen and did not recognize any cytoplasmic antigen.

If these results can be confirmed in humans, the detection of nonhistone nuclear antigens in biopsy material might have the potential of being an early marker of bowel cancer development.

5.3. Antigens Immunogenic in the Original Tumor Host

There is evidence of the expression of both individually unique and common tumor associated antigens in bowel carcinomas induced with either DMH or N-methyl-N'-nitroso-guanidine (MNNG). The individually unique antigens have been demonstrated by isograft rejection tests (Steele, 1975; Sjögren, 1978), but they have not yet been analyzed serologically in relation to the antigens shared by most or all bowel cancers of the rat. Stronger isograft rejection responses were induced than by shared antigens. The antigens appear to be analogous to the individually unique antigens demonstrated in other chemically induced experimental neoplasms (Sjögren, 1965).

The existence of antigens shared by most colorectal carcinomas of the rat was first indicated by lymphocyte cytotoxicity analysis (Steele and Sjögren, 1974b). Lymph node cells from rats bearing colon carcinomas induced by DMH or MNNG were cytotoxic to target cells of 15 different rat colon carcinomas, but not to normal adult rat colon mucosa or to other tumor types. Spleen cells of tumor bearers or of immunized rats contain large numbers of NK cells, which makes it difficult to analyze selective antitumor reactivity. Peripheral blood lymphocytes also showed a considerable NK activity, but selective antitumor effects could still usually be demonstrated. However, a technique has been established by which the NK cells can be eliminated, so that one can demonstrate selective tumor reactivity of spleen cells, too (Malmström et al., 1978). This technique is also applicable to human blood lymphocytes (Malmström et al., 1980a). An organ specificity of tumor-associated antigens analogous to that of colorectal carcinomas has not usually been demonstrated with experimental neoplasms. However, such shared antigens have been found among urinary bladder carcinomas (Taranger et al., 1972) and among breast carcinomas (Baldwin and Embleton, 1974).

Sera of colon carcinoma-bearing rats were shown to block the tumor-selective lymphocyte cytotoxicity but did not affect the NK activity or the selective immune lymphocyte effect on target tumor cells unrelated to the bowel cancers (Sjögren and Steele, 1975). These results are quite analogous to those of similar studies on human large bowel carcinoma (Hellström et al., 1971b). The blocking activity could be absorbed out with protein A and with insolubilized rabbit anti-rat IgG (Steele et al., 1974; Steele, 1975). This indicated that the blocking phenomenon was associated with antibodies with specificity for colon carcinoma cells, most likely in the form of circulating immune complexes.

Sera of rats developing primary DMH-induced bowel carcinomas have been shown to contain antibodies reacting with syngeneic colon carcinoma cells and with cells of 13–15 day old fetuses. These antibodies were demonstrated in assays for complement-dependent cytotoxicity (Sjögren, 1978), antibody-dependent cellular cytotoxicity (Sjögren, 1979), and binding assays with viable target cells (Brodin, Nilsson, Sjögren, unpublished) or colon cancer extract preparations bound to agarose beads (Nelson et al., 1977). Studies on sequential sera of DMH-treated rats in the course of the latency period before detection of visible bowel cancer have revealed antibodies several months before detection of tumor by X-ray or laparotomy (Sjögren, 1979). Although high antibody activity was recorded, it was often transient and the complement-dependent cytotoxicity was usually lower or sometimes undetectable at the time of tumor appearance. At least some of the antibodies appear to be directed against the embryonic antigens associated with rat colon carcinoma cells. It is not yet clear whether there are antibodies to other tumor-associated antigens. The results indicate that humoral antibody responses to tumor-associated antigens might occur early in the development of primary tumor, long before the tumor mass is detectable by X-ray examinations or has given any symptoms.

5.4. Expression of Embryonic Antigens on Rat Colon Carcinoma Cells

There are three lines of evidence for the expression of embryonic antigens on rat colon carcinoma cells: (1) Immunization with colon carcinoma cell antigens has been shown to result in immune reactivity to antigens of fetal cells; (2) immunization with antigens of fetal cells results in reactivity to colon carcinoma cells; (3) papain- and $3M$ KCl-solubilized cell preparations of rat colon carcinoma contain embryonic antigens.

Lymph node cells of rats bearing primary, chemically induced bowel carcinomas or isografts of such tumors are cytotoxic to freshly explanted fetal gut cells, but not to explanted normal adult fibroblasts or colon mucosa cells. Similarly, sera of rats bearing primary or isografted colorectal carcinomas contain antibodies reacting with cells of 13–15 day old fetuses in cytotoxicity tests or in a binding assay using agarose beads to which extracted fetal antigens were bound (Nelson et al., 1977). Furthermore, as mentioned above, appropriately absorbed rabbit antisera to rat colon carcinoma tissue show reactivity to fetal cells and rat colon carcinoma cells as well, but not to various types of normal adult cells (Martin et al., 1975).

Lymph node cells of multiparous pregnant rats have been shown to be cytotoxic to syngeneic colon carcinoma cells and embryonic cells, but not to normal adult cells (Steele and Sjögren, 1974a). Cocultivation of normal spleen cells with syngeneic embryonic cells in vitro makes them cytotoxic to colon carcinoma cells and embryonic cells (Nelson and Sjögren, 1978). Implantation of intact large bowel of 13–14-day-old fetuses was recently shown to induce isograft resistance (Hedlund and Sjögren, 1980).

Antibodies reactive in complement dependent cytotoxicity with colon carcinoma cells, but not with adult normal cells have been demonstrated in sera of multiparous, pregnant rats (Steele and Sjögren, 1974a). Such sera were often capable of blocking the cytotoxicity of lymphocytes from rats with colon carcinoma on fetal gut cells and often also on colon carcinoma target cells. This blocking activity could be absorbed out specifically by colon carcinoma or fetal gut cells, indicating that it owed to antibodies or circulating immune complexes. Admixture of papain- and $3M$ KCl preparations of rat colon carcinoma isografts to the effector lymphocytes in cytotoxicity tests results in specific inhibition of the effect of colon carcinoma bearers' lymphocytes on fetal gut cells, and also an inhibition of the effect of lymphocytes from multiparous rats on fetal cells (Steele et al., 1975).

Some of the antigens shared among rat colorectal carcinomas induce tumor rejection, as detected by isograft rejection tests (Sjögren, 1978), and immunoprevention of carcinogenesis by DMH. Isograft rejection tests have also demonstrated the existence of individually unique antigens, which tend to induce stronger rejection responses than the shared antigens.

5.5. Conclusions

Rat colorectal carcinomas are characterized by common membrane antigens, at least some of which are also expressed by gut cells of 13–15-day-old fetuses. In addition, individually unique antigens distinguish the various bowel carcinomas from each other. The antigens induce tumor rejection responses. Cell-mediated immunity, as well as humoral antibodies against these antigens can be demonstrated in vitro by various assays. Humoral antibodies to shared antigens of the bowel cancer cells and embryonic cells often appear in the serum of DMH-treated rats several months before any primary bowel carcinoma can be detected by X-ray examination or laparotomy. The antigens have not yet been characterized chemically and their possible presence in the circulation has not been investigated.

The fact that these antigens are proven immunogenic in the host of origin makes them interesting as possible targets for immunotherapeutic action and also as diagnostic markers. They might form a useful model for analogous antigens in human gastrointestinal cancers. The tissue-type specific, shared antigens associated with human colorectal carcinomas, against which immunosensitization seems to occur, might be the human counterpart to the shared embryonic antigens of the rat model. It is still conceivable that these antigens are present also on some normal cells of humans as well as of adult rats. If so, this does not seem to prevent them from inducing a rejection response in the animal model, although this response is often weaker than the corresponding response to the individually unique antigens.

Acknowledgments

The research of the authors and the preparation of this manuscript were supported by Public Health Service Grant CA-14924 from the National Cancer Institute through the National Large Bowel Cancer Project and by grants from the Swedish Cancer Society, John and Augusta Persson's Foundation, and Cancerföreningen in Stockholm.

References

Abdelfattah-Gad, M., and H. Denk (1980), *J. Natl. Cancer Inst.* **64**, 1025.

Alexander, Jr., J. C., P. B. Chretien, A. L. Dellon, and J. Snyder (1978), *Cancer* **42**, 1492.

Alm, T., and B. Wahren (1975), *J. Gastroent.* **10**, 875.

Al-Sarraf, M., L. Baker, R. W. Talley, K. Kithier, and V. K. Vaitkevicius (1979), *Cancer* **44**, 1222.

Baldwin, R. W., and M. J. Embleton (1974), *Int. J. Cancer* **13**, 1801.

Baldwin, R. W., M. J. Embleton, J. S. P. Jones, and M. J. S. Langman (1973a), *Int. J. Cancer* **12**, 73.

Baldwin, R. W., M. J. Embleton, and M. G. Price (1973b), *Int. J. Cancer* **12**, 84.

Balinsky, D. (1980), in *Cancer Markers: Diagnostic and Developmental Significance* (Sell, S., ed.), Humana Press, Clifton, New Jersey, p. 191.

Bara, J., A. Paul-Gardais, F. Loisillier, and P. Burtin (1978), *Int. J. Cancer* **21**, 133.

Beck, P. R., A. Belfield, R. J. Spooner, L. H. Blumgart, and C. B. Wood (1979), *Cancer* **43**, 1772.

Blasecki, J. W., and S. S. Tevethia (1973), *J. Immunol.* **110**, 590.

Bloom, E. T., J. L. Fahey, I. A. Peterson, G. Geering, M. Bernhard, and G. Trempe (1973), *Int. J. Cancer* **12**, 21.

Brooks, W. S., T. Hersh, E. C. Hall, and C. Moore (1979), in *Carcinoembryonic Proteins: Chemistry, Biology, Clinical Application,* (Lehmann, F., ed.), Elsevier, Amsterdam, p. 557.

Bull, D. M., J. R. Leibach, M. A. Williams, and R. A. Helms (1973), *Science* **1818**, 957.

Burtin, P., G. Chavanel, and H. Hirsch-Marie (1973), *J. Immunol.* **111**, 1926.

Burtin, P., E. Martin, M. C. Sabine, and S. von Kleist (1972), *J. Natl. Cancer Inst.* **48**, 25.

Burtin, P., S. von Kleist, and M. C. Sabine (1971), *Cancer Res.* **31**, 1038.

Chiu, J. F., D. Pumo, and D. Gootnick (1980), *Cancer* **45**, 1193.

Chu, T. M., E. D. Holyoke, B. Cedermark, J. Evans, and D. Fischer (1976), in *Onco-Developmental Gene Expression* (Fishman, W. H., and S. Sell, eds.) Academic Press, New York, p. 427.

Davidsohn, I. (1972), *Am. J. Clin. Pathol.* **57**, 715.

Davidsohn, I., S. Kovarik, and C. L. Lee (1966), *Arch. Path.* **81**, 381.

Dean, J. H., J. S. Silva, J. L. McCoy, C. M. Leonard, M. Middleton, G. B. Cannon, and R. B. Herberman (1975), *J. Natl. Cancer Inst.* **54**, 1295.

Denk, H., G. Tappeiner, A. Davidovits, R. Eckerstorfer, and J. H. Holzner (1974), *J. Natl. Cancer Inst.* **53**, 933.

Denk, H., G. Tappeiner, R. Eckerstorfer, and J. H. Holzner (1972), *Int. J. Cancer* **10**, 262.

Deutsch, E., C. A. Apffel, H. Mori, and J. E. Walker (1973), *Cancer Res.* **33**, 112.

Dhar, P., T. Moore, N. Zamcheck, and H. Kupchick (1972), *JAMA* **221**, 31.

Doos, W. G., W. I. Wolff, H. Shinya, A. DeChabon, R. J. Stenger, L. S. Gottlieb, and N. Zamcheck (1975), *Cancer* **36**, 1996.

Doos, W. G., C. Saravis, G. Pusztaszeri, B. Burke, S. K. Oh, N. Zamcheck, and L. S. Gottlieb (1978), *J. Natl. Cancer Inst.* **60**, 1375.

Drewinko, B., and L. -Y. Yang (1980), *Oncology* **37**, 89.

Dykes, P. W., K. R. Hine, A. R. Bradwell, J. C. Blackburn, T. A. Reeder, Z. Drolc, and S. N. Booth (1980), *Brit. Med. J.*, 220.

Edgington, T. S., R. W. Astarita, E. F. Plow (1975), *New Engl. J. Med.* **293**, 103.

Elias, E. G., and L. L. Elias (1975), *Surgery, Gynecol. Obstet.* **141**, 715.

Elias, E. G., E. D. Holyoke, and T. M. Chu (1974), *Dis. Colon Rect.* **17**, 38.

Ellis, D. J., C. Speirs, R. D. Kingston, V. S. Brookes, J. Leonard, and P. W. Dykes (1978), *Cancer* **42**, 623.

Field, E. J., and E. A. Caspary (1970), *Lancet* **2**, 1337.

Fujimoto, S., Y. Kitsukawa, and K. Itoh (1979), *Cellular and Molecular Biol.* **25**, 153.

Fuks, A., J. Shuster, and P. Gold (1980), in *Cancer Markers: Diagnostic and Developmental Significance* (Sell, S., ed.), Humana Press, Clifton, New Jersey, p. 315.

Gadler, H., K. Bremme, and B. Wahren (1980), *Int. J. Cancer* **25**, 91.

Gold, D., and D. M. Goldenberg (1980), in *Cancer Markers: Diagnostic and Developmental Significance* (Sell, S. ed.), Humana Press, Clifton, New Jersey, p. 329.

Gold, D., and F. Miller (1974), *Immunochemistry* **11**, 369.

Gold, D., and F. Miller (1975), *Nature* **255**, 85.

Gold, D., and F. Miller (1978), *Cancer Res.* **38**, 3204.

Gold, P., and S. O. Freedman (1965a), *J. Exptl. Med.* **122**, 467.

Gold, P., and S. O. Freedman (1965b). *J. Exptl. Med.* **121,** 439.

Gold, P., J. M. Gold, and S. O. Freedman (1968), *Cancer Res.* **28,** 1331.

Gold, P., T. Wilson, R. Romero, J. Shuster, and S. O. Freedman (1973), *Dis. Colon Rect.* **16,** 358.

Goldenberg, D. M. (1976), in *Current Topics in Pathology* (Grundmann, E., and W. H. Kirsten, W. H. eds.), Vol. 63, Pathology of the Gastro-Intestinal Tract, Springer-Verlag, p. 290.

Goldenberg, D. M., F. DeLand, E. Kim, S. Bennett, F. Primus, J. van Nagell, N. Estes, P. DeSimone, and P. Rayburn (1978), *New Engl. J. Med.* **298,** 384.

Goldenberg, D. M., K. D. Pant, and H. L. Dahlman (1976a), *Cancer Res.* **36,** 3455.

Goldenberg, D. M., R. M. Sharkey, and F. J. Primus (1976b), *J. Natl. Cancer Inst.* **57,** 11.

Griffing, G., and J. Vaitukaitis (1980), in *Cancer Markers: Diagnostic and Developmental Significance* (Sell, S. ed.), Humana Press, Clifton, New Jersey, p. 169.

Giullou, P. J., and G. R. Giles (1973), *Gut* **14,** 733.

Hager, J. C., D. V. Gold, J. A. Barbosa, Z. Fligiel, F. Miller, and D. L. Dexter (1980), *J. Natl. Cancer Inst.* **64,** 439.

Hahn, W. V., M. F. Kagnoff, and L. H. Hatleu (1978), *J. Natl. Cancer Inst.* **60,** 779.

Hakamori, S., S. -M. Wang, and W. W. Young (1977), *Proc. Natl. Acad. Sci.* **74,** 3023.

Häkkinen, I. (1966), *Scand. J. Gastroent.* **1,** 28.

Häkkinen, I. (1974), *Cancer Res.* **34,** 3069.

Häkkinen, I. (1979), in *Compendium of Assays for Immunodiagnosis of Human Cancer* (Herberman, R. B., ed.), Elsevier, New York, p. 241.

Häkkinen, I., O. Järvi, and J. Grönroos (1968a), *Int. J. Cancer* **3,** 572.

Häkkinen, I., L. K. Korhonen, and L. Saxén (1968b), *Int. J. Cancer* **3,** 582.

Halliday, W. J., A. Malnish, and W. H. Isbister (1974), *Brit. J. Cancer* **29,** 31.

Halliday, W. J., A. Malnish, P. M. Stephenson, N. C. Davis (1977), *Cancer Res.* **37,** 1962.

Hammarström, S., T. Svenberg, A. Hedin, and G. Sundblad (1978), *Scand. J. Immunol.* **7,** 33.

Hansen, H. J., J. J. Snyder, E. Miller, J. P. Vandevoorde, O. N. Miller, L. R. Hines, and J. J. Burns (1974), *Human Pathology* **5,** 139.

Hedlund, G., and H. O. Sjögren (1980), *Int. J. Cancer* **26,** 71.

Hellström, K. E., and I. Hellström (1970), in *Carcinoma of the colon and antecedent epithelium* (Burdette, W. J., ed.), Charles C. Thomas, Springfield, Ill., p. 176.

Hellström, I., K. E. Hellström, H. O. Sjögren, and G. A. Warner (1971), *Int. J. Cancer* **7,** 1.

Hellström, I., K. E. Hellström,, and T. H. Shepard (1970), *Int. J. Cancer* **6,** 346.

Hellström, I., H. O. Sjögren, G. A. Warner, and K. E. Hellström (1971b), *Int. J. Cancer* **7,** 226.

Herberman, R. B., and H. T. Holden (1978), *Adv. Cancer Res.* **27,** 305.

Herlyn, M., Z. Steplewski, D. Herlyn, and H. Koprowski (1979), *Proc Natl. Acad. Sci.* **76**, 1428.

Herlyn, D. M., Z. Steplewski, M. F. Herlyn, and H. Koprowski (1980), *Cancer Res.* **40**, 717.

Herrera, M. S., T. M. Chu, and E. D. Holyoke (1976), *Ann. Surg.* **183**, 5.

Hirsch-Marie, H., G. Chavanel, and P. Burtin (1973), *Digestion* **9**, 193.

Hollinshead, A. C., D. Glew, B. Bunnag, P. Gold, and R. Herberman (1970), *Lancet* **7**, 1191.

Hollinshead, A. C., C. McWright, T. Alford, and D. Glew (1972), *Science* **177**, 887.

Isaacson, P., and H. P. Le Vann (1976), *Cancer* **38**, 1348.

Kim, E. E., F. H. DeLand, S. Casper, R. L. Corgan, F. J. Primus, and D. M. Goldenberg (1980), *Cancer* **45**, 1243.

Koldovsky, P., and J. Weinstein (1972), *Natl. Cancer Inst. Monograph.* **37**, 33.

Koprowski, H., Z. Steplewski, K. Mitchell, M. Herlyn, D. Herlyn, and P. Fuhrer (1979), *Somatic Cell Genet.* **5**, 957.

Laurence, D. J. R., U. Stevens, R. Bettelheim, D. Darcy, C. Leese, C. Turberville, P. Alexander, E. W. Johns, and A. M. Neville (1972), *Brit. Med. J.* Sept. 9, 605.

Lindgren, J. (1980), *Acta Path. Microbiol. Scand.*, Sect. A, **88**, 49.

Loewenstein, M. S., and N. Zamcheck (1978), *Cancer* **42**, 1412.

Lo Gerfo, P., and F. P. Herter (1975), *Ann. Surg.* **181**, 81.

Mach, J. -P., M. Forni, J. Ritschard, F. Buchegger, S. Carrel, S. Widgren, A. Donath, and P. Alberto (1980), *Oncodevelopmental Biol. Med.* **1**, 49.

Mach, J. -P., P. Jaeger, M. -M. Betholet, C. -H. Ruegsegger, R. M. Loosli, and J. Pettavel (1974), *Lancet* **2**, 535.

Mach, J. P., and G. Pusztaszeri (1972), *Immunochemistry* **9**, 1031.

Mach, J. P., S. Carrel, C. Merenda, B. Sorbat, and J. C. Cerottini (1974), *Nature* **248**, 704.

Malmström, P., Å. Jönsson, T. Hallberg, and H. O. Sjögren (1980a), *Cell Immunol.* **53**, 39.

Malmström, P., Å. Jönsson, and H. O. Sjögren (1980b), *Cell Immunol.* **53**, 50.

Malmström, P., K. Nelsson, Å. Jönsson, H. O. Sjögren, H. Walter, and P. -Å. Albertsson (1978), *Cell Immunol.* **37**, 409.

Martin, E. W., M. Cooperman, G. King, and J. Noltimier (1979), in *Carcinoembryonic proteins II*, (Lehmann, F. G., ed.), Elsevier/North Holland, p. 81.

Martin, E. W., K. K. James, P. E. Hurtubise, P. Catalano, and J. P. Minton (1977), *Cancer* **39**, 440.

Martin, F., F. Knobel, M. Martin, and M. Bordes (1975), *Cancer Res.* **35**, 333.

Martin, F., and M. Martin (1972), *Int. J. Cancer* **9**, 641.

Matsuoka, Y., M. Hara, K. Takatsu, and M. Kitagawa (1973), *Gann* **64**, 203.

Matsushima, T., S. Kawabe, M. Shibuya, and T. Sugimura (1968), *Biochem. Biophys. Res. Commun.* **30**, 565.

Mavligit, G. M., J. U. Gutterman, C. M. McBride, and E. M. Hersh (1972), *Proc. Soc. Exptl. Biol. Med.* **140**, 1240.

Mavligit, G. M., E. M. Hersh, C. M. McBride (1973), *J. Natl. Cancer Inst.* **51**, 337.

Mayer, R. J., M. B. Garnick, G. D. Steele Jr., and N. Zamcheck (1978), *Cancer* **42**, 1428.

McIllmurray, M. B., M. R. Price, and M. J. S. Langman (1974), *Brit. J. Cancer* **29**, 305.

McIntire, K. R., T. A. Waldman, C. G. Moertel, and V. L. W. Go (1975), *Cancer Res.* **35**, 991.

Moertel, C. G., A. J. Schutt, and V. L. W. Go (1978), *JAMA* **239**, 1065.

Müller, M., J. Irmscher, H. Grossmann, M. Kotzsch, G. Heidl, H. Wagner, and R. Fischer (1978), in *Modern Trends in Cell Electrophoresis*, Schriften der Med. Akad., Dresden, Band 15, p. 7.

Nairn, R. C., A. P. P. Nind, E. P. G. Guli, D. J. Davies, J. M. Rolland, A. R. McGiven, and E. S. R. Hughes (1971), *Brit. Med. J.* **4**, 706.

Nelson, K., and H. O. Sjögren (1978), *Int. J. Cancer* **21**, 108.

Nelson, K., H. O. Sjögren, and J. E. Rosengren (1977), *Int. J. Cancer* **20**, 227.

Nind, A. P., R. C. Navrin, J. M. Rolland, E. P. Guli, and E. S. Hughes (1973), *Brit. J. Cancer* **28**, 108.

Pant, K. D., H. L. Dahlman, and D. Goldenberg (1978), *Cancer* **42**, 1626.

Papapetrou, P., N. Sákarelou, H. Braouzi, and P. Fessas (1980), *Cancer* **45**, 2583.

Parvinen, M., M. Kormano, and I. Häkkinen (1979), *Cancer Treat. Rept.* **63**, 2121.

Pasternak, G., B. v. Broen, S. Albrecht, T. Le Thanh, G. Gryschek, and B. Sclott (1978), in *Modern Trends in Cell Electrophoresis*, Schriften der Med. Akad., Dresden, Band 15, p. 18.

Perlmann, P., and O. Broberger (1963), *J. Exptl. Med.* **117**, 717.

Picard, J., D. W. Edward, and T. Feizi (1978), *J. Clin. Lab. Immunol.* **1**, 119.

Pihl, E., J. McNaughtan, J. Ma, H. A. Ward, and R. C. Nairn (1980), *Pathology* **12**, 7

Plow, E. F., and T. S. Edgington (1975), *Int. J. Cancer* **15**, 748.

Potter, V. R. (1969), *Canad. Cancer Cont.* **8**, 9.

Powell, A. E., A. M. Sloss, R. N. Smith, J. T. Makley, and C. A. Huley (1975), *Int. J. Cancer* **16**, 905.

Pusztaszeri, G., C. Saravis, and N. Zamcheck (1976), *J. Natl. Cancer Inst.* **56**, 275.

Rieger, Å., B. Wahren (1975), *Scand. J. Gastroent.* **10**, 869.

Rittgers, R. A., G. Steele Jr., N. Zamcheck, M. S. Loewenstein, P. H. Sugarbaker, R. J. Mayer, J. J. Lokich, J. Maltz, and R. E. Wilson (1978), *J. Natl. Cancer Inst.* **61**, 315.

Saito, H., and J. Hokkaido (1975), *J. Med. Sci.* **50**, 540.

Saravis, C., H. Kupchik, M. O'Brien, and N. Zamcheck (1979), in *Compendium of Assays for Immunodiagnosis of Human Cancer* (Herberman, R. B., ed.), Elsevier, New York, p. 237.

Saravis, C. A., S. K. Oh, G. Pusztaszeri, W. G. Doos, and N. J. Zamcheck (1978), *J. Natl. Cancer Inst.* **60**, 1371.

Schwartz, M. K. (1976), *Cancer* **37**, 542.

Schultz, R. M., W. A. Woods, and M. A. Chirigos (1975), *Int. J. Cancer* **16**, 16.

Shively, J. E., and C. W. Todd (1980), in *Cancer Markers: Diagnostic and Developmental Significance* (Sell, S., ed.), Humana Press, Clifton, New Jersey, p. 295.

Sjögren, H. O. (1965), *Progr. Exptl. Tum. Res.* **6**, 289.

Sjögren, H. O. (1978), in *Carcinoma of the Colon and Rectum* (Enker, W. E., ed.), The Year Book Med. Publ. Inc., p. 247.

Sjögren, H. O. (1979), in *Immunodiagnosis and Immunotherapy of Malignant Tumors*, (Flad, Herfarth, and Betzler eds.), Springer Verlag, Berlin, p. 20.

Sjögren, H. O. (1980), in *Inhibition of Tumor Induction and Development* (M. Zedeck and M. Lipkin, eds.), Plenum, New York.

Sjögren, H. O., and G. Steele (1975), *Ann. NY Acad. Sci.* **259**, 404.

Staab, H. J., F. A. Anderer, E. Stumpf, and R. Fischer (1978), *Am. J. Surg.* **136**, 322.

Steele, G. (1975), Immunologic Studies of Chemically Induced Rat Bowel Tumors. Doctoral thesis, Lund.

Steele, G., J. Ankerst, and H. O. Sjögren (1974), *Int. J. Cancer* **14**, 83.

Steele, G., and H. O. Sjögren (1974), *Int. J. Cancer* **14**, 435.

Steele, G., and H. O. Sjögren (1974), *Cancer Res.* **34**, 1801.

Steele, G., H. O. Sjögren, and M. R. Price (1975), *Int. J. Cancer* **16**, 33.

Steele, G., S. Sonis, P. Stelos, R. Rittgers, N. Zamcheck, D. Finn, J. Maltz, R. Mayer, J. Lokich, and R. E. Wilson (1978), *Surgery* **83**, 648.

Steele, G., N. Zamcheck, R. Wilson, R. Mayer, J. Lokich, P. Rau, and J. Maltz (1980), *Am. J. Surgery* **139**, 544.

Taranger, L. A., W. H. Chapman, I. Hellström, and K. E. Hellström (1972), *Science* **176**, 1337.

Thomson, D. M. P., J. E. Rausch, J. C. Weatherhead, P. Friedlander, R. O'Connor, N. Grosser, J. Shuster, and P. Gold (1978), *Brit. J. Cancer* **37**, 753.

Thomson, D. M. P., D. N. Tataryn, J. C. Weatherhead, P. Friedlander, J. Rausch, R. Schwartz, P. Gold, and J. Shuster (1980), *Europ. J. Cancer* **16**, 539.

Timonen, T., E. Saksela, A. Ranki, and P. Häyry (1979), *Cellular Immunol.* **48**, 133.

Vanky, F., E. Klein, J. Stjernswärd, and U. Nilssonne (1974), *Int. J. Cancer* **14**, 277.

von Kleist, S., G. Chavanel, and P. Burtin (1972), *Proc. Natl. Acad. Sci.* **69**, 2992.

von Kleist, S., M. King, and P. Burtin (1974), *Immunochemistry* **11**, 249.

von Kleist, S., S. Troupel, M. King, and P. Burtin (1977), *Br. J. Cancer* **35**, 875.

Vuento, M., E. Engvall, M. Seppälä, and E. Ruoslahti (1976a), *Int. J. Cancer* **18**, 156.

Vuento, M., E. Ruoslahti, H. Pihko, T. Svenberg, T. Ihamäki, and M. Siurala (1976b), *Immunochemistry* **13**, 313.

Wahren, B. (1976). *Skandia Int. Symp. Health Control in Detection of Cancer* Almqvist & Wiksell International, Stockholm, p. 61.

Wahren, B., P. Esposti, and R. Zimmerman (1977), *Cancer* **40**, 1511.

Wahren, B., J. Harmenberg, F. Edsmyr, P. Jakobsson, and S. Ingimarsson (1979), *Scand. J. Gastroent.* **14,** 361.

Wanebo, H. J., B. Rao, C. M. Pinsky, R. G. Hoffman, M. Stearns, M. K. Schwartz, and H. F. Oettgen (1978), *New Engl. J. Med.* **299,** 448.

Wasserman, E., and C. Levine (1961), *J. Immunol.* **87,** 290.

Wood, C. B., J. G. Ratcliffe, R. W. Burt, A. J. H. Malcolm, and L. H. Blumgart (1980). *Br. J. Surg.* **67,** 46.

Zamcheck, N. (1978). in *Colon Cancer, Cancer Campaign* (Grundmann, E., ed.), Vol. 2 Gustav Fisher Verlag, Stuttgart, p. 149.

6

Hepatocellular Carcinoma Markers

Stewart Sell

Department of Pathology, University of California Medical School, San Diego, La Jolla, California

1. Introduction

Primary hepatocellular carcinomas (PHC) are derived from parenchymal liver cells. Since the liver is the major metabolic factory of the body, a number of products of the abnormal cells of PHC are potential diagnostic markers. However, because PHC has such a relatively low incidence in the United States, markers for PHC have not attracted as much clinical attention in North America as those for some other cancers, such as lung, breast, or gastrointestinal tract. On the other hand, there is a wide range in incidence of PHC in different parts of the world (Szmuness, 1978). In the United States, the incidence in autopsy studies ranges from 0.2 to 0.6% (Hoyne and Kernohan, 1947; MacDonald, 1957; Mosher, 1960; Patton and Horn, 1964; San Jose et al., 1965) with evidence for an increasing incidence from 0.17% during the period 1918–1953, to 0.96% in 1964–1973 as determined at the University of Southern California Medical Center (Peters, 1976). In Europe, the incidence ranges from approximately 0.25% in Germany to 1.65% in France (Szmuness, 1978). In many parts of Africa, primary liver cell cancer is the most common cancer in males (up to 90%), and there is a generally high incidence found in Asia (10–40%) (Ezraty and Gauthier, 1977). There is a greater interest in the clinical use of markers of PHC in Africa and Asia, in particular in Japan and China.

133

The relationship of PHC to environmental influences is of particular interest to oncologists. Hepatocellular carcinoma is frequently associated with cirrhosis and one of three other factors: hepatitis B infection, alcoholism, or aflatoxin exposure (Popper, 1979). For instance, the extremely high incidence of PHC among Bantu of South Africa may be related to dietary consumption of aflatoxin (Higginson and Oettle, 1960; Purves, 1973; Berman, 1951; Wogan, 1976); the generally high incidence of PHC in many countries is associated with a high incidence of infection with hepatitis B virus (Szmuness, 1978), and an unexpectedly high incidence of PHC in Geneva, Switzerland is thought to be related to high alcohol consumption (Tuyns and Obradovic, 1975).

The early diagnosis of hepatocellular carcinoma is exceedingly difficult. Owing to the large size and functional reserve of the liver, PHC is often far advanced and metastases are frequently present before symptoms of the disease are noted (Ihde et al., 1974; Al-Sarraf et al., 1974). About one-third of patients with PHC present with abdominal discomfort related to a right upper quadrant mass, and/or weight loss and ascites. Others exhibit malaise, anorexia, jaundice, etc. (Ihde et al., 1974; Al-Sarraf, 1974; Okuda, 1976).

The high incidence of cirrhosis preceding PHC makes separation of symptoms and tests for PHC from those of underlying cirrhosis difficult (Peters, 1976; Shikata, 1976). The application of laboratory tests to the diagnosis of PHC reflects this basic problem. There is no single serum marker for PHC. The clinician must weigh the results of a number of tests, along with the clinical symptoms, physical findings, radiographic analysis, and pathologic examination in order to make the diagnosis. In this review, the value of serum markers for liver cancer will be presented. These include tests for liver function, isozymes, serum hormone levels, specific serum protein changes (alphafetoprotein, ferritin), and the presence of hepatitis B antigen (HBsAg).

2. Liver Function Tests

A list of commonly used tests of liver function is given in Table 1. The cells of the liver normally perform a number of metabolic functions including intermediate metabolism of proteins, carbohydrates, and lipids; storage of nutrients and minerals; detoxification of various biologically active hormones, drugs, and other compounds; synthesis and secretion of a variety of serum proteins; and secretion of bile. The standard laboratory tests include measurement of intracellular enzymes that enter the blood when liver cells are injured, products of diseased liver cells, and antibodies against liver antigens released during injury.

Examination of Table 1 clearly illustrates that there is no easily identifiable combination of test results that leads to a diagnosis of PHC. This conclusion becomes even more obvious in view of the fact that at least 50% of PHC occur in livers with preexisting cirrhosis. Slight elevations of liver cell enzymes or changes in serum albumin/globulin ratios will, in the great majority of cases, not differentiate PHC from normal or from cirrhosis of the liver. In a review of 65 cases of PHC at Grace Hospital, Detroit, MI, elevations of 2 to 5 times normal of serum alkaline phosphatase (88%), SGOT (78%), SGPT (34%), and LDH (66%) were found in many of these patients. However, two-thirds of the patients with PHC also had liver cirrhosis, which could account for these abnormal enzyme levels (Al-Sarraf et al., 1974). A recently described biliary glycoprotein (BGPI) is elevated in the sera of patients with inflammatory diseases of the liver, but its usefulness in diagnosis of PHC has not yet been established (Svenberg et al., 1979). The diagnosis of PHC is most frequently made by detection of single or multiple intrahepatic masses by physical examination, isotopic liver scan, or celiac arteriography (Ihde et al., 1974). However, the association of PHC with more specific serum abnormalities, such as elevations in alphafetoprotein, may aid considerably in making the diagnosis.

3. Alphafetoprotein

Alphafetoprotein (AFP) is the single most useful marker for the diagnosis and management of PHC. However, elevation of serum AFP above normal by itself is not diagnostic of PHC since elevations may occur in other diseases of the liver or in association with tumors arising in other organs.

AFP is a serum protein normally found in low concentrations in the serum of normal adults (5–10 ng/mL), but in high concentrations in fetal serum (up to 10 mg/mL at 12 weeks of gestation). Elevations of serum AFP in mice with hepatocellular carcinomas were first observed by Abelev et al. in 1963 and in humans with PHC by Tatarinov in 1964. Since that time, a large number of studies have demonstrated elevations of serum AFP in patients with PHC. The early data were confused by the use of insensitive assays. It is now generally accepted that up to 80–90% of patients with PHC have serum AFP concentrations above normal (regardless of race or area of habitation). The association of serum AFP elevations with PHC and other tumors as well as other diseases in various experimental models has been the subject of many recent reviews; Abelev, 1968; Abelev, 1971; Sell and Wepsic, 1974; Alpert, 1976; Abelev, 1974; Adinolfi et al., 1975; Sell and Becker, 1978; Delpre and Gilat, 1978; Sell, 1980; Seppälä and Ruoslahti, 1976; Ruoslahti et al., 1974a). A number of important aspects of AFP, such as physicochemical properties, fetal

Table 1
Laboratory Tests for Liver Function[a]

Test	Normal values	Values expected in					Comments
		Liver cell injury	Obstructive disease	Alcoholic cirrhosis	Primary or secondary cancer	
Enzymes						
Serum glutamic oxalacetic transaminase (SGOT)	10–40 Units	400–4000	100–300	100–300	200	Also elevated in heart disease
Serum glutamine pyruvic transaminase (SGPT)	5–40 Units	400–4000	100–300	100–300	200	More specific for liver cell injury than SGOT
Lactic dehydrogenase (LDH)	24–78 International units	400	100–300	200	200	More elevated in myocardial infarct and hemolysis
Alkaline phosphatase	2.0–4.5 Units (Bodansky)	Normal or slight elevation	3× Normal	Normal or slight increase	Moderate to 2× normal	Also elevations in bone disease and pregnancy
Proteins						
Serum bilirubin	1.2 mg/100 mL	2–40	3–15	3–15	Normal	
Urine urobilinogen	0.3–10.0 Units	Slight increase	Variable	Variable	Normal	

Total serum proteins	6.0–8.0 g/100 mL	Normal	Normal	Decrease	Usually normal	A/G ratio may be reversed in cirrhosis
Albumin	3.5–4.5 g/100 mL	Normal	Normal	Decreased	May be decreased	
Globulin	3–4 g/100 mL	Normal	Normal	Increase	Normal	
Ceruloplasmin	20–40 mg/100 mL	—	—	—	Normal	Under 10 mg/100 mL in Wilsons Disease
Vitamin B_{12}	200–800 mg/100 mL	Marked increase	Normal or moderate increase	Moderate increase	Rare increase	High in leukemia
Prothrombin time	100% (of normal)	10–80%	40–100%	80–100%	Normal	
Others						
Serum copper	90–120 g/100 mL	Normal	Normal	Normal	Normal	10–70 g/mL in Wilsons Disease
Serum iron	60–190 g/100 mL					Elevated in hemochromatosis
Blood ammonia	50–150 g/mL (arterial)	Terminal elevation				Elevated in hepatic coma
Serum cholesterol total	150–250 mg/100 mL	Decrease	Increase	Slight increase	Normal	
Esters	60–70% of total					

[a]Modified from: Edmondson, H. A., and R. L. Peters, in *Pathology* (Anderson, W. A. D., Anderson, and J. M. Kissane, Eds.). St. Louis, Mosby, 7th ed. pp. 1330–1331.

production, biological activities, and production in experimental models will not be covered in the present chapter (see Sell, 1980 for a recent review of these topics). The relevance of AFP as a marker for PHC in humans will be emphasized.

Determination of serum AFP concentrations has been extensively evaluated as a diagnostic test for PHC in humans (see above reviews). The normal concentration of AFP in adult humans is 10 ng/mL. Elevations of AFP above 3000 ng/mL are essentially diagnostic of PHC. Elevations between 30 and 400 ng/mL occur frequently in nonmalignant liver disease. The significance of values between 400 and 3000 ng/mL is controversial. In a recent large series of patients, Chen and Sung (1977) found the results shown in Table 2. Using a normal upper level of 10 ng/mL, AFP elevations were found in many patients with a variety of different liver diseases, however, 69% (86/125) of patients with PHC had elevations above 400 ng/mL; only 1/60 patients with chronic aggressive hepatitis had an elevation of serum AFP above 400 ng/mL. From their results, it could be concluded that serum AFP concentrations above 400 ng/mL are diagnostic of PHC if other types of AFP producing tumors, such as teratocarcinoma, can be ruled out. This conclusion is consistent with that arrived at earlier by other workers (see Ruoslahti et al., 1974b).

However, not all studies indicate such a low diagnostic AFP concentration. A comparison of the results of Lehmann and Wegener (1979) with those of Chen and Sung (1977) exemplifies the differences in the range of AFP concentrations associated with different liver diseases. 18/19 patients with serum AFP between 400 and 1000 ng/mL had PHC in the series studied by Chen and Sung. On the other hand, of 15 individuals with serum AFP concentrations between 400 and 3000 ng/mL reported by Lehmann and Wegener, 12 did not have PHC. In a statistical evaluation of data on

Table 2

Alphafetoprotein in 402 Patients with Liver Diseases and Nongerminal Tumors[a]

Diagnosis	Percent of cases with AFP		
	>10 ng/mL	>320 ng/mL	>400 ng/mL
Hepatocellular carcinoma	90	74	69
Other nongerminal tumors	20	1.5	0
Cirrhosis	34	1.4	0
Chronic aggressive hepatitis	58	6.7	1.7
Chronic persistent hepatitis	42	8.3	0
Subacute hepatitis	69	0	0
Acute viral hepatitis	47	5.6	0
HBsAg carriers	23	0	0

[a]Modified from Chen and Sung, 1977.

the relationship of serum concentration of AFP in PHC, Phillips et al. (1977) conclude that low elevations of serum AFP (30–50 ng/mL) result in misdiagnosis of PHC; only 10% of patients with such values have liver cancer. Serum AFP concentrations of 500 ng/mL or more are diagnostic of PHC and detect 59% of all patients with PHC. Although elevated concentrations below 500 ng/mL diagnose a larger number of cases, the costs of excluding false positives are considerable. Thus, the final diagnosis of hepatoma can often be made on the basis of an elevated serum AFP alone (perhaps 50%).

Differentiation of elevations of serum AFP associated with nonmalignant disease from those associated with PHC may be possible by serial evaluation of serum AFP concentrations. In animal models, elevations of serum AFP associated with hepatocyte proliferation stimulated by a single event (partial hepatectomy, chemical injury) are transient (Sell, et al., 1976b; Sell et al., 1974a). (Figure 1). Similarly in humans, elevations of serum AFP associated with hepatitis or cirrhosis are generally transitory, whereas those associated with PHC are persistant or increase upon serial determinations (Kew et al., 1973, Delmont et al., 1974; Ruoslahti et al., 1974b; Karvountis and Redeker, 1974; Silver et al., 1974; Endo et al., 1975; Murray-Lyon et al., 1976; Dedieu et al., 1978; Lehmann and Wegener, 1979). An additional procedure that may differentiate serum AFP elevations associated with PHC from those associated with nonmalignant liver disease is the effect of administration of pyridoxine and ATP on subsequent serum AFP concentrations. The studies of Watanabe et al. (personal communication) suggest that twice daily injections of pyridoxine (200 mg) and ATP (60 mg) decrease serum AFP concentrations if nonmalignant liver disease is the cause; this challenge has no effect on elevations associated with PHC. There has not been an opportunity to confirm this interesting relationship and the effect of such treatment on hepatocyte regeneration is not known.

The degree of elevation of AFP following acute liver injury, such as chemically induced hepatocellular necrosis in the rat (Sell et al., 1976) or acute viral hepatitis in humans (Kew et al., 1973; Ruoslahti et al., 1974b; Silver et al., 1974; Endo et al., 1975; Murray-Lyon et al., 1976) appears to reflect the degree of liver cell regeneration. Elevations of serum AFP occur after the peak elevation of liver cell enzymes (SGOT, SGPT, etc.) during the time that proliferation occurs (Fig. 1). In general, the extent of AFP elevation correlates with the extent of the elevation of serum enzymes that occur earlier during the course of the disease. However, if the serum liver cell enzyme and AFP determinations are performed on single serum samples, no such correlation is found. Little or no AFP elevation following massive liver cell damage as determined by SGOT of SGPT values over 500 mIU/mL indicates a poor prognosis. Although conflicting reports ex-

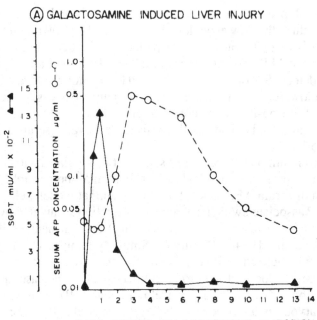

Fig. 1. Serial determination of serum AFP in rats following chemically induced liver injury (A) and during growth of a transplantable hepatoma (B). Panel A illustrates SGPT and AFP elevations occurring following a sublethal dose of galactosamine (Sell et al., 1976). Within 12 h SGPT rises sharply, falling back to normal levels within 3–4 days. Serum AFP elevation is first seen on day 2, reaches a maximum on day 3, and gradually falls to normal (<0.06 μg/mL) during the next week. Panel B depicts AFP elevations following transplantation of Morris hepatoma 7777 (Sell et al., 1974b). The shaded area illustrates the range of

ist, elevations of AFP occur with near equal frequency in hepatitis patients with or without serum hepatitis B antigen (Tong et al., 1971; Ruoslahti et al., 1973; Silver et al., 1974; Kew et al., 1973; Chen and Sung, 1979). In patients with AFP elevations associated with alcoholic cirrhosis, serum AFP concentrations decrease in abstinent patients; continued elevations above 100 ng/mL in such circumstances strongly suggest the development of PHC (Dedieu et al., 1978).

Patients with primary malignancies other than PHC may also have elevations of serum AFP. This is most frequently seen with gonadal teratocarcinomas containing yolk sac elements (see Chapter 11) and with other tumors. In the case of teratocarcinomas, AFP is produced by cells that resemble yolk sac endoderm (endodermal-sinus tumors, Nørgaard-Pedersen, 1976). Since yolk sac endoderm normally produces AFP, it is not surprising that AFP is produced by tumors containing such cellular structures. AFP elevation also rarely occurs with tumors of the gastrointes-

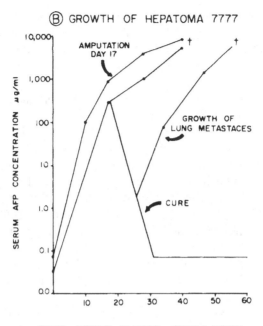

Ⓑ GROWTH OF HEPATOMA 7777

DAYS AFTER TUMOR INOCULATION

serum AFP concentrations in eight rats inoculated intramuscularly with 5×10^6 hepatoma cells. The sigmoidal elevation reflects the growth kinetics of the tumor with death (†) of all animals occurring by day 40. If the tumor is removed surgically the serum AFP falls with a half-life of approximately 1 day. Complete removal results in a return to normal levels, but development of recurrence or lung metastasis results in reelevation of AFP. The ordinate of panel A covers two logs for AFP whereas that of Panel B covers six logs.

tinal tract with or without metastasis to the liver (Boureile et al., 1971; Kozower et al., 1971; Mehlman et al., 1971; Bernades et al., 1971; Alpert et al., 1971; Ruoslahti et al., 1972; Akai and Koto, 1973; McIntire, 1975). In most cases, nonhepatic, nonteratomatous tumors associated with serum AFP elevations are derived from the upper gut, which is embryologically closely related to yolk sac and liver. In metastatic cancer to the liver, AFP has been localized, in some cases, to the tumor itself (Montplaisir et al., 1973) and, in other cases, to adjacent nontumorous liver (Bierfeld et al., 1973; Tsung, 1975). In instances of AFP elevations associated with lung cancer, it is not clear whether AFP may be produced by bronchogenic carcinoma or is produced by liver cells as the result of secondary hepatic lesions. Reports of AFP elevations associated with leukemia, malignant melanoma (Mihalev et al., 1976), and rhabdomyosarcoma (Mori et al., 1979) raise the possibility that AFP may be produced by nongut-associated tumors. Unequivocal synthesis of AFP by such tumors has not been demonstrated by incorporation of labeled amino acids into AFP by the tumor. In instances where elevations of serum AFP occur in association with tumors derived from nonhepatic or nongonadal tissues, the serum concentration usually is below 400 ng/mL (McIntire et al., 1975; Ruoslahti et al., 1974b).

Differentiation of elevations caused by PHC from those arising from other tumors may be possible by characterization of the proportion of AFP that binds to concanavalin A (con A). AFP arising from the yolk sac early in development contains a high proportion of molecules that do not bind to con A (15–45%), whereas AFP produced by fetal liver later in development contains a much higher percentage of AFP that binds to con A (Ruoslahti et al., 1978). Although the sera of rats with chemically induced PHC contain AFP that binds to con A at different ratios (11–64%; Smith et al., 1977), AFP in human serum found with PHC usually binds to con A at a high percentage (>90%), whereas that produced by yolk sac tumors (Ruoslahti et al., 1978), or that associated with nonliver gastrointestinal tumors or metastatic tumors to the liver (Endo, personal communication) binds to a lesser extent (<50%).

The possibility that screening of human populations for AFP may be useful for early detection of PHC or identification of individuals at high risk for development of PHC has been considered. The observation that rats fed hepatocarcinogens demonstrate marked elevations of serum AFP many months prior to appearance of PHC (Becker and Sell, 1974; Sell and Becker, 1978) provides support for the idea that humans exposed to hepatocarcinogens may also exhibit elevated serum AFP before developing PHC. Some evidence that such effects may be observed in humans was reported by Purves et al., 1973. The serum AFP concentrations in Bantu males and males from Mozambique and Malaysia, who have an extremely high incidence of PHC, are higher that those in Caucasians who have a low PHC incidence. In Bantu diamond miners of South Africa, evidence for an environmental influence on serum AFP concentration was found. Some Bantu males leave their homelands and sign on to work for 1 year in diamond mines in South Africa. During the time they work, they live at the mine and do not return home until their contract expires. Purves et al. 1973, found that Bantu, upon first arriving at the mines, had higher serum AFP concentrations than did Caucasians at the mine. After 1 year, the serum AFP concentrations in the Bantu were no longer elevated. Thus, it is possible that elevated serum AFP in the Bantu may be related to the presence of an hepatocarcinogen in their native diet or to another environmental factor not present at the mines, but present in their native habitat. On the other hand, a systematic survey of males from seven populations with different incidences of PHC by Sizaret et al. (1975) did not reveal a difference in serum AFP concentrations. In an extensive study carried out in the Peoples Republic of China from 1972 to 1974, 417,644 asymptomatic individuals were screened for elevations of serum AFP (see Terry, 1978). Fifty-seven sera had levels greater than 500 ng/mL. All 57 of these patients had liver cancer. At the Shanghai Tumor Institute, 115,000 people were surveyed in 1974. Twenty patients with PHC were identified by the presence of high serum AFP. Of 270 additional patients with persistent low-level elevations, 233 had normal values on later examination and 9 developed PHC during a 2-year followup. Thirty-eight people continued to have elevations with evidence of abnormal liver function. Similar results were obtained at other Chinese institutions (Terry, 1978). These data suggest that screening of PHC high risk populations for AFP elevations may be effective in early detection of PHC, but the effectiveness in low risk populations, such as in the United States, remains to be determined.

The presence of elevated serum AFP in children with hereditary tyrosinemia most likely owes to continued proliferation of hepatocytes that express fetal characteristics. Hereditary tyrosinemia is a rare autosomal recessively inherited disease characterized by developmental retardation, neurologic symptoms, and a defective ability to convert parahydroxyphenylpyruvic acid to homogentisic acid owing to increased activity of p-hydroxyphenol pyruvate hydroxylase in the liver and kidney (Halvorsen et al., 1966; Gentz et al., 1967; Hill et al., 1972). These children maintain higher fetal levels of serum AFP (Mawas et al., 1970; Buffe and Rimbaut, 1973; Belanger et al., 1973) and prolonged expression of fetal liver isozymes (Guguen et al., 1979). They have a high incidence of PHC and marked increases of AFP may be associated with development of PHC (Rimbaut et al., 1979). The relationship of the high incidence and early development of PHC to continued production of AFP remains unclear. The possibility that the metabolic abnormality that results in continued expression of fetal characteristics may be the same that results in PHC is deserving of further study. A correlation exists between serum bilirubin levels and AFP concentrations in neonatal hyperbilirubinemia (Ikonen et al., 1980).

Serial determinations of AFP may be used to evaluate the effects of therapy of an AFP-producing PHC. By using transplanted hepatocellular carcinomas in experimental animals, it has been demonstrated that serum AFP concentrations accurately reflect tumor growth and the effects of therapy (see Fig. 1). Following surgical removal of PHC by partial hepatectomy, serum AFP will fall. If re-elevations occur, recurrence and/or development of metastases are likely. If surgery is curative, the serum AFP falls to normal. In humans, if the serum AFP does not return to normal or if the serum concentration declines with a half-life longer that 7–8 days, incomplete removal must be considered (Lin et al., 1972; Sugawara et al., 1973; McIntire et al., 1972; Matsumoto et al., 1974; Purtilo et al., 1973). In one interesting case, removal of a non-AFP-producing tumor from an infant was followed by a transient increase in serum AFP. Subsequently, serum

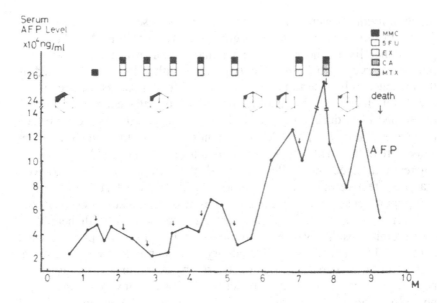

Fig. 2. Sequential serum AFP concentrations in a patient with hepatocellular carcinoma during chemotherapy. This patient, a 68-year-old male, was first noted to have an impairment of liver function in 1968 when he had a gastrectomy for a polyp. He first noted epigastric discomfort in January 1973 and was hospitalized on April 16th because of upper abdominal pain and hepatomegaly. The liver was palpated four finger-breadths below the right costal margin in the midclavicular line. Laboratory data: alkaline phosphatase, 65 units (KA); SGOT, 83 units (karmen); LDH, 340 units (Isozyme 1, 40.6%; 2, 39.5%; 3, 12.3%; 4, 1.9%; 5, 5.8%); total bilrubin, 1.75 mg/100 mL; total protein, 7.0 g/100 mL; BSP test 10%

AFP returned to normal and no tumor recurrence occurred (Matray et al., 1972). The transient AFP increase was most likely caused by production of AFP by regenerating liver, as occurs in experimental animals (Sell et al., 1974a). Such increases have not been reported in adult humans following partial hepatectomy.

Sequential determinations of AFP may be used to evaluate the effectiveness of chemotherapy of PHC (Purves et al., 1970; McIntire, 1972; Matsumoto et al., 1974; Kubo and Shimokawa, 1976; Nagasue et al., 1977). Although the response of patients with PHC to chemotherapy is usually not good, some beneficial effects are seen in individual patients. An example of such a patient is shown in Fig. 2. Administration of therapeutic chemicals resulted in temporary decline in serum AFP. Re-elevations become more frequent as the tumor became more refractory to treatment. Failure of a patient to exhibit a decrease in serum AFP indicates a poor response to therapy. The results of Kubo and Shimokawa (1976) are presented in Table 3.

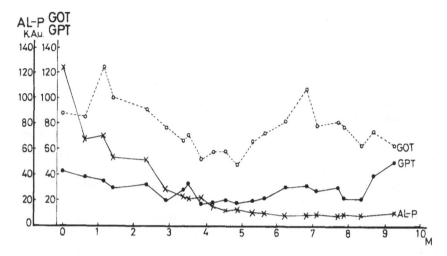

at 45 min; and AFP 23,200 ng/mL). Diagnosis of PHC associated with cirrhosis was made by liver scan, laparoscopy, biopsy, and angiography. He had one shot therapy eight times, the first dose being Mitomycin C alone (MMC). A cocktail of 10 mg MMC, 500 mg cyclophosphamide (Endoxan, Ex), and 500 mg 5-fluorouracil (5-FU) was given thereafter. Following the first several shots, severe pain subsided the tumor regressed with a concomitant decrease in serum alkaline phosphatase and AFP. Despite reduction in tumor size after the fourth injection, the serum AFP continued to rise. Combination of chemotherapeutic agents was changed to 10 mg MMC, 500 mg Ex and 10 mg cytosine arabinoside (CA) or MMC, CA, and 100 mg methotrexate (MTX) after the fourth shot. Pancytopenia developed after the eighth injection and the patient died of pneumonia (from Kubo and Shimokawa, 1976).

Table 3

Relationship of Serum AFP Concentration to Hepatocellular Carcinoma Size Following Chemotherapy

	Number of Cases	Range of serum AFP, ng/mL	Response of Serum AFP[a]		
			Decreased	Unchanged	Increased
Decrease in size	12	20,000–340,000	9 (26–93%)	3 (± 5%)	0
No change or increase in size	15	20,000–1,600,000	4 (14–48%)	3 (± 5%)	8 (19–582%)

[a]Maximum change in serum concentration as percentage of pretreatment level. Modified from Kubo and Shimokawa, 1976.

Attempts to localize AFP-producing tumors in vivo using radiola-beled antibody to AFP have produced promising results. Following the work of Pressman and Korngold (1953), radiolabeled antibodies have been used to localize metastases of CEA-producing tumors in animals and in man (Goldenberg et al., 1979). Since AFP is a secreted protein, in con-trast to CEA, which is largely a cell surface molecule, localization of AFP-producing tumors may not be possible owing to formation of anti-body–antigen complexes when radiolabeled anti-AFP is injected into an individual with an AFP-producing tumor. However, immune complex for-mation does not appear to prohibit localization of CEA producing tumors in patients with circulating CEA (Primus et al., 1980). Radiolabeled horse anti-rat AFP has been used to localize transplanted hepatomas in rats by to-tal body scintigraphy (Koji et al., 1980). In addition, 16 human patients with known metastatic lesions were studied for tumor localization by radioimmunodetection. Twelve metastatic sites in five patients with AFP-producing PHC or teratocarcinomas were identified. Six of 16 lesions in patients with non-AFP-producing tumors were also identified (Kim et al., 1980). Although these results are encouraging, several important ques-tions remain unanswered. First, it has never been demonstrated that tumor localization by radiolabeled anti-CEA or anti-AFP involves binding of radiolabeled antibody to the tumor; localization could be the result of nonspecific effects owing to increased vascularity of tumors. Second, the diagnostic efficiency of radioimmunodetection is low. Of 200 patients studied by Goldenberg's group using labeled anti-CEA (personal commu-nication), radioimmunodetection missed 30 lesions detected by standard radiologic techniques, whereas 6 lesions were detected by radioimmune scintigraphy that were not found by other methods. Thus, radioimmune detection does not appear to be suitable for extensive diagnostic applica-tion. Its usefulness is most likely in localizing an occult lesion in selected patients who have a rising serum marker (such as CEA or AFP) and in whom a tumor cannot be localized by other techniques.

The passive administration of anti-AFP as a therapeutic technique has had differing effects on the growth of AFP producing PHC in vivo. Partial reduction in growth rate or decreased takes of transplanted AFP-producing tumors have been noted in some, but not all, animals treated with anti-AFP (Sell et al., 1976a; Mizejewski and Dillon, 1979; Wepsic et al., 1980). This effect is noted in 10–25% of treated animals. In animals actively im-munized to their own AFP by breaking of tolerance, a similar effect on growth of a transplantable hepatoma is noted by some investigators (Gousev and Yasova, 1974; Sell et al., 1976a) but not by others (Engvall et al., 1977). In a single human patient, no effects of passive anti-AFP on an inoperable hepatoma were noted (Koji et al., 1980). Further studies are underway in animals and humans using anti-AFP conjugated to daunomy-cin in an attempt to focus delivery of this toxic chemical to AFP-producing tumors. No definitive results are yet available (Hirai et al., unpublished data). Autoimmunization to AFP in mice did not inhibit the development of chemically induced PHC in a study by Jalanko et al. (1978).

In summary, serum AFP elevations may be used as an aid in the diagnosis and management of PHC. Serum concentrations between 10 and 400 ng/mL are associated with nonmalignant liver diseases, such as hepatitis and cirrhosis, and with gastrointestinal cancer, metastatic tumors of the liver, and in pregnancy as well as with PHC. The significance of serum concentrations between 400 and 1000 ng/mL is controversial, but a PHC must be given first consideration. Serum concentrations above 1000 ng/mL are essentially diagnostic of PHC. On the other hand, approximately 10–20% of patients with PHC will not have an elevation of serum AFP. Serum elevations of AFP associated with cirrhosis or hepatitis are usually transient; continued elevations upon serial determinations strongly suggest PHC. Successful therapy of an AFP-producing tumor is usually reflected in a fall in serum AFP concentration; constant or rising concentrations indicate failure of therapy. AFP produced by PHC usually binds to con A at a high percentage (>90%), whereas that produced by other tumors binds less (<50%). This difference may be useful in differentiating tumors that make AFP. Screening of populations at high risk for development of PHC may be effective in early detection of such tumors, but the effectiveness in low risk populations remains to be determined. The use of antibody to AFP for tumor localization or tumor therapy is being examined experimentally with promising results; further study is needed to determine whether these procedures will be of general applicability.

4. Enzymes and Isozymes

An excellent review of the association of enzymatic changes in cancer by Balinsky (1980) in the first volume of this series points out two basic abnormalities of expression of enzymes in cancer; reappearance of "fetal" forms of an enzyme, and "ectopic" expression of enzymes not normally found in the liver (see also Potter, 1968; Weinhouse, 1972; Schapira, 1973; Knox, 1976; Goldfarb and Pitot, 1976; Weber, 1977; Schapira et al., 1979). A partial listing of some enzymatic forms not normally found in adult liver but present in PHC tissue is given in Table 4. Most of the enzymes listed are normally found in fetal liver, and thus their presence in PHC represents first-level expression of an oncodevelopmental marker (Sell, 1978). Others may be ectopic in that they are normally produced by other developmentally related tissues and represent second or third level expression (Table 5).

Extensive analysis of the enzyme content of transplantable "Morris" hepatomas and studies of human PHC tissue reveal a number of abnormal-

Table 4
Some Fetal Type Isozymes Found "Abnormally" in Hepatomas[a]

		Normal distribution	
Enzyme	Form	Fetal	Adult
Aldolase	A	Liver	Muscle etc.
Aldolase	C	Liver	Brain
Pyruvate kinase	$M_2(K)$	Liver	Multiple
Hexokinase	II	Liver	Muscle
Phosphorylase	III	Liver	Brain, kidney
Hexosaminidase	A	Liver	Brain
Glutaminase	K	Liver	Brain, kidney
Alcohol dehydrogenase	Anodic	Liver	Stomach
Lactic dehydrogenase	H(B)	Liver	Heart, brain, kidney
Esterase		Liver	
Uridine kinase		Liver	
Thymidine kinase		Liver	
Alkaline phosphatase	Regan	Placenta	
Diaphorase	P	Placenta	
Branched chain amino acid transaminase	III	Placenta	Brain
Fructose diphosphatase		Other tissue	Muscle
Glycogen synthetase		Other tissue	Muscle

[a]Modified from Shapira et al., 1979.

ities in the tumor cells. In addition to the presence of fetal isozymes, enzymes of nucleic acid metabolism and carbohydrate metabolism (glycolytic pathway) may be elevated in PHC. This is not surprising since PHC tissue generally grows rapidly in comparison to normal adult liver and requires enzymes for generation of energy (glycolytic) and for nucleic acid synthesis. In contrast, gluconeogenic enzymes used for synthesis of glycogen (energy storage) are reduced in PHC compared to normal tissue (Balinsky, 1980).

Isozymes are multiple molecular forms of enzymes that differ in physiological and/or physiochemical properties, but have the same enzymatic activity (Fig. 3). A particular form of an enzyme predominates in a particular organ so that optimal metabolic function of that tissue occurs. The isozymes most extensively studied are lactate dehydrogenase, pyruvate kinase, aldolase, hexokinase, and alkaline phosphatase. For a more detailed review of the expression of developmental forms of these enzymes, as well as others in liver tumors, please consult Balinsky (1980).

The application of measurement of serum enzymes and isozymes to the diagnosis of liver cancer is complicated by the fact that most tumors do

Table 5
Expression of Some Oncodevelopmental Markers by Tumors[a]

Product	Fetal or adult tissue normally producing it	Level of expression by tumors		
		Embryologically closely related	Embryologically more distantly related	Different
CEA	Colonic carcinoma	Gastric, pancreatic, liver CA	Lung, breast CA	Sarcoma, lymphoma
AFP	Hepatoma, yolk sac, teratocarcinoma	Colonic, gastric, pancreatic CA	Lung CA?	Sarcoma?
Hormone (APUD) (e.g., serotonin)	Carcinoid	Adrenal (pheochromocytoma)	Oat cell CA (lung)	Lung CA
Placental isoenzymes	Choriocarcinomas, seminoma	Testicular-ovarian teratocarcinoma	Hepatomas	Lung CA

[a]From Sell, S., ed. (1980), *in Cancer Markers*, Humana Press.

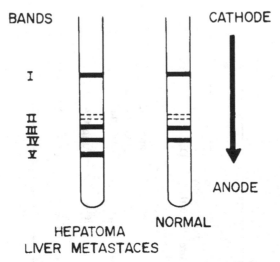

Fig. 3. Isozymes of 5'-nucleotide phosphorylase. Four or five bands of 5'-nucleotide phosphorylase may be visualized on polyacrylamide gels. Four bands are found in sera from normal patients, but a fifth band, 5'-nucleotide phosphodiesterase isoenzyme V, may be seen in sera from patients with primary hepatocellular carcinomas or with metastatic cancer in the liver.

not release the enzymes, and enzymes may be released from noncancerous tissue damaged by tumor growth. Bodansky (1961) and Schwartz (1973) have pointed out the difficulties in distinguishing between benign and malignant lesions on the basis of elevation of various serum enzymes. Some enzymes, such as amino acid glutamyl transferase (GGT) and 5'-nucleotidase, have been proposed as having the potential to indicate liver metastases (Neville and Cooper, 1976). In a recent study by Tsou and Lo (1980) 5'-nucleotide phosphodiesterase, isozyme V (5'-NDPase V) was present in 79% of the cases with PHC and in 88% of patients with metastatic disease of the liver. Since AFP elevations occur frequently in PHC and much less frequently with liver metastases, elevations of both 5'-NPDase V and AFP suggest PHC; whereas elevated 5'-NPDase V alone was found in 59% of patients with a variety of nonmalignant liver diseases and in 13% of patients with other nonmalignant diseases. Beck et al. (1978) did not find that GGT or 5'-nucleotidase were valuable tests since these enzymes were only elevated when widespread metastases were present and a high incidence of false positives was found. The placental D variant of alkaline phosphatase may be elevated in up to 30% of patients with hepatocellular carcinoma (Higashino et al., 1975; Suzuki et al., 1975), but its usefulness as a diagnostic test for PHC has not been clearly demonstrated. Alpha$_1$-antitrypsin deficiency has been found in association with PHC (Zwi et al., 1975; Schleissner and Cohen, 1975), but it is such a rarity that it is not a useful diagnostic marker.

Ligandin (glutathione S-transferase B; Kamisaka et al., 1975), an enzyme present in large amounts in adult hepatocytes, but in much lower amounts in neonatal hepatocytes (Fleischner et al., 1975; Leffert et al., 1978) may appear in the serum of patients with PHC. Ligandin binds bilirubin, anionic dyes, steroid hormone metabolites, and a variety of drugs and carcinogens (Kamisaka et al., 1975; Morey and Litwack, 1969; Smith, G., et al., 1977; Tipping et al., 1976). The level of ligandin in the cytosol of liver, kidney, and intestine of phenobarbital-treated animals is elevated, but this treatment does not affect serum concentrations of ligandin (Reyes et al., 1971; Bass et al., 1977). Ligandin appears to play a role in transfer of bilirubin from plasma into liver (Wolkoff et al., 1979). Preliminary measurements of ligandin indicate normal adult human serum concentration of 80–100 μg/mL. However, in 11/15 patients with PHC, serum concentrations of 100–560 μg/mL were found (Arias, personal communication). Further studies are needed to determine whether serum ligandin is a useful marker for PHC and whether or not elevations are associated with other tumors.

5. Systemic Manifestations of Hepatoma and Ectopic Hormone Production

Systemic manifestations in patients with PHC include a number of abnormalities that could be explained by increased levels of hormones or the effects of other biologically active materials that might serve as markers for PHC (Margolis and Homcy, 1972; Cochrane and Williams, 1976). See Table 6. If hormones such as insulin, erythropoietin, or parathormone were produced by PHC, these might be considered examples of "ectopic" hormone production (see Chapter 14; also Griffing and Vaitukaitis, 1980).

Table 6
Some Systemic Manifestions of Primary
Hepatocellular Carcinoma[a]

Finding	Possible marker
Erythrocytosis	Erythropoietin
Hypercalcemia	Parathormone
Hypoglycemia	Insulin
Gynecomastia	Chorionic gonadotropin
Hyperlipidemia	Beta-lipoprotein
Porphyria cutania tarda	Porphyrin
Dysfibrinogenemia	Abnormal fibrinogens

[a]Modified from Margolis and Homcy, 1972.

A hormone produced by tumors arising from tissues that normally produce that hormone at some stage of development is termed "eutopic." Ectopic hormone production refers to production of hormone by a tumor that arises from a tissue that normally does not produce that hormone. It is reasoned that since all cells have the genetic information to produce all cellular products, expression of ectopic products by a tumor results from changes in the control of gene expression associated with malignant change. Different levels of ectopic production are listed in Table 5.

The concept of "ectopic" hormone production has been challenged by Skrabanek (1980a, b) who argues that production of hormones by tumors actually occurs only when the tumor arises from a tissue that normally has the capacity to produce those hormones. He further states that the concept of ectopic production of hormones has arisen from a misunderstanding of the origin of hormone-producing tumors. According to Skrabanek, hormone-producing tumors arise from either of two cellular lineages, the enterochromatic (Kultschnitzky) cells or chromatin cells.

Erythrocytosis—an increase in the production of red blood cells—may result from the production of erythropoietin by PHC, or erythropoietic activity may be a secondary effect of PHC. Erythropoietin is usually produced by the kidney. The liver and PHC have been shown to produce a protein that is activated to form erythropoiesis stimulating factor (ESF) which, in turn, is activated by a proteolytic enzyme secreted by the kidney (renal erythropoietic factor; Gordon et al., 1970). In addition, erythropoietin may be produced by normal liver cells (Reissman and Nomura, 1962), therefore, its production by PHC may not really be ectopic.

Hypercalcemia associated with PHC suggests the ectopic production of parathormone (Samuelsson and Werner, 1963) and is referred to as a form of pseudohyperparathyroidism (Fry, 1962; Nadie et al., 1968; Knill-Jones et al., 1970). However, hypercalcemia may also be caused by destruction of bone by metastatic lesions. The differentiation of hypercalcemia arising from increased parathormone activity and that from bone absorption is not always clear (Nadie et al., 1968). More direct evidence that parathormone (PTH) is produced by PHC is the finding of PTH-like material in PHC tissue and a drop in elevated plasma PTH levels upon resection of PHC in one patient (Knill-Jones et al., 1970). Demonstration of synthesis of PTH by PHC tissue by methods such as incorporation of radiolabeled amino acids in vitro has not been reported. Skrabanek et al., (1980), point out that other factors such as prostaglandins and osteoclast-activating factors may also be responsible for tumor-associated hypercalcemia, and they are not convinced that PTH production directly by tumors other than those of the parathyroid has been demonstrated. Thus, hypercalcemia associated with PHC may be an example of pseudo-pseudohyperparathyroidism.

Table 7
Characteristics of Two Types of Hypoglycemia Associated with Hepatocellular Carcinoma[a]

	Type A	Type B
Relative frequency	87%	13%
Appetite	Reduced	Normal
Weight loss	Profound	Slight
Histology	Undifferentiated, glycogen absent	Well-differentiated, glycogen abundant
Time of onset	Shortly before death	2–10 Months before death
Control of hypoglycemia	Easy	Difficult

[a]Modified from Margolis and Homcy, 1972.

Hypoglycemia, one of the more frequent systemic manifestations of PHC, could indicate ectopic production of insulin. However, PHC-associated hypoglycemia is not caused by insulin production, but by depletion of normal liver enzyme systems or by rapid growth of the tumor (Margolis and Homcy, 1972). Two types of hypoglycemia are associated with PHC (McFadzean and Young, 1969, see Table 7). Type-A hypoglycemia results when the liver is replaced by tumor to the extent that the remaining liver is unable to synthesize glucose in sufficient quantity to meet the demands of the other organs. Type-B hypoglycemia is caused by development of abnormal gluconeogenic enzyme patterns (reduction of phosphorylase activity needed for glycogen breakdown and of glucose 6-phosphatase required for synthesis of glucose) resulting in an acquired form of glycogen storage disease.

Gonadotropin activity may lead to sexual precocity in children with liver tumors or to gynecomastia in adult males with PHC. Chorionic gonadotropin has been reported to be found in the sera of up to 17% of patients with PHC or hepatoblastoma (Braunstein et al., 1973) and chorionic somatotropin in 2 of 15 patients with hepatoma (Weintraub and Rosen, 1971). Given the close developmental relationship of the liver to the yolk sac, as evidenced by the commonality of AFP production, production of chorionic hormone by liver tumors should not be unexpected. Furthermore, symptoms such as gynecomastia may occur in terminal states of liver disease because of the inability of the liver to catabolize sex hormones normally.

Hyperlipidemia, an increase in total blood lipids and hypercholesterolemia has been reported in patients with PHC (Santer et al., 1967; Viallet et al., 1962) with an incidence as high as 33% (Alpert et al., 1969). Suggested mechanisms of hyperlipidemia include production of an abnormal lipoprotein, obstruction of biliary secretion, or loss of feedback inhibitors of cholesterol synthesis (Margolis and Homcy, 1972).

Other rare systematic manifestations of PHC include porphyria cutanea tarda, presumably owing to production of porphyrins by the tumor (Thompson et al., 1970) and dysfibrinogenemia or cryofibrinogenemia caused by abnormal protein production by the liver (Bell et al., 1966). Extremely high serum levels of a vitamin B_{12}-binding protein produced by PHC may result in extraordinary elevations of serum vitamin B_{12}, but this does not result in megaloblastosis (Waxman and Gilbert, 1973).

Although the systemic manifestation of PHC are of considerable clinical and theoretical interest, these occur rarely, are much more obvious at advanced stages of the disease, are found with other malignant and non-malignant conditions, and are associated with a diagnostic marker so infrequently that the presence of such markers is more remarkable as a clinical curiosity than as a generally useful diagnostic test.

6. Ferritin

Ferritin, the major iron-binding protein of serum, becomes elevated in relationship to the quantity of iron in the tissues (Reissman and Dietrich, 1956). A protein termed β-fetoprotein, found in fetal serum and in patients with PHC, has been identified as ferritin (Alpert et al., 1973). Increased serum concentrations of ferritin are not only found with PHC, but also in Hodgkins disease, leukemia, breast cancer, and other diseases (Jones et al., 1973; Niitsu et al., 1975; Hazard and Drysdale, 1977; Kew et al., 1978). Therefore, elevated serum ferritin is not useful as a specific marker of PHC. When elevations are associated with a particular cancer, serial determinations may be useful in determining the effects of therapy (Hann et al., 1980).

7. Hepatoma-Associated Antigens

The presence of tumor antigens on transplantable rat hepatomas has been studied extensively by Baldwin and his coworkers using serological and cellular assays. In selected hepatomas, they demonstrated tumor specific transplantation antigens as well as serologically detected tumor-specific and embryonic antigens (Baldwin et al., 1972, 1973, 1974; Jones et al., 1978). They report that sera and lymph node cells of pregnant rats react against transplantable hepatomas by fluorescence and cytotoxicity (Baldwin et al., 1974). In addition, lymph node cells from animals immunized with embryo tissue retarded the growth of a hepatoma at ratios of 3000/1 prior to transplantation (Shah et al., 1976). However, this effect was significant in only 3/7 experiments with one hepatoma and ineffective with another. In general, the results are inconsistent and the assays are difficult to quantitate and control. It does not seem likely that PHC-associated antigens, other than AFP, will be useful as tumor markers until more reliable techniques are developed and better characterization of such antigens has been performed (see reviews by Sell, 1980; Chism, 1980; Chism et al., 1978).

The presence of ribosomal antigens in PHC has also been reported. Wikman-Coffelt et al. (1972) found two antigenic differences between the proteins of 60-S ribosomes from PHC cells and those from normal liver by absorbing antisera prepared to 60-S ribosomal proteins of Novikoff hepatoma cells with ribosomal proteins of normal liver. The molecular weights of these proteins were 30,000 and 60,000; further characterization and evidence for these proteins in other PHC has not appeared.

"Preneoplastic antigen" was identified by Okita et al. (Okita and Farber, 1975; Okita et al., 1975) using rabbit antisera raised against microsomal preparations of "neoplastic" nodules induced in rats by N-2-acetylaminofluorene feeding. This antigen was found by immunofluorescence in neoplastic nodules and PHC carcinomas, but not in normal liver cells. In neoplastic nodules, this antigen was localized to the smooth endoplasmic reticulum (Lin et al., 1977). Preneoplastic antigen was isolated by Griffin and Kizer (1978) and shown to be present in solubilized microsomes from normal liver. Treatment of normal tissue with deoxycholate is required for demonstration of this antigen, whereas treatment of nodular tissue with deoxycholate does not alter reactivity. They estimate that nodular microsomes contain about four times as much preneoplastic antigen as do normal liver microsomes and that the antigen is present in nodules in different form owing to an altered state of the membranes of the endoplasmic reticulum. In more recent studies, Levin et al. (1977) have identified preneoplastic antigen as epoxide hydrase.

An antigen designated SF (carcinoma supernate fraction) was identified by rabbit antisera using immunofluorescence and immunodiffusion (Carruthers et al., 1977) to be present in PHC and cholangiocarcinomas induced by 3-methyl-dimethylaminoazobenzene and shown not to be AFP or neoplastic antigen. Further developments are needed to determine if any of these "antigens" could be useful tumor markers.

8. Hepatitis B Virus

A number of studies have suggested that PHC in man may result from hepatitis B infection (see review by Szmuness, 1978). This hypothesis is based on three major observations: (1) the close correlation of geographic distribution of PHC and hepatitis B, (2) the unusually high frequency with which evidence of persistent hepatitis B infection is detected in patients with PHC, and (3) the presence of hepatitis B viral DNA in some PHC.

Table 8

Comparison of HBsAg Prevalence and Incidence of PHC in Different Areas of the World[a]

Geographic region	HBsAg prevalence, %	Incidence of PHC in males, %
USA and Canada	0.25	0.4
North and Western Europe	0.25	0.3
South and Eastern Europe	1.5	1.5
Southeast Asia	10.0	2.5
Japan	1.5	3.0
Central and South Africa	10.0	4.0
China	7.5	7.0

[a]Data extracted from Szmuness (1978).

Evidence for persistent hepatitis B infection is the presence in the serum of hepatitis B surface antigen (HBsAg) and/or antibody to the hepatitis core antigen (anti-HBc). Evidence for past self-limited infection is the presence of antibody to surface (anti-HBs). A comparison of HBsAg prevalence and incidence of PHC in autopsies from different parts of the world is given in Table 8. The frequency of HBsAg detection in patients with PHC and controls from different parts of the world is shown in Table 9. The correlation of persistent hepatitis B infection with PHC is striking; the frequency of HBsAg in patients with PHC is 10–20 times higher than in in-

Table 9

Comparison of HBsAg in PHC Patients and Controls From Different Parts of the World[a]

Country	PHC, % positive	Controls, % positive
USA	21.4	1.2
Finland	4.3	0.2
Greece	57.1	5.0
Bantu (S. Africa)	59.5	9.0
Mozambique	66.0	14.3
Senegal	61.2	11.0
Uganda	78.9	7.0
Zambia	63.1	7.5
Japan	37.3	2.6
Taiwan	80.0	14.6
Vietnam	80.3	24.0

[a]Data from Szmuness (1978).

Table 10
Prevalence of Anti-HBs in Patients with PHC and Controls

Country	Patients with PHC, % positive	Controls, % positive
Bantu (S. Africa)	11.6	33.4
Japan	7.5	18.3
Uganda	26.0	45.4
Senegal	18.2	42.1

dividuals without PHC. In contrast, the frequency of anti-HBs, evidence of self-limited previous infection with hepatitis B, is higher in controls than in patients with PHC (Table 10).

Computation of the relative risk of individuals with HBsAg and those without, for developing PHC, is 1–1.5 in high incidence areas, 10–15 in low incidence areas. Although the percentage of PHC patients who are HBsAg positive is much reduced in some areas of the world (compare USA with Africa or Asia), the relative difference between HBsAg positivity in PHC patients and controls is greater (20/1 vs 6/1). This argues against the interpretation that the lower percentage of HBsAg positive patients in low incidence areas indicates weaker association between PHC and hepatitis B infection. Szmuness (1978) has calculated that in low incidence areas, the chance of dying from PHC is 50–100 times greater in HBsAg positive than in HBsAg negative individuals.

Although the above data can be analyzed statistically and a clear association found, these data do prove a cause and effect relationship between HBV infection and PHC. In a recent report of a prospective study, Obata et al. (1980) found that 7/20 patients (23%) with HBsAg developed PHC during the 4-½ year period of observation, wheres 5/85 (5.9%) of HBsAg negative individuals developed PHC.

Further evidence for a possible causative relationship has been obtained by identification of integrated HBV–DNA in tumor tissue using molecular probes and recombinant DNA technology. Integration of viral DNA into the host cell genome has been found in various cell lines malignantly transformed by animal viruses. Similar results have been found for HBV–DNA in a human hepatocellular carcinoma cell line that synthesizes HBsAg (Marion et al., 1980; Chakraborty et al., 1980; Edman et al., 1980). HBV–DNA has also been identified in some, but not all, human PHC examined (Shouval et al., 1980; Shafritz and Kew, 1981). This analysis can be performed on material obtained by precutaneous liver biopsy and may serve as a possible test for malignant transformation of hepatocytes.

9. Summary

Laboratory tests that are potentially useful in the differential diagnosis of PHC include serum enzyme and isozyme changes, abnormal hormone production, elevated serum proteins, and the presence of hepatitis B surface antigen or antibody to hepatitis core antigen. Except for exceedingly high elevations of alphafetoprotein (above 1000 ng/mL), no single test is diagnostic for PHC. Approximately 50% of patients with PHC have cirrhosis; many commonly used tests are unable to differentiate PHC from cirrhosis. Systemic manifestations of PHC and altered enzyme levels in the serum are frequently associated with other conditions. Extensive analysis of serum AFP demonstrates that testing for AFP is useful in the diagnosis and management of patients with PHC; in up to about 50% of patients the diagnosis be based on elevated AFP alone. In the other cases elevations fall below 400 ng/mL where elevations owing to nonmalignant diseases are frequent. If elevation of a serum protein, hormone, or enzyme is caused by hepatocellular production, serial determinations may be useful in evaluating the effects of therapy. Tumor antigens, other than AFP, are not useful as yet in detecting liver cell cancer. The relatively high incidence of PHC in individuals with evidence of persistent hepatitis B infection and the finding of hepatitis B viral DNA integrated into tumor tissue have suggested a causative relationship between hepatitis B infection and development of PHC.

References

Abelev, G. I. (1968), *Cancer Res.* **28**, 1344.
Abelev, G. I. (1971), *Adv. Cancer Res.* **14**, 1295.
Abelev, G. I. (1974), *Transplant Rev.* **20**, 3.
Abelev, G. I., S. D. Perova, N. I. Khramokova, Z. A. Prostnikova, and I. S. Irin (1963), *Transplant* **1**, 1974.
Adinolfi, A., M. Adinolfi, and M. H. Lessof (1975), *J. Med. Genet.* **12**, 138.
Akai, S., and K. Koto (1973), *Gann Monogr.* **14**, 149.
Alpert, M. E., M. S. Hutt, and C. S. Davidson (1969), *Am. J. Med* **46**, 794.
Alpert, E., K. W. Pinn, and J. Isselbacher (1971), *New England J. Med.* **285**, 1058.
Alpert, E., K. J. Isselbacher, and J. W. Drysdale (1973), *Lancet* **1**, 43.
Alpert, E. (1976), in *Hepatocellular Carcinoma*, in (Okuda, K., and R. L. Peters, eds.) Wiley, New York, p. 353.
Al-Sarraf, M., T. S. Go, K. Kithier, and V. K. Vaitkevicius (1974), *Cancer* **33**, 574.
Baldwin, R. W., D. Glaves, and B. M. Voss (1972), *Int. J. Cancer* **10**, 233.
Baldwin, R. W., M. J. Embleton, and R. A. Robins (1973), *Int. J. Cancer* **11**, 1.

Baldwin, R. W., M. J. Embleton, M. R. Price, and B. M. Voss (1974), *Transplant Rev.* **20,** 77.

Balinsky, D. (1980), in *Cancer Markers* (Sell, S., ed.), Humana Press, Clifton, N.J., p. 191.

Bass, N. M., R. E. Kirsch, S. A. Tuff, and S. J. Saunders (1977), *Biochim. Biophys. Acta* **494,** 131.

Beck, P. R., A. Belfield, R. J. Spooner, L. H. Blumgart, and C. B. Wood (1978), *Clin. Chem.* **24,** 839.

Becker, F. F., and S. Sell (1974), *Cancer Res.* **34,** 2489.

Belanger, L., M. Belanger, and L. Prive (1973), *Path Biol.* **21,** 449.

Bell, W., R. Bahr, T. A. Waldman, and P. P. Carbone (1966), *Ann. Int. Med.* **64,** 658.

Berman, C. (1951), *Primary Cancer of the Liver,* Lewis, London.

Bernades, P., M. Smadja, B. Rueff, R. Bonnefond, T. Tursz, E. Martin, C. Bognel, J. Barge, and J. Uriel (1971), *Presse Med.* **79,** 1585.

Bierfeld, J. L., M. I. Scheiner, D. R. Schulta, M. D. Moral, and A. I. Rogers (1973), *Am. J. Dig. Dis.* **18,** 517.

Bodansky, O. (1961), *Adv. Cancer Res.* **6,** 1.

Boureile, J., P. Metayer, and F. Sauger (1970), *Presse Med.* **78,** 1277.

Braunstein, G. D., J. L. Vaitukaitis, P. P. Carbone, and G. T. Ross (1973), *Ann. Int. Med.* **78,** 39.

Brechot, C., C. Pourcel, A. Louise, B. Rain, and P. Tiollais (1980), *Nature* **286,** 533.

Buffe, D., and C. Rimbaut (1973), *Biomedicine* **19,** 172.

Carruthers, C., A. Baumler, and A. Neilson (1977), *Oncology* **34,** 47.

Chakraborty, P. R., N. Ruiz-Opazo, D. Shouval, and D. A. Shafritz (1980), *Nature* **286,** 531.

Chen, D.-S., and J.-L. Sung (1977), *Cancer* **40,** 779.

Chen, D.-S., and J.-L. Sung (1979), *Cancer* **44,** 984.

Chism, S. E. (1980), in *Cancer Markers: Development and Diagnostic Significance* (Sell, S. ed.), Humana Press, Clifton, N.J., p.115.

Chism, S. E., R. C. Burton, and N. L. Warner (1978), *Clin. Immunol. Immunopath.* **11,** 346.

Cochrane, M., and R. Williams (1976), in *Hepatocellular Carcinoma* (Okuda, K., and R. L. Peters, eds.) Wiley, New York, p.333.

Dedieu, P., J. Simon, J. F. Chatal, F. Buzelin, J. Le Portz, and P. Minicont (1978), *Gastroentrol. Clin. Biol.* **2,** 7.

Delmont, J., J. Kermarec, J. Lafon, C. Bonet, J. P. Cassuto, and R. Masseyeff (1974), *Digestion* **10,** 29.

Delpre, G., and T. Gilat (1978), *Gastroentrol. Clin. Biol.* **2,** 87, 193.

Edman, J. C., P. Gray, P. Valenzuela, L. B. Rail, and W. J. Rutter (1980), *Nature* **286,** 535.

Endo, Y., K. Kanai, T. Oda, K. Mitamura, S. Iino, and H. Susuki (1975), *Ann. NY Acad. Sci.* **259,** 234.

Engvall, E., H. Pihko, H. Jalanko, and E. Ruoslahti (1977), *J. Natl. Cancer Inst.* **59,** 277.

Ezraty, A., and P. Gauthier (1977), *Rev. Prat.* **27,** 3409.

Fleishner, G., K. Kamisaka, W. H. Habig, W. B. Jakoby, and I. M. Arias (1975), *Gastroenterol* **69**, 229.

Gentz, J., B. Lindblad, S. Lindstedt, L. Levy, W. Shasten, and R. Zetterström (1967), *Amer. J. Dis. Child.* **113**, 31.

Goldenberg, D. M. F. J. Primus, and F. Deland (1979), in *Immunodiagnosis of Cancer* (Herberman, R. B., and K. R. McIntire, eds.) Vol. 1, Dekker, New York, p. 265.

Goldfarb, S., and H. C. Pitot (1976), *Front. Gastroentest Res.* **2**, 194.

Gordon, A. S., E. D. Zajanai, and R. Zalusky (1970), *Blood* **35**, 151.

Gousev, A., and A. Yazova (1974), *Colloques L'Inserm L'Alpha Foetoproteine*, (Masseyeff, R., ed.), Editions Inserm, Paris, France, p. 255.

Griffin, J. J., and D. E. Kizer (1978), *Cancer Res.* **38**, 1136.

Griffing, G., and J. L. Vaitukaitis (1980), in *Cancer Markers: Developmental and Diagnostic Significance* (Sell, S., ed.), Humana Press, Clifton, NJ, p. 169.

Guguen, C., Szajnert, M. F., Schapira, F., Belanger, L., and Grenier, A. (1979), *Europ. J. Cancer* **15**, 1131.

Halvorsen, S., H. Pande, A. C. Loken, and L. R. Gjessing (1966), *Arch. Dis. Child.* **41**, 238.

Hann, H. W., H. M. Levy, and A. E. Evans (1980), *Cancer Res.* **40**, 1411.

Hazard, J. T., and J. W. Drysdale (1977), *Nature* **265**, 755.

Higashino, K., R. Ohtahi, S. Kudo, M. Hashinotsume, T. Hada, K. Y. Kang, T. Ohkochi, Y. Takahashi, and Y. Yamaura (1975), *Ann. Int. Med.* **83**, 74.

Higginson, J., and A. G. Oettle (1960), *J. Natl. Cancer Inst.* **24**, 589.

Hill, A., G. N. Hoag, and W. A. Zaleski (1972), *Clin. Chim. Acta* **77**, 455.

Hoyne, R. M., and J. W. Kernohan (1947), *Arch. Intern. Med.* **79**, 532.

Ihde, D. C., D. Sherlock, S. S. Winawer and J. G. Fortner (1974), *Am. J. Med.* **56**, 83.

Ikonen, R. S., J. Lindgren, E. Niemi, A. E. Sorto, M. Seppälä, and E. Ruoslahti (1980), *Acta Paediatr. Scand.* **69**, 59.

Jalanko, H., E. Engvall, and E. Ruoslahti (1978), *Immunol. Comm.* **7**, 209.

Jones, J. A., G. Robinson, R. C. Rees, and R. W. Baldwin (1978), *Int. J. Cancer* **21**, 171.

Jones, P. A. E., F. M. Miller, M. Worwood, and A. Jacobs (1973), *Brit. J. Cancer* **27**, 212.

Kamisaka, K., W. H. Habig, J. N. Ketley, I. M. Arias, and W. B. Jakoby (1975), *Eur. J. Biochem.* **60**, 153.

Karvountis, G. G., and A. G. Redeker (1974), *Ann. Int. Med.* **80**, 156.

Kew, M. C., L. R. Purves, and I. Berson (1973), *Gut* **14**, 939.

Kew, M. C., J. D. Torrance, D. Derman, M. Simon, G. M. MacNab, R. W. Charlton, and T. H. Bothwell (1978), *Gut* **19**, 294.

Kim, E. E., F. H. Deland, M. O. Nelson, S. Bennett, G. Simmons, E. Alpert, and D. M. Goldenberg (1980), *Cancer Res.* **40**, 3008.

Knill-Jones, R. P., R. M. Buckle, V. Parsons, R. Y. Calme, and R. Williams (1970), *New Engl. J. Med.* **285**, 1059.

Knox, W. E. (1976), *Enzyme Patterns in Fetal, Adult and Neoplastic Rat Tissues*, 2nd ed., Karger, Basel.

Koji, T., N. Ishii, T. Munehisa, Y. Kusumoto, S. Nakamura, A. Tamenishi, A. Hara, K. Kobayashi, Y. Tsukada, S. Nishi, and H. Hirai (1980), *Cancer Res.* **40**, 3013.

Kozower, M., K. A. Fawaz, H. M. Miller, and M. M. Kaplan (1971), *N. Eng. J. Med.* **285**, 1059.

Kubo, Y., and Y. Shimokawa (1976), in *Hepatocellular Carcinoma* (Okuda, K., and R. L. Peters, eds.) New York, p. 477.

Leffert, H., T. Moran, S. Sell, H. Skelly, K. Ibsen, M. Mueller, and I. M. Arias (1978), *Proc. Natl. Acad. Sci.* **75**, 1834.

Lehmann, F. C., and T. Wegener (1979), *J. Toxicol. Environ. Health* **5**, 281.

Levin, W., A. Y. Lu, P. E. Thomas, D. Ryan, D. E. Kizer, and M. J. Griffin (1978), *Proc. Nat'l. Acad. Sci.* **75**, 3240.

Lin, T., S. Chu, M. Chen, and C. Chen (1972), *Cancer* **30**, 435.

MacDonald, R. A. (1957), *Arch. Int. Med.* **99**, 532.

Margolis, S., and C. Homcy (1972), *Medicine* **51**, 381.

Marion, P. L., F. A. Salazar, J. J. Alexander, and W. S. Robinson (1980), *J. Virol.* **33**, 795.

Matray, F., F. Sauger, J. Borde, P. Mitrofanoff, M. Grosley, M. Bourg, R. Laumonier, and J. Hemet (1972), *Pathol. Biol.* **20**, 353.

Matsumoto, Y., T. Suzuki, H. Ono, A. Nakase, and I. Honjo (1974), *Cancer* **34**, 1602.

Mawas, C., O. Buffe, and O. Schweisguth (1970), *Rev. Europ. Et. Clin. Biol.* **16**, 430.

McFadzean, A. J. S., and R. T. T. Yeung (1969), *Am. J. Med.* **47**, 220.

McIntire, K. R., C. L. Vogel, G. L. Princler, and I. R. Patel (1972), *Cancer Res.* **32**, 1941.

McIntire, K. R., T. A. Waldmann, C. G. Moertel, and V. L. W. Go (1975), *Cancer Res.* **35**, 991.

Mehlman, D. J., B. H. Bulkley, and P. H. Wiernik (1971), *N. Engl. J. Med.* **285**, 1060.

Mihalev, A., D. Tzingilev, and L. M. Sirakov (1976), *Neoplasma* **23**, 103.

Mizejewski, G. L., and W. R. Dillon (1979), *Arch. Immunol. Therapy Exp.* **27**, 655.

Morey, S., and G. Litwack (1969), *Biochemistry* **8**, 4813.

Mori, H., N. Matsubara, M. Fujii, T. Kawai, T. Tanaka, and M. Takahashi (1979), *Acta Path. Jap.* **29**, 485.

Mosher, L. (1960), *Stanford Med. Bltn.* **18**, 59.

Murray-Lyon, I. M., A. H. Orr, B. Gazzard, J. Kohn, and R. Williams (1976), *Gut* **17**, 576.

Nagasue, N., K. Inokuchi, M. Kobayaski, and M. Saku (1977), *Cancer* **40**, 615.

Nadie, W., R. Matz, and P. W. Spear (1968), *Am. J. Digest Dis.* **13**, 705.

Neville, A. M., and E. H. Cooper (1976), *Ann. Clin. Biochem.* **13**, 283.

Niitsu, Y., S. Ohtsuka, Y. Kohgo, N. Watanbe, J. Koseki, and I. Urushizaki (19759, *Tumor Res.* **10**, 31.

Nørgaard-Pedersen, B. (1976), *Scand. J. Immunol. Suppl.* **4**, 1.

Obata, H., N. Hayashi, Y. Motoike, T. Hisamitsu, H. Okuda, S. Kobayaski, and K. Nishioka (1980), *Int. J. Cancer* **25**, 741.

Okita, K., and E. Farber (1975), *Gann Monogr.* **17**, 283.

Okita, K., L. H. Kligmon, and E. Farber (1975), *J. Natl. Cancer Inst.* **54**, 199.

Okuda, K. (1976), in *Hepatocellular Carcinoma* (Okuda, K., and R. L. Peter, eds.) Wiley, New York, p. 387.

Patton, R. B., and R. C. Horn (1964), *Cancer* **17**, 757.

Peters, R. L. (1976), in *Hepatocellular Carcinoma* (Okuda, K., and R. L. Peters, eds.) Wiley, New York, p. 107.

Phillips, P. J., R. Rowland, D. P. Reid, and M. E. Coles (1977), *J. Clin. Pathol.* **30**, 1129.

Popper, H. (1979), *Environ. Res.* **19**, 482.

Potter, V. R. (1968), *Canad. Cancer Conf.* **8**, 9.

Pressman, D., and L. Korngold (1953), *Cancer* **6**, 619.

Primus, F. J., S. J. Bennett, E. E. Kim,, F. H. DeLand, M. C. Zahn, and D. M. Goldenberg (1980), *Cancer Res.* **40**, 497.

Purtillo, D. T., J. H. Kersey, H. M. Hallgren, K. R. Fox, and E. J. Yunis (1973), *Am. J. Clin. Pathol.* **59**, 295.

Purves, L. R. (1973), *S. Afr. J. Sci.* **69**, 173.

Purves, L. R., I. Bersohn, E. W. Geddes, G. Falkson, and L. Cohen (1970), *S. Afr. Med. J.* **44**, 590.

Purves, L. R., W. R. Branch, E. W. Geddes, C. Manso, and M. Portugal (1973), *Cancer* **31**, 578.

Reissman, K. R., and M. R. Dietrich (1956), *J. Clin. Invest.* **35**, 588.

Reissman, K. R., and T. Nomura (1962), in *Proceedings of the Conference on Erythrophoresis* (Jacobson, L., and M. Doyle, eds.) Grune and Stratton, New York, pp. 72.

Reyes, M., A. J. Levi, Z. Gatmaitan, and I. M. Arias (1971), *J. Clin. Invest.* **50**, 2242.

Rimbaut, C., A. Hoffenbach, C. Rudant, and D. Buffe (1979), *Protides of the Biological Fluids* **27**, 293.

Ruoslahti, E., M. Seppälä, P. Vuopio, E. Saksela, and P. Peltokallio (1972), *J. Natl. Cancer Inst.* **49**, 623.

Ruoslahti, E., M. Seppälä, J. A. Rasanen, P. Vuopio, and T. Helske (1973), *Scand J. Gastroenterol.* **8**, 197.

Ruoslahti, E., H. Pihko, and M. Seppälä (1974a), *Transplant. Rev.* **20**, 38.

Ruoslahti, E., M. Salaspuro, H. Pihko, L. Andersson, and M. Seppälä (1974b), *Brit. Med. J.* **2**, 527.

Ruoslahti, E., E. Engvall, A. Pekkala, and M. Seppälä (1978), *Int. J. Cancer* **22**, 515.

Samuelsson, S. M., and I. Warner (1963), *Acta. Med. Scand.* **173**, 539.

San Jose, D. S., A. Cady, M. West, B. Chomet, and H. S. Zimmerman (1965), *Am. J. Dig. Dis.* **10**, 657, 1965.

Santer, M. A., T. A. Waldmann, and H. J. Fallon (1967), *Arch. Int. Med.* **120**, 735.

Schapira, F. (1973), *Adv. Cancer Res.* **18**, 77.

Schapira, F., A. Hatzfeld, A. Weber, and A. Guillouzo (1979), in *Carcinoembryonic Proteins*, Vol. 1, (Lehmann, F. G., ed.) Elsevier/North Holland, Amsterdam, p. 411.

Schleissner, L. A., and A. H. Cohen (1975), *Am. Rev. Resp. Dis.* **111**, 863.

Schwartz, M. K. (1973), *Clin. Chem.* **19**, 10.

Sell, S. (1980a) in *Cancer Markers: Developmental and Diagnostic Significance.* (Sell, S., ed.) Humana Press, New Jersey, p. 249.

Sell, S. (1980b), *Cancer Biology Rev.* **1**, 251.

Sell, S. (1978), in *Handbook of Cancer Immunology* (Walters, H., ed.) Vol. 3, Garland STM Press, New York, p. 1.

Sell, S., and F. F. Becker (1978), *J. Natl. Cancer Inst.* **60**, 19.

Sell, S., and H. T. Wepsic (1974), in *The Liver: The Molecular Biology of its Diseases,* (Becker, F., ed.) Dekker, New York, p. 773.

Sell, S., M. Nichols, F. F. Becker, and H. Leffert (1974a), *Cancer Res.* **34**, 865.

Sell, S., H. T. Wepsic, R. Nickel, and M. Nichols (1974b), *J. Natl. Cancer Inst.* **52**, 133.

Sell, S., H. W. Sheppard, Jr., R. Nickel, D. Stillman, and M. Michaelsen (1976a), *Cancer Res.* **36**, 476.

Sell, S., D. Stillman, and N. Gochman (1976b), *Am. J. Clin. Path.* **66**, 847.

Sell, S., D. Stillman, M. Michaelsen, J. Alaimo, and C. Von Essen (1977), *Rad. Res.* **69**, 54.

Seppälä, M., and E. Ruoslahti (1976), *Contr. Gynec. Obstet.* **2**, 143.

Shafritz, D. A., and M. C. Kew (1981), *Hepatology,* **1**, 1.

Shah, L. P., R. C. Rees, and R. W. Baldwin (1976), *Brit. J. Cancer* **33**, 577.

Shikata, T. (1976), *Hepatocellular Carcinoma* (Okuda, K., and R. L. Peters, eds.) Wiley, p. 53.

Shouval, D., P. R. Chakraborty, N. Ruiz-Opazo, S. Baum, I. I. Spigland, E. Muchmore, M. A. Gerber, S. N. Thung, H. Popper, and D. A. Shafritz (1980), *Proc. Natl. Acad. Sci.* **77**, 6147.

Silver, H. K. B., J. Deneault, P. Gold, W. G. Thompson, J. Shuster, and S. O. Freedman (1974), *Cancer Res.* **34**, 244.

Sizaret, T., A. Tuyns, N. Martel, A. Jouvenceaus, A. Levin, Y. W. Dng, and J. Rive (1975), *Ann. NY Acad. Sci.* **259**, 136.

Skrabanek, P. (1980a), *Irish J. Med. Sci.* **149**, 181.

Skrabanek, P. (1980b), *Medical Hypotheses* **6**, 437.

Skrabanek, P., J. McParlin, and D. Powell (1980), *Medicine* **59**, 262.

Smith, C. J., H. P. Morris, and P. C. Kelleher (1977), *Cancer Res.* **37**, 2651.

Smith, C. J., V. S. Ohl, and G. Litwack (1977), *Cancer Res.* **37**, 8.

Sugawara, K., A. Kashii, H. Kogure, J. Manaka, T. Shjirakura, and S. Mitani (1973), *Arch. Surg.* **106**, 63.

Suzuki, H., S. Iino, Y. Endo, M. Torii, K. Miki, and T. Oda (1975), *Ann. NY Acad. Sci.* **259**, 307.

Svenberg, T., B. Wahren, and S. Hammarström (1979), *Clin. Expl. Immunol.* **36**, 317.

Szmuness, W. (1978), *Prog. Med. Virology* **24**, 40.

Tatarinov, Y. (1964), *Vopr. Med. Khim.* **10**, 90.

Terry, W. D. (1978), in *Cancer in China* (Kaplan, H. S., and P. J. Tsuchitani, eds.) Alan R. Liss, New York, pp. 101.

Thompson, R. P., D. C. Nicholson, T. Farnan, D. N. Whitmore, and R. Williams (1970), *Gastroenterol.* **59**, 779.

Tipping, E., B. Ketterer, L. Christodoulides, and G. Enderby (1976), *Eur. J. Biochem.* **67**, 583.

Tong, M. J., S.-C. Sun, B. T. Schaeffer, N.-K. Chang, J.-J. Lo, and R. L. Peters (1971), *Ann. Int. Med.* **75,** 687.

Tsou, K. S., and K. W. Lo (1980), *Cancer* **45,** 209.

Tsung, S. H. (1975), *Arch. Pathol.* **99,** 267.

Tuyns, A. J., and M. Obradovic (1975), *J. Natl. Cancer Inst.* **54,** 61.

Viallet, A., J. P. Benhamow, and R. P. Feauvert (1962), *Canad. Med. Assn. J.* **85,** 1118.

Waxman, S., and H. S. Gilbert (1973), *New Engl. J. Med.* **289,** 1053.

Weber, G. (1977), *New Engl. J. Med.* **296,** 486.

Weinhouse, S. (1972), *Cancer Res.* **32,** 2007.

Weintraub, B. D., and S. W. Rosen (1971), *J. Clin. Endocrin. Metab.* **32,** 94.

Wepsic, H. T., Y. Tsukada, N. Takeichi, S. Nishi, and H. Hirai (1980), *Int. J. Cancer* **25,** 655.

Wikman-Coffelt, J., G. A., Howard, and R. R. Traut (1972), *Biochim. Biophys. Acta* **277,** 671.

Wogan, G. N. (1976), in *Hepatocellular Carcinoma* (Okuda, K., and R. L. Peters, eds.) Wiley, New York, p. 25.

Wolkoff, A. W., C. A. Goresky, J. Cellin, Z. Gatmaitin, and I. M. Arias (1979), *Amer. J. Physiol.* **236,** E638.

Zwi, S., S. S. Hurwitz, C. Cohen, I. Prinsloo, and E. Kagan (1975), *S. Afr. Med. J.* **49,** 1887.

7

Pancreatic Tumor Markers

John R. Hobbs

Department of Chemical Pathology, Westminster Medical School, London, Great Britain

1. Introduction

Adenocarcinoma of the pancreas has shown a real increase in recent years, accounting for 4.5% of all deaths certified as owing to malignancy, and has always created serious problems for clinicians, because current 5–10 year survivals following attempts at curative therapy are abysmally low at 1–5% (Silverberg, 1977). Careful postmortem examination in a Norwegian series showed that, although 3% of the deaths certified as resulting from cancer were correctly indicated to be of pancreatic origin, a further 2% needed to be added after postmortem examination, producing a true figure of 5% from autopsy studies (Hartveit, 1979). Cancer of the pancreas is thus now among the fourth or fifth commonest of killing cancers. This increase is probably the result of smoking (Krain, 1970).

The reasons for the failure of surgery are almost certainly that some 80% of patients already have regional or distant metastases at initial diagnosis, but it is not clear whether this results from late presentation or inherent early spread pancreatic cancers. What can be said is that the few patients who have been cured by surgery seem to have been diagnosed early by chance, and therefore a simple test that might improve earlier diagnosis is greatly needed.

Older methods for detecting cancers of the pancreas included testing the feces for occult blood, which was useful in the rare carcinoma of the ampulla of Vater. When one has seen a silver stool, one will not forget the association of bleeding with obstructive jaundice, rare symptoms that can point to a similar diagnosis. More often, however, there was simply the insidious onset of jaundice, which biochemically appeared typically obstructive in type, and for something like 40% of tumors large enough to obstruct the common bile duct, there was an elevated level of lactate dehydrogenase (LDH) in the serum of the patient. This usually showed a pattern with a predominance of type-3 isoenzyme, but, since such patients usually came to surgery anyway, the additional expense of such enzyme studies seemed unnecessary. With the advent of endoscopic retrograde cholangiopancreatography (ERCP), it became possible to look directly at the ampulla and to demonstrate obstructions in this region. The important new advance was the ability to sample pancreatic juice directly under visual control. We found that such pancreatic juice rapidly became activated by sampling and that the proteases would then destroy any proteins the juice contained. We therefore found it necessary to line the sampling tube with an equal mixture of Trasylol (5000 kallikrein units/mL) and 10% w/v epsilon-aminocaproic acid (EACA). This combination successfully preserved both pancreatic oncofetal antigen (POA) and CEA (v.i.). For rarer tumors of the pancreas, such as the mucoprotein-secreting cystadenocarcinoma, a marker could be found in the urine (Hobbs et al., 1974). And, of course, where the tumor produced secretion products, such as gastrin, insulin, somatostatin, pancreatic polypeptide, and glucagon, these could also be detected by radioimmunoassay of the serum or of the urine.

2. Pancreatic Oncofetal Antigen

The discovery of this tumor marker was reported by Banwo et al. in 1974. They introduced antiproteases to stabilize homogenates of fetal pancreas or adult carcinoma of pancreas, and these were then used to raise antisera in rabbits. The antisera were adsorbed with similarly stabilized homogenates of normal adult pancreas, and cleaned further with fetal liver and human plasma to identify an antigen present in both fetal and carcinomatous pancreas. Its existence was denied by Hegelund et al.(1976), but reconfirmed by Gelder et al. (1978) and by Arndt et al. (1978). At the 1979 meeting of the International Society for Oncodevelopmental Biology and Medicine, these two latter groups agreed with us to use the one name "pancreatic oncofetal antigen" (POA) for this new, confirmed tumor marker. POA has since been isolated by affinity chromatography (Knapp and Hobbs, 1980) from homogenates of either fetal pancreas or adult carcinoma of the pancreas. From these extracts, it fractionates as a small protein of molecular weight 40,000 daltons, which is unaffected by neuraminidase treatment and does not bind to several lectins, confirming an apparent absence of carbohydrate. This appears to make it distinct from those tumor antigens representing variants of the heavy chain of HLA present on the membranes of some neoplasms. In the serum of patients with pancreatic cancer, however, we confirm the finding of Gelder et al. (1978) that it exists as a large molecular weight complex of 900,000 daltons. In our own studies we were able to reduce this with SDS to its 40,000 component and were unable to detect any known carrier protein similar to 84 known plasma proteins. Monomer POA was unaffected by DNase or RNase, but was completely destroyed by trypsin, papain, or pepsin.

Gelder's group and Thiele's group have exchanged apparently monospecific antisera with us, and all three antisera yield only a single peak with purified POA. Each of the three antisera can remove POA reactivity from either extracts of tissue or of the sera of patients and prevent it being developed with the other antisera. When used in Ouchterlony gel diffusion, these antisera produce lines of fusion, and therefore appear to be detecting the identical antigen. Arndt et al. (1978) isolated their POA from fetal pancreas and find a molecular weight of 36,000 daltons. All three antisera can be used for rocket immunoassay. In our own hands, the within-batch CV is 4%, while the between-batch CV is 6%. We have adopted a serum with a high content of POA as a working standard and assigned to it a unitage of 15 units/mL. We then find that 7 µg of affinity-purified POA appears to be the immunological equivalent of 1 unit.

This indicates a recovery of POA from either serum or homogenate of about 25%, which may not fully be representative of the original 100% reactive material. Even so, absorption with this POA does remove all reactivity of the antiserum with the original material. We can, therefore, be reasonably certain that the purified POA contains the material that is antigenic in serum, pancreatic juice, pancreatic extracts, or histological sections. Mihas (1978) is studying a similar protein called POP, and Nishida et al. (1980) claim to have developed an enzyme immunoassay for POA.

2.1. Tissue Localization of POA

Using an immunoperoxidase sandwich, POA has been studied throughout fetal tissues, and normal and carcinomatous pancreas, and has been sought in some other neoplasms, notably carcinoma of the stomach, colon, and liver (Hobbs et al., 1980). POA was localized in the cytoplasm of the secretory cells of adenocarcinoma of the pancreas, and positive staining also occurred nearby in the stroma and in the lumen of the ducts (see Fig. 1). This is compatible with POA being secreted by carcinoma cells and may explain its relatively high levels in the serum, where it does not appear to be necessary to use radioimmunoassay, but instead the more robust and reliable rocket immunoassay (v.i.). POA was also well localized in the adenomatous parts of fetal pancreas and was quite clearly negative in the islets. We were unable to detect POA in fetal liver, lung, stomach, colon,

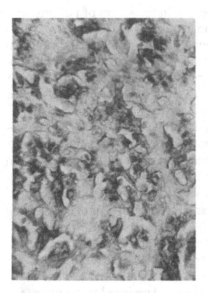

Fig. 1. On the right is an H and E section from a carcinoma of the pancreas, and on the left is a comparable field stained by the immunoperoxidase method to develop anti-POA (magnification, × 300). The dark staining areas show the presence of POA mainly in the cytoplasm of the acinar cells.

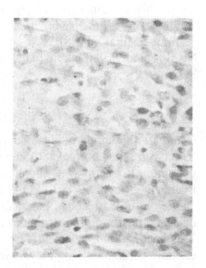

Fig. 2. On the right is an H and E stained section of carcinoma of the stomach, and on the left a similar field has been developed with anti-POA. The virtual absence of any dark staining is consistent with no POA being detected (magnification, × 300).

or small intestine. We have not yet had an opportunity to examine the fetal biliary tree. Among other human cancers, we have detected no positive staining in 20 each of primary hepatoma, gastric carcinoma (see Fig. 2), adenocarcinoma of the lung, and carcinoma of the rectum. However, 1 of 20 colonic carcinomata did stain—albeit weakly, but quite definitely and quite specifically, as if it contained POA (see Fig. 3). Among other patients with biopsy-proven clinical diagnoses of carcinoma of the stomach, liver, colon, and lung where POA levels had been detected in the serum of the patient, the commonest explanation was that the patient had probably had both cancers, i.e., some other specific tumor that had already been diagnosed, together with a carcinoma of the pancreas. This was especially true for the cases of lung cancer, where among 50 patients who had survived four years from their initial diagnosis, no fewer than 15 have now had proven independent carcinoma of the pancreas. One cannot but be impressed in this situation with a common causal agent, such as smoking. Thus, from these immunohistochemical studies, it appears at the moment that POA may be more specific at biopsy level than it is in the serum (v.i.), but that it has definitely been identified in one colonic carcinoma, and of course it may be identified in some other cancers when the numbers are increased in the future.

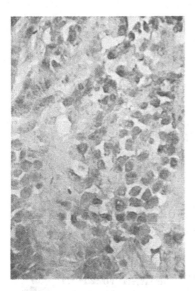 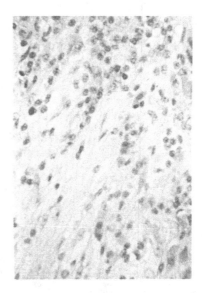

Fig. 3. On the right is the H and E section of a carcinoma of the colon from a patient with a serum level of POA of 4 U/mL. On the left a similar field has been developed with anti-POA and "brown" staining can be seen in cells equivalent to epithelial cells. It was of about half the intensity of that seen in fetal or adult carcinoma of the pancreas (magnification, × 700).

2.2. Serum Levels of POA in Malignant Diseases

From these cross-sectional studies, an arbitrary level of 7 units of POA/mL was chosen as likely to differentiate well between carcinoma of the pancreas and other malignant diseases (see Fig. 4). With this chosen level, serum levels at presentation have been measured in 288 patients with malignant diseases, all eventually proven by biopsy, with the results that are shown in Table 1. From this it becomes apparent that in our assay a positive level (> 7 units/mL) is detected in 95% of patients with carcinoma of the pancreas, whose tumors were detected clinically and proven by biopsy.

Positive levels are only occasionally found in patients proven to have other cancers, and whereas it cannot be excluded at present that such tumors might produce POA, or an antigenically related substance, intensive investigation of such false positives most often reveals that the two cancers are present in the same patient (see Hobbs et al., 1980). In the borderline gray area, however, the frequency of values up to 6 units among other cancers, especially stomach and colon, does suggest that in the absence of a common carcinogenic cause, embryological overlap in oncofetal antigen production is more likely to prove to be the explanation. The concentra-

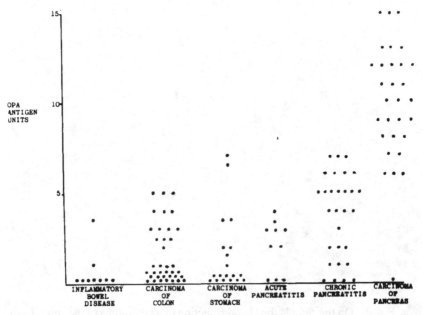

Fig. 4. Serum POA levels in U/mL as found in the sera of 30 patients with biopsy-proven carcinoma of the pancreas, and 104 patients with other conditions, all at first clinical presentation. At a level of 7 U/mL the only overlap here is seen between carcinoma of the stomach and chronic pancreatitis.

Table 1
POA Serum Levels from New Consecutive Patients with
Biopsy-Proven Malignant Diseases

Totals	Primary diagnosis	< 6 U/mL	> 7 U/mL	Percent positive
100	Carcinoma of the pancreas	5	95	95
11	Primary hepatoma	11	0	0
2	Bile duct carcinoma	2	0	—
50	Carcinoma of the stomach	47	3	6
50	Carcinoma of the colon	49	1	2
25	Lung cancer	23	2	8
25	Breast cancer	25	0	0
25	Myelomatosis	25	0	0
288				

tions of POA-like materials in such tumors may not be high enough to demonstrate with the presently available immunohistochemistry, but a clinical-sized tumor might be big enough to contaminate the serum. The other possibility is that cancers near the pancreas may by local invasion, or by local influence of humoral substances released from the cancers, induce the production of POA by the pancreas itself. We ourselves cannot agree with Gelder et al. that there is a 14% overlap with other cancers at our chosen level of 7 units/mL. We have not yet been able to compare our standard with their standard. Now that carcinoma of the pancreas has increased to an almost comparable frequency with these other cancers, it would not, for instance, be surprising to eventually find an overlap of up to 5% owing to the concurrence of both cancers. This is certainly true for carcinoma of the lung, where a common carcinogenic action of smoking seems to be present. It is worth mentioning here that the patient whose colonic tumor stained weakly positive for POA in fact only had a serum level of 4 units/mL. However, the overlap with chronic pancreatitis (v.i.) does seem to represent a problem.

To date, two small tumors have been detected, one at a level of 7 units/mL where only 2 g of tumor was found at surgery and resected, after which the level of POA became undetectable, and another at 9 units/mL where a 3 g tumor was removed from the tail of the pancreas, also with the rapid disappearance of a detectable level of POA. These anecdotal experiences do offer hope for the earlier detection of at least some cancers of the pancreas, and for their possible subsequent cure by surgery. The two patients described are alive and well, with negative serum POA, at 23 and 39 months, respectively.

2.3. POA in Pancreatic Juice

We have only a limited experience of POA detected in pancreatic juice that was carefully collected with antiproteases during ERCP. In our few cases, the pancreatic juice level of POA has always been found to be higher than the concurrent serum level, and this is in agreement with previous experience for CEA (v.i.). It therefore does seem that, in those patients coming to ERCP, determining POA levels in the pancreatic juice may offer a more sensitive and reliable means of cancer detection than its measurement in serum. In this respect, two other approaches have been fruitful; there is that of DiMagno et al. (1977), where the CEA level has been elevated following stimulation with cholecystokinin-pancreozymin (CCK-PZ) which is confirmed by Lindstedt et al. (1978). The second has been the observation by Fedail et al. (1978) that the lactoferrin level in carcinoma of the pancreas is not much higher than normal, whereas this is markedly raised in chronic pancreatitis. The tandem use of these two approaches is being explored to see whether they will conjointly sharpen diagnostic discrimination for carcinoma of the pancreas.

2.4. Differential Diagnostic Value of POA in Obstructive Jaundice

From the results in Table 2, and again using a level of 7 units/mL as positive, it can be seen that in obstructive jaundice of unknown etiology the POA level seems to be extremely valuable in recognizing just when the jaundice results from carcinoma of the pancreas. It must be admitted that our experience of carcinomata of the biliary duct and gall bladder is not

Table 2
Serum POA Levels Under Conditions Contributing to the
Differential Serum POA Diagnosis of Jaundice

Totals	Patients with Jaundice	< 6 U/mL	> 7 U/mL	Percent positive
30	Carcinoma of the pancreas	1	29	97
18	Gallstones only	18	0	0
22	Cirrhosis of the liver	22	0	0
4	Primary hepatoma	4	0	0
9	Metastases in liver (not from pancreas)	9	0	0
2	Carcinoma of the bile duct	2	0	0
75				

[a]It can be seen that as yet there have been no false positives and only one false negative.

large enough to indicate whether or not there will be overlap, but in either event the surgeon would have some forewarning of any malignancy becoming evident at laparotomy. Certainly detection of very high levels of POA would argue against attempts at curative surgery.

2.5. The Differentiation Between Carcinoma of the Pancreas and Chronic Pancreatitis

Table 3 shows our results in this difficult situation. Those patients labeled as having carcinoma of the pancreas are all biopsy-proven. Unfortunately it has not been possible to say that carcinoma of the pancreas was not also present in all those patients given the diagnosis of chronic pancreatitis. This is only natural because of the present reluctance to biopsy the pancreas in conditions of apparent inflammation. However, it is true to say that some 60% of the patients with chronic pancreatitis had a history of its presence for longer than 5 years' duration, and that among the group the false positive rate was only 8%. We still do not know whether the reason for the high false positive rate (15% overall, and higher in cases with shorter histories) is the coexistence of a carcinoma as the underlying cause of recurrent pancreatitis, or whether the condition itself has resulted in tissue regeneration with a concomitant re-expression of the oncofetal antigen POA. Certainly among cases of undoubted postmortem diagnosed pancreatitis, whereby biopsy material has been available, we have not been able to satisfy ourselves that regeneration is common. It is not as easy to detect POA as it is to find CEA in ulcerative colitis. Again our ERCP studies are at present too limited for comment, but the approaches outlined above for interpreting pancreatic juice results may well help in the future. It is also

Table 3
Serum POA Levels in the Distinction between Inflammatory
and Carcinomatous Lesions of the Pancreas

Totals		< 6 U/mL	> 7 U/mL	Percent positive
100	Carcinoma of the pancreas	5	95	95
48	Chronic pancreatitis	41	7	15
21	Acute pancreatitis	21	0	0
7	Fibrocystic disease	7	0	0
6	Tyrosinosis	6	0	0
6	Hemochromatosis	6	0	0
18	Diabetes mellitus	18	0	0
206				

worth pointing out that Gelder et al. (1978) did notice an association of POA with post-alcoholic pancreatitis.

Following acute pancreatitis, when tissue regeneration might be expected to occur, we have not yet detected any elevation of POA in the serum, though we have now had an opportunity to look at three patients who suffered such pancreatitis following the use of very high doses of corticosteroids (2 g/day) in an attempt to control graft-vs-host disease; in those patients, we failed to detect any POA. In other more chronic destructive diseases of the pancreas, such as fibrocystic disease, tyrosinosis, hemochromatosis, and diabetes mellitus, we have again found no increased incidence of raised POA levels. It may, therefore, be that only certain kinds of regeneration, possibly in the presence of a carcinogen or cocarcinogen, encourages the re-expression of POA.

2.6. Longitudinal Studies of POA

As has been mentioned above, two of our patients have now had the benefit of attempts at curative surgery, and POA, which was detectable before the operation, has disappeared within three months (see Fig. 5). It has also been possible to follow the progress of patients who have had bypass operations for incurable cancer of the pancreas causing obstructive jaundice, and a representative example of such a patient is also shown in Fig 5. A few such patients have now received intensive courses of chemotherapy, and it would still be anecdotal to give full details. It can be said that some of our patients have enjoyed 2–4 years of very full and useful life following such an approach, and during this time the level of POA was reduced below 3 U/mL and remained there in a plateau phase to rise slowly, predicting the clinical relapse by about 6–12 months. Nishida et al., using their own unitage, have also seen elevations with progression, and reductions by appropriate treatment. It can therefore be said that POA shows promise as a marker suitable for monitoring the response of carcinoma of the pancreas to treatment.

2.7. The Future for POA

Overall, the overlap in chronic pancreatitis is too large at 15% to encourage sole reliance on POA levels above 7 units/mL for the diagnosis of carcinoma of the pancreas. Unfortunately, the kind of patient where this diagnosis comes to mind is one with a subacute history of abdominal pain, which must in itself overlap with the diagnosis of chronic pancreatitis. For that class of patient it would seem that the approach of ERCP, with its collateral diagnostic investigations, may be improved in the future by including at the time a POA level in pancreatic juice, coupled with a lactoferrin level. Where the lactoferrin level is markedly raised, the balance is in favor of a diagnosis of chronic pancreatitis; where the POA level

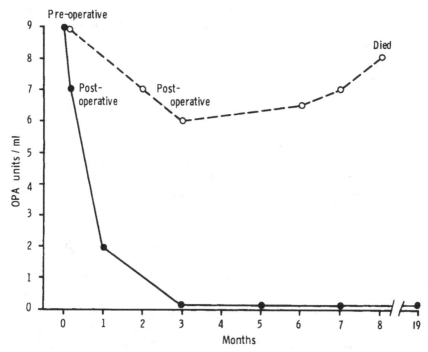

Fig. 5. POA levels found in the sera from two patients who started with similar levels pre-operatively. The solid line shows the progress of a patient who had a 3-g tumor, apparently confined to the tail of the pancreas, which was removed; the POA level was undetectable at 3 months and has remained there for 39 months. The other patient was less fortunate, the tumor was inoperable, so was bypassed, and chemotherapy from 10 to 80 days post-operatively temporarily reduced the level of POA, which then climbed back with the patient dying at 8 months from the operation.

is raised by itself, its appearance would tend to favor a diagnosis of carcinoma of the pancreas. This approach would, therefore, be used in selected patients, and needs to be further evaluated, but most certainly would not offer a means of screening the general population.

In patients who present with insidious onset of jaundice, we would consider a serum estimation of POA to be a valuable help in the differential diagnosis.

In the screening of populations aged 40–60 years (Hobbs, 1974) who have smoked heavily, POA levels may turn out to be valuable. However, there seems to be about an equal chance of dying of a lung cancer, even should an early carcinoma of the pancreas be successfully resected. At least the use of CEA estimations to prevent unnecessary surgery for cancer of the lung (Concannon et al., 1978) will reduce the number of patients surviving a lung cancer who might need screening for POA.

Finally, in patients who present with metastases that are available for easy biopsy, the use of immunohistochemistry could identify the primary lesion as being within the pancreas.

Longitudinal studies in patients known to have carcinoma of the pancreas may well be able to guide the early introduction of adjuvant chemotherapy with a rising serum level of POA, or indeed lack of its disappearance following surgery, and might also enable the development of optimal drug schedules to treat patients who first present with more extensive disease.

The use of antibody against POA, coupled to either radioactive tracers (for diagnostic localization; Goldenberg et al., 1978) or cytotoxic drugs (for therapy: Oon et al., 1975) offers further hope for the future.

3. Comparison with Carcinoembryonic Antigen

The FDA (1974) has ruled against the use of CEA for mass screening in the early diagnosis of cancer, the major reason for this being the high false positive rate that would lead to the further unnecessary investigation of too many subjects (Hobbs, 1974). In a population of patients known to have pancreatic cancer, plasma CEA was elevated in 85% (Zamcheck, 1976), but in an unselected population Wood and Moossa (1977) found that CEA gave a positive result in their tests in only 57% of all tested patients who had pancreatic cancer. This contrasted with a sensitivity of 91% for POA. When they looked at the predictive value of a positive CEA test (true positive), they found that in the population they tested only 48% of the patients with a positive test in fact had pancreatic cancer. This contrasted with 60% for POA. When they looked at the predictive value of a negative test (true negative: patients without pancreatic cancer who had a negative test as a percentage of all patients with a negative test), they found for CEA a value of 75%, whereas for POA it was 94%. On the basis of the Wood and Moossa results, one is forced to conclude that POA is much better in the accurate diagnosis of pancreatic cancer than is CEA.

Acknowledgments

I am indebted to my coworkers O. Banwo, Dr. J. Versey, M. L. Knapp, and Dr. A. C. Branfoot; to many clinical colleagues, especially Mr. C. Wastell and Dr. B. Gazzard; to Miss Carol Marshall for secretarial assistance; to the Westminster Photographic Department, and to the Cancer Research Campaign for financial support.

References

Arndt, R., K. Nishida, W.-M. Becker, and H.-G. Thiele (1978), *Proceedings of the 6th Meeting of the International Society for Oncodevelopmental Biology and Medicine*, Abstract 229.

Banwo, O., J. Versey, and J. R. Hobbs (1974), *Lancet* **1**, 643.

Concannon, J., M. H. Dalbow, S. E. Hodgson, J. J. Headings, E. Markopoulos, J. Mitchell, W. J. Cushing, and G. A. Liebler (1978), *Cancer* **42**, (3 Suppl.), 1477.

DiMagno, E. P., J.-R. Malagelada, C. G. Moertel, and V. L. W. Go (1977), *Gastroenterology* **73**, 457.

FDA Drug Bulletin (January, 1974).

Fedail, S. S., R. Harvey, P. R. Salmon, and A. E. Read (1978), *Brit. Med. J.* **1**, 304.

Gelder, F. B., C. J. Reese, A. R. Moossa, T. Hall, and R. Hunter (1978), *Cancer Res.* **38**, 313.

Goldenberg, D. M., F. DeLand, E. Kim, S. Bennett, F. J. Primus, J. R. van Nagell, N. Estes, P. DeSimone, and P. Rayburn (1978), *New Eng. J. Med.* **298**, 1384.

Hartveit, F. (1979), *J. Pathol.* **129**, 111.

Hegelund, H., N. H. Axelsen, E. Bock, B. Nørgaard-Pedersen, and O. C. Røder (1976), *Protides of the Biological Fluids* **24**, 525.

Hobbs, J. R. (1974), *Lancet* **2**, 1305.

Hobbs, J. R., O. Banwo, and J. M. B. Versey (1976), *Die Untersuchung der Bauchspeicheldrüse*, 45.

Hobbs, J. R., D. J. Evans, and O. M. Wrong (1974), *Brit. Med. J.* **2**, 87.

Hobbs, J. R., M. L. Knapp, and A. C. Branfoot (1980), *Oncofetal Biol. Med.* **1**, 37.

Knapp, M. L., and J. R. Hobbs (1980), *Protides of the Biological Fluids* **27**, 63.

Krain, L. S. (1970), *J. Surg. Oncol.* **2**, 115.

Lindstedt, G., P.-A. Lundberg, and P. Rolny (1979), *Cancer* **43**, 2465.

Mihas, A. A. (1978), *J. Natl. Cancer Inst.* **60**, 1439.

Nishida, K., M. Sugiura, T. Yoshikawa, and M. Kondo (1980), *Lancet* **1**, 262.

Oon, C.-J., M. Apsey, H. Buckleton, K. B. Cooke, I. Hanham, A. Hazarika, J. R. Hobbs, and B. McLeod (1975), *Behring Inst. Mitt.* **56**, 228.

Silverberg, E. (1977), *Ca-A Cancer J. Clin.* **27**, 26.

Wood, R. A. B., and A. R. Moossa (1977), *Brit. J. Surg.* **64**, 718.

Zamcheck, N., (1976), *Clinics Gastroenterol.* **5**, 625.

8
Prostate Cancer Markers

T. Ming Chu, Ming C. Wang, Ching-li Lee, Carl S. Killian, Manabu Kuriyama, Lawrence D. Papsidero, Luis A. Valenzuela, and Gerald P. Murphy

Department of Diagnostic Immunology Research and Biochemistry, Roswell Park Memorial Institute, Buffalo, New York

1. Introduction

According to the American Cancer Society, this year an estimated 57,000 new cases of prostate cancer (1979) will be diagnosed among American males (American Cancer Society, 1979). The Society also estimates that 20,000 lives will be lost to this form of cancer. One of the major reasons for this high mortality is that many cases are not detected until after metastases have occurred (Gittes and Chu, 1976). Therefore, markers that may serve as aids for early diagnosis of this disease and in monitoring the effectiveness of therapies have long been investigated. The purpose of this chapter is to review the prostate tumor markers that have been shown to be of significant value in diagnosis and treatment of this disease. It will include new information for old markers such as prostatic acid phosphatase, and data on new markers under investigation, such as prostate antigen. Other known markers that have been shown to be associated with cancer of the prostate are also described briefly.

2. Prostatic Acid Phosphatase

Acid phosphatase may be the oldest marker for all forms of tumor, and in fact the assay of acid phosphatase activity has been used in diagnosis of prostate cancer for over five decades (Gutman and Gutman, 1936). Excellent general reviews on acid phosphatase are available elsewhere (Yam, 1974; Schwartz et al., 1969) and will not be discussed. Only new information reported in the last few years is summarized in this chapter.

Prostatic acid phosphatase has now been purified (Chu et al., 1978b; Lee et al., 1978; Choe et al., 1978a; Vihko et al., 1978a; Van Etten and Saini, 1978). Chemical analysis revealed that prostatic acid phosphatase is composed of approximately 95% polypeptides and 5% carbohydrates. It has a molecular weight of approximately 100,000, with two identical subunits of 50,000 each (Ostrowski, 1968; Chu et al., 1975). Purified prostatic acid phosphatase was demonstrated by the isoelectric focusing technique, among others, to contain at least several isoenzymes with their isoelectric points ranging from 4.2 to 5.5 (Chu et al., 1978a). This microheterogeneity of prostatic acid phosphatase cannot be attributed to sialic acid content alone, since treatment of neuraminidase did not yield a single isoenzyme (Chu et al., 1978a; Mahan and Doctor, 1979). Data are available to suggest that prostatic acid phosphatase is different biochemically from acid phosphatases of other tissues or blood cellular components (Chu et al., 1978a).

Antiserium raised against purified prostatic acid phosphatase (PAP) has been shown to exhibit immunologic specificity since extracts of other tissues do not react with antiPAP antiserum (Shulman et al., 1964; Chu et al., 1978b; Lee et al., 1978; Choe et al., 1978b). Chemical modification studies have revealed some information on the interaction between prostatic acid phosphatase and its substrate at the enzyme active site (McTigue and Van Etten, 1978a). At least two arginine residues of prostatic acid phosphatase have been shown to be involved in binding to a negatively charged phosphate group of the substrate. In addition, a histidine has been postulated to be a nucleophile in the formation of the covalent phosphoenzyme intermediate. It appears that prostatic acid phosphatase possesses a quite different type of phosphate transfer reaction from that of alkaline phosphatase (McTigue and Van Etten, 1978b; Lee et al., 1980c). By means of immunoprecipitation techniques, with partial trypsin digestion, prostatic acid phosphatase has been shown to contain at least three different antibody-binding sites, which seem to be distant from the enzyme active sites (Cooper and Foti, 1974). Furthermore, the antibody-bound prostatic acid phosphatase has a better stability than free prostatic acid phosphatase (Lee et al., 1978). These properties have been the basis for the development of recent immunoassays for the specific measurement of circulating prostatic acid phosphatase. Four sensitive, yet specific, immunoassays for prostatic acid phosphatase are available, namely: radioimmunoassay, counterimmunoelectrophoresis, immunofluoroassay, and immunoenzyme assay.

The radioimmunoassay (RIA) for prostatic acid phosphatase was first described in 1974 (Cooper et al., 1978). Acid phosphatase was partially purified from normal prostatic fluid by gel filtration on Sephadex G-100. Rabbit antiserum raised against this preparation of enzyme, after absorption with normal female serum, was shown to be specific to acid phosphatase of prostate origin. With this immunological reagent, a double antibody RIA was developed and improved a year later, resulting in a solid-phase radioimmunoassay (Foti et al., 1975). The specificity and sensitivity of this new solid-phase radioimmunoassay was shown to be superior to that of conventional chemical methods. In a group of 109 patients with prostate cancer, elevated prostatic acid phosphatase as detected by RIA was found in 73% of patients (Foti et al., 1977). According to the clinical stages of their prostate cancers, approximately one-half of the patients with stage I and II were found to have an elevated prostatic acid phosphatase and more than 90% of the patients with stages III and IV diseases had elevated prostatic acid phosphatase levels. Other similar radioimmunoassays for prostatic acid phosphatase have been developed by using enzyme purified from ejaculated human seminal plasma or benign hypertrophic prostate (Bellville et al., 1978; Choe et al., 1978b; Vihko et al., 1978b).

Although the RIA technique for prostatic acid phosphatase has been reported for almost 6 years, no clinical information from extensive evaluation has been reported. With the recent availability of RIA kits from commercial sources, such data can be expected in the near future. Basically, the RIA technique is a sound procedure that provides good sensitivity, but also has some disadvantages, such as the instability of the labeled enzyme, the difficulty and requirement of purified enzyme as the primary standard, and the possible contamination of radioactive materials.

A simple and practical immunoassay for serum prostatic acid phosphatase is the so-called counterimmunoelectrophoresis (CIEP) assay, as described by this laboratory over four years ago (Chu et al., 1976). Rabbit specific antiprostatic acid phosphatase antiserum was produced against purified prostatic acid phosphatase isolated from human malignant prostate. The principle of this technique is the movement of prostatic acid phosphatase and its antiserum in opposite directions under an electric field to form an immune prostatic acid phosphatase–antiprostatic acid phosphatase complex. The antibody-complexed enzyme was then detected by a sensitive histochemical staining technique at the nanogram level of sensitivity (Chu et al., 1978b). Using similar approaches, two other laboratories have described a specific CIEP asssay for the measurement of serum prostatic acid phosphatase (McDonald et al., 1978; Romas et al., 1978).

Our original CIEP technique was evaluated in a national trial study that essentially confirmed our preliminary study (Wajsman et al., 1979). In this national trial, a total of 962 serum specimens from patients with prostate cancer were analyzed. Results indicated that 38% of 64 patients with stage A prostate cancer, 35% of 178 samples from stage B patients,

59% of 235 samples from stage C patients, and 69% of 485 samples from patients with stage D were shown to be positive for serum prostatic acid phosphatase by the CIEP technique. Data were also obtained from this study indicating that CIEP was a more sensitive technique than the conventional chemical methods with simultaneous measurement.

Our original semiquantitative CIEP recently has been modified and improved to become a quantitative method by means of densitometry and fixed-point kinetic spectrophotometries (Killian et al., 1980b). Furthermore, the sensitivity has been improved to detect 1 ng of prostatic acid phosphatase per mL of specimen, which is comparable with that of radioimmunoassay currently available. Using the improved CIEP, the levels of serum prostatic acid phosphatase in normal healthy age-matched controls and patients with nonprostatic tumor were shown to be similar, and those in patients with early stages of prostatic cancer who were originally shown by chemical methods to have normal acid phosphatase activities were shown to be significantly elevated. Theoretically, the CIEP technique measures the prostatic acid phosphatase protein both by antigenicity and hydrolytic activities of the enzyme, and therefore may be superior to the conventional method, which measures enzyme activity alone, or radioimmunoassay, which measures protein (antigenicity) alone. In addition, a large number of specimens can be run simultaneously, which makes CIEP suitable for use as an initial screening method for serum prostatic acid phosphatase measurement.

Lee et al. of this laboratory reported a solid-phase fluorescent immunoassay (SPIF) for serum prostatic acid phosphatase (Lee et al., 1978). This assay utilizes the immunologic specificity of antiprostatic acid phosphatase antibody prepared on solid-phase support. The fluorescent property of α-naphthol, the hydrolytic product of the enzyme, was measured by use of a spectrophotofluorometer. The sensitivities of this new immunoassay for prostatic acid phosphatase was 20–60 pg of prostatic acid phosphatase protein/mL of specimen, more sensitive than CIEP or RIA. It requires no isotope, and hence may provide advantages in some laboratories. Initial clinical evaluation indicated that prostatic acid phosphatase was found by this technique to be elevated in a great majority of patients with early prostate cancer and in almost all patients with advanced stage D prostate cancer. Patients with carcinomas of other origins had a normal range of values for serum prostatic acid phosphatase. A larger scale testing of this SPIF was recently completed (Lee et al., 1980a), and essentially confirmed the results from the initial study. Patients with early stages of prostate cancer, such as A_2 surgically staged, had elevated levels of serum prostatic acid phosphatase. Although the number of patients studied was limited, the data indicate that patients with encapsulated tumor within the prostate have elevated circulating prostatic acid phosphatase. These observations may profoundly change the classic concepts of and approaches to the staging and treatment of prostate cancer.

Most recently, two new non-isotopic immunocolorimetric assays for serum prostatic acid phosphatase were reported (Lee et al., 1980b; Choe et al., 1980). Neither technique requires the use of a sophisticated spectrophotofluorometer or gamma-spectrometer. A major advantage of these two assays is the use of a spectrophotometer, which is widely available in most clinical laboratories. Clinical evaluation, although still in its early stages, has shown a sensitivity and specificity similar to those of previous immunoassays (Lee et al., 1978; Choe et al., 1978b).

The comparative diagnostic value of various prostatic acid phosphatase immunoassays is not at present available. However, results from various papers on radioimmunoassay and the other non-isotopic procedures can be compiled. Results from two radioimmunoassays (Mahan and Doctor, 1979; Griffiths, 1980) and the original CIEP (Chu et al., 1978b) were quite similar, but were different from the report of another RIA (Foti et al., 1977). Data from the solid-phase immunofluoroassay and immunoadsorbent assay appear to agree to a large degree with each other (Lee et al., 1978; Lee et al., 1980b). One should be cautious, though, in making this kind of comparison, since the practice of staging in prostate cancer may vary from investigator to investigator, and some patients may have received treatment that could effect the results at the time of blood testing.

In addition to the study of serum prostatic acid phosphatase, there has been an abundance of data and experience in recent years regarding the use of bone marrow acid phosphatase in the management of prostate cancer. Many reports have indicated that greater accuracy in detecting metastatic prostatic cancer can be achieved by the determination of bone marrow acid phosphatase (Reynolds et al., 1973; Gursel et al., 1974; Marshall et al., 1974; Yarrison et al., 1976). With the availabilities of immunochemical assays for prostatic acid phosphatase, the precise role of bone marrow acid phosphatase determination has recently been re-investigated. The majority of reports using immunoassays for prostatic acid phosphatase have indicated that the measurement of bone marrow acid phosphatase activity is not of additional value in detecting bony metastasis originating from prostate cancer (Catane et al., 1978; Cooper et al., 1978; Drucker et al., 1978; Pontes et al., 1978).

3. Prostate Antigen

A new potential biological marker for prostate cancer was recently reported from this laboratory. A prostate-specific antigen, distinct biochemically and immunologically from prostatic acid phosphatase, has been identified in normal, benign hypertrophic, and cancerous prostate by means of immunologic techniques.

This prostate antigen also has been purified from human prostate tissues (Wang et al., 1979). The purified prostate antigen was shown to be a glycoprotein in nature, with a molecular weight of 34,000 and an isoelectric point of 6.9. Amino acid composition studies revealed that approximately one molecule of prostate antigen contains 300 amino acid residues (Li et al., 1981). Antiserum against prostate antigen reacts only with prostate antigen and does not react with prostatic acid phosphatase, as shown by immunodiffusion, counterimmunoelectrophoresis, or a sensitive enzyme immunoassay (Wang et al., 1979; Kuriyama et al., 1980a). By rocket immunoelectrophoresis with a sensitivity of 0.05 mg, prostate antigen was shown to be present only in human prostate, and not in other tissues examined, either normal or cancerous (Papsidero et al., 1980). By a more sensitive enzyme immunoassay, with a sensitivity of 0.01 ng, and using cultured human cells and spent cultured media as samples, only cells and media of human prostate tumor origin expressed prostate antigen (Papsidero et al., 1981). Furthermore, with in vitro animal systems, only serum from nude mice bearing human prostate tumors contained a significant amount of prostate antigen.

By immunocytochemical staining technique, prostate antigen is localized at the epithelium lining of the prostate gland and ducts, as well as in prostate secretions and concretions (Papsidero et al., 1981; Nadji et al., 1981). Also, prostate antigen has been shown to be primarily of cytoplasmic origin. Tissue specificities of this newly discovered prostate antigen are further confirmed by this highly sensitive immunocytochemical technique. Prostate antigen is indeed found only in prostate tissue, regardless of the pathological origin of the tissue. No other tissues or cells contain this prostate antigen at the sensitivity levels of this immunocytochemical procedure.

In addition, only tumors of prostate origin, both primary and secondary, are found to express the prostate antigen. In this report (Nadji et al., 1981), the antigen was detected in 79/79 of primary prostatic tumors and 49/49 metastatic prostate tumors. Other tumors, 79 of nonprostatic origin, contain no prostate antigen, including 17 of urinary bladder tumor with extension to the prostate gland.

Using immunological peak enhancement experiments, the immunological relationship between prostate antigen in prostate tissue and serum from prostate cancer patients has been studied (Papsidero et al., 1980b). The immunological identity of serum and tissue prostatic antigen has been shown. A single immunoprecipitin line from mixed specimens of prostate tissue and serum from prostate cancer patients was also obtained by a two-dimensional immunoelectrophoresis and isoelectric focusing technique. Using antibody affinity chromatography and radioimmunoprecipitation techniques, the antigen in sera from prostatic cancer patients was purified and subjected to sodium dodecyl sulfate electrophoresis. Results revealed that the serum-borne antigen exhibited a molecular weight of approximately 36,000, similar to that of the antigen isolated from prostate tissues.

Therefore, it can be concluded that the serum-borne prostate antigen is immunologically identical and biochemically similar to that of prostate tissue origin.

A sensitive sandwich-type enzyme immunoassay technique using cyanogen bromide-activated Sepharose 4B-conjugated antiprostate antigen IgG antibodies and peroxidase-conjugated antiprostate antigen IgG antibodies has been developed (Kuriyama et al., 1980a). Sensitivity of the assay is 0.01 ng/mL. With this sensitive enzyme immunoassay technique, the distribution of prostate antigen in extracts from prostate and other tissues was investigated. Since the enzyme immunoassay technique can detect prostatic acid phosphatase at the concentration of 0.01 ng, it is much more sensitive than immunodiffusion or rocket immunoelectrophoresis. And unlike the immunoperoxidase technique, the enzyme immunoassay also is quantitative. Again, significant amounts of prostate antigen are found only in prostate tissue, regardless of pathological origin. Normal, benign, and malignant prostate appear to contain a similar amount of prostate antigen. No other tissues examined, including normal kidney and bladder, contain this antigen as detected at the sensitivity of 0.01 ng.

Using the sensitive enzyme immunoassay technique, serum prostate antigen levels from normal controls, from patients with prostate cancer and from patients with cancers of nonprostatic origin have been determined. Values obtained with normal male subjects showed an upper limit of 1.792 ng of prostate antigen/mL of serum. No prostate antigen was detected in serum of normal females or female cancer patients, and antigen in the normal range was found in patients with cancers other than prostate. The majority of patients with prostate cancer was found to contain an elevated circulating prostate antigen, although some patients with benign prostatic hypertrophy also had an elevated level. From an initial clinical evaluation, results indicated that elevated prostate antigen was found in 69% of patients with benign prostatic hypertrophy, 63% of clinical stage A prostate cancer, 80% of stage B, 77% of stage C, and 86% of stage D, with only 4% of patients with nonprostatic cancer showing an elevated prostate antigen level. Statistical analysis revealed no significant difference between nonprostate cancer patients and normal males, but patients with benign prostatic hypertrophy and all stages of prostate cancer showed significant differences ($p < 0.001$). In comparison with benign prostatic hypertrophy, stage A prostate cancer showed no difference, whereas stage B revealed a suggestive difference ($p < 0.010$), and stage C or D prostate cancer showed an apparent statistically significant difference ($p < 0.01$ and <0.001, respectively).

Potential prognostic value of circulating prostate antigen was studied in patients with stage D_2 prostate cancer. These patients all were resistant to hormone therapy and showed no response to other chemotherapeutic agents. Results revealed that the lower the mean value of prostate antigen before treatment, the longer the survival time (Kuriyama et al., 1980b). For example, prostate antigen levels in patients who survived no longer than 5 months were statistically higher than those of other groups who survived more than 5 months. Therefore, the pretreatment circulating prostate antigen value appears to be of prognostic value. In addition, serial prostate antigen measurements can be used to monitor the efficacy of treatment with stage D prostate cancer. In patients with stage B prostate cancer, after radical prostatectomy, elevation of prostate antigen can proceed months before disease recurrence.

Therefore, data obtained so far indicate that prostate antigen is a new marker for prostate cancer, although it is a histotypic product of the human prostate. Furthermore, it has been found that the prostate antigen level in the serum is unrelated to serum prostatic acid phosphatase level. Therefore, simultaneous determinations of circulating prostate antigen and prostatic acid phosphatase levels may provide a more sensitive measurement than either test alone in detecting patients with prostate cancer.

4. Alkaline Phosphatase

The potential value of the activities of serum alkaline phosphatase and its isoenzymes in prostate cancer has been reported. In a series of randomly selected patients with prostate cancer, stage D_2, who underwent various treatment protocols, the pretreatment levels of total alkaline phosphatase were found to be of prognostic significance for treatment response (Wajsman et al., 1978). Patients with total alkaline phosphatase values less than 150 mU/mL have a more favorable response than those having values of 150 or greater. Similarly, pretreatment levels of bone alkaline phosphatase isoenzyme and liver alkaline phosphatase isoenzyme were analyzed in respect to patients' responses to treatment. Again, those patients who had normal levels of liver alkaline phosphatase or only slightly elevated values were found to have a better response rate than those who had abnormal liver alkaline phosphatase activities. Patients with normal bone alkaline phosphatase isoenzyme activities also showed a favorable response to chemotherapy. Patients with normal pretreatment levels of alkaline phosphatase also had a significantly longer survival time. Patients with a poor survival rate were those who had the most highly elevated total alkaline phosphatase activities. From studies of survival rate versus bone alkaline phosphatase isoenzyme activity, it has been shown that patients at highest risk were those with the most highly elevated pretreatment bone alkaline phosphatase activities (Killian et al., 1981). Similarly, pretreatment liver alkaline phosphatase isoenzyme activity also demonstrated a similar effect.

The carcinoplacental isoenzyme called Regan alkaline phosphatase also has been found in some patients with advanced prostatic cancer (Slack et al., 1981). Approximately 18% of patients exhibited an elevated level of Regan isoenzyme of alkaline phosphatase, a frequency similar to those reported by other investigators for most other tumor types. Serial Regan isoenzyme activities of alkaline phosphatase were found to have no correlation with the patient's general disease characteristics or response to chemotherapy.

5. Ribonuclease (RNase)

RNase has been reported to be associated with many types of cancers, particularly with cancer of the pancreas. Over 70% of patients with advanced prostate cancer exhibited elevated serum RNase activities (Chu et al., 1975). RNase of human prostatic origin has been isolated (Lee et al., 1979). Four proteins exhibiting RNase activities were purified from human seminal plasma. Although the study of substrate specificities revealed that prostate RNase is similar to that of pancreatic RNase, the prostate RNase appeared to exhibit different immunologic characteristics from pancreatic RNase, since antisera produced against the prostatic RNase do not cross-react with pancreatic RNase. Whether or not a specific immunoassay can be developed that reveals a diagnostic value for prostatic RNase remains to be determined.

6. Polyamines

Elevation of polyamines in erythrocytes in cancer patients has been reported to be associated with increased cell proliferation and correlated with nucleic acid concentrations in rapidly growing tissues (Russell et al., 1973). Polyamines, therefore, may be sensitive biochemical markers for monitoring therapies of prostate cancer patients. Automated methods using high performance liquid chromatography or amino acid analyzer to determine polyamines in blood specimens have been developed (Russell et al., 1973; Killian et al., 1980a). Serial polyamines in erythrocytes from prostatic cancer patients have been analyzed. Clinico-pathological correlations indicated that polyamine levels in erythrocytes, as determined serially from prostate cancer patients undergoing treatment, have been shown to be useful in following the therapeutic response of these patients (Killian et al., 1980a).

7. Conclusions

The most promising markers for prostate cancer, at the present stage of development, are prostate acid phosphatase and the newly identified prostate antigen. Clinical application of prostatic acid phosphatase in the diagnosis of prostate cancer is well known. Several new immunoassay procedures, developed recently, are being investigated extensively and shown to be of possible use in early detection of this malignancy. Although prostatic acid phosphatase has been reported for several decades, knowledge of its biological function in prostate gland is totally lacking. Biological studies of this enzyme, therefore, should be the next logical extension of investigation. Data available to date have shown the new prostate antigen to be a great potential marker for prostate cancer. It should be noted that both prostatic acid phosphatase and prostate antigen are tissue type-specific proteins for the prostate, and are of cytoplasmic origin. These characteristics are somewhat different from those of other tumor markers. Physiology and pathology of the prostate now can be be studied with the aid of these markers for prostatic gland epithelium.

Acknowledgment

The work reported here has been supported in part by Research Grants CA-15126, CA-15437, and CA-23990, awarded by the National Cancer Institute.

References

American Cancer Society, (1979), *Facts on Prostate Cancer*, p. 3
Belville, W. D., H. D. Cox, D. E. Mahan, J. P. Olmert, B. T. Mittenmayer, and A. W. Bruce (1978), *Cancer* **41**, 2286.
Catane, R., Z. Wajsman, T. M. Chu, and G. P. Murphy (1978), *N. Y. State J.Med.* **78**, 1060.
Choe, B. K., E. J. Pontes, S. Bloink, and N. R. Rose (1978a), *Arch. Androl.* **1**, 236.
Choe, B. K., E. J. Pontes, M. K. Morrison, and N. R. Rose (1978b), *Arch. Androl.* **1**, 227.
Choe, B. K., E. J. Pontes, N. R. Rose, M. Koral, and E. J. Pontes (1980), *Proc. Soc. Exptl. Biol. Med.* **162**, 396.
Chu, T. M., W. Ostrowski, M. J. Varkarakis, C. Merrin, and G. P. Murphy, (1975), *Cancer Chemotherapy Rept.* **59**, 97.
Chu, T. M., M. C. Wang, R. Kajdasz, R. Kucil, and G. P. Murphy (1976), *Proc. Am. Assoc. Cancer Res.* **17**, 191.
Chu, T. M. (1977), *Antibiot. Chemother.* **22**, 121.

Chu, T. M., M. C. Wang, L. Valenzuela, C. Merrin, and G. P. Murphy (1978a), *Oncology* **35**, 198.

Chu, T. M., M. C. Wang, W. W. Scott, R. P. Gibbons, D. E. Johnson, J. D. Schmidt, S. A. Leoning, G. R. Prout, and G. P. Murphy (1978b), *Invest. Urol.* **15**, 319.

Cooper, J. F., and A. G. Foti (1974), *Invest. Urol.* **12**, 98.

Cooper, J. F., A G. Foti, and P. W. Shank (1978), *J. Urol.* **119**, 392.

Drucker, J. R., C. W. Moncure, C. L. Johnson, M. J. Smith, and W. W. Kootz (1978), *J. Urol.* **119**, 94.

Foti, A. G., H. Herschman, and J. F. Cooper (1975), *Cancer Res.* **35**, 2446.

Foti, A. G., H. Herschman, J. F. Cooper, and H. Imfeld (1976), *Arch. Biochem. Biophys.* **176**, 154.

Foti, A. G., J. F. Cooper, H. Herschman, and R. R. Malbaez (1977), *New Engl. J. Med.* **297**, 1357.

Gittes, R. F., and T. M. Chu (1976), *Semin. Oncology* **3**, 123.

Griffiths, J. C. (1980), *Clin. Chem.* **26**, 433.

Gursel, E. O., M. Rezvan, F. A. Sy, and R. J. Veenema (1974), *J. Urol.* **111**, 53.

Gutman, A. B., and E. N. Gutnam (1938), *J. Clin. Invest.* **17**, 473.

Killian, C. S., F. P. Vargas, S. Beckley, Z. Wajsman, G. P. Murphy, and T. M. Chu (1980a), *Clin. Chem.* **26**, 983.

Killian, C. S., F. P. Vargas, C. L. Lee, M. C. Wang, G. P.. Murphy, and T. M. Chu (1980b), *Invest. Urol.* **18**, 219.

Killian, C. S., F. P. Vargas, E. J. Pontes, N. Slack, G. P. Murphy, and T. M. Chu (1981), *Prostate* (in press).

Kuriyama, M., M. C. Wang, L. D. Papsidero, C. S. Killian, T. Shimano, L. A. Valenzuela, T. Nishuira, G. P. Murphy, and T. M. Chu (1980a), *Cancer Res.* **40**, 4658.

Kuriyama, M., M. C. Wang, L. D. Papsidero, G. P. Murphy, and T. M. Chu (1980b), *Proc. Amer. Assoc. Center Res.* **21**, 207.

Lee, C. L., M. C. Wang, G. P. Murphy, and T. M. Chu (1978), *Cancer Res.* **38**, 2871.

Lee, C. L., G. P. Murphy, and T. M. Chu (1979), *Fed. Proc.* **38**, 498.

Lee, C. L., T. M. Chu, Z. Wajsman, N. H. Slack, and G. P. Murphy (1980a), *Urol.* **15**, 338.

Lee, C. L., C. S. Killian, G. P. Murphy, and T. M. Chu (1980b), *Clin. Chim. Acta* **101**, 209.

Lee, C. L., G. P. Murphy, and T. M. Chu (1980c), *Fed. Proc.* **39**, 413.

Li, S., M. C. Wang, and T. M. Chu (1981), unpublished data.

Mahan, D. E., and D. P. Doctor (1979), *Clin. Biochem.* **12**, 10.

Marshall, S., R. P. Lyon, and M. P. Scott (1974), *Urol.* **4**, 435.

MacDonald, I., N. R. Rose, E. J. Pontes, and B. K. Choe (1978), *Arch. Androl.* **1**, 225

McTigue, J. J., and R. L. Van Etten (1978a), *Biochim. Biophys. Acta* **523**, 422.

McTique, J. J., and R. L. Van Etten (1978b), *Biochim. Biophys. Acta* **523**, 407.

Nadji, M., S. Z. Tabei, A. Castro, T. M. Chu, M. C. Wang, and A. R. Morales (1981), *Cancer* (in press).

Ostrowski, W. (1968), *Acta Biochem Polonica* **15**, 213.

Papsidero, L. D., M. Kuriyama, M. C. Wang, J. S. Horoszewicz, J. J. Leong, L. A. Valenzuela, G. P. Murphy, and T. M. Chu (1981), *J. Natl. Cancer Inst.* **66,** 37.

Papsidero, L. D., M. C. Wang, L. A. Valenzuela, G. P. Murphy, and T. M. Chu (1980), *Cancer Res.* **40,** 2428.

Pontes, E. J., B. K. Choe, N. R. Rose, and J. M. Pierce (1978), *J. Urol.* **119,** 772.

Reynolds, R. D., B. R. Greenberg, C. D. Martin, R. N. Lucas, C. N. Gaffney, and L. Hawn (1973), *Cancer* **32,** 181.

Romas, A. N., K. C. Hsu, P. Tomashefsky, and M. Tannenbaum (1978), *Urol.* **12,** 79.

Russell, D. (1973), In *Polyamines in Normal and Neoplastic Growth* (Russell, D., ed.), Raven Press, New York.

Schwartz, M. K., M. Fleisher, and D. Bodansky (1969), *Ann. N.Y. Acad. Sci.* **166,** 775.

Shulman, S., L. Mamrod, M. J. Gonder, and W. A. Soones (1964), *J. Immunol.* **93,** 474.

Slack, N. H., T. M. Chu, Z. Wasjman, and G. P. Murphy (1981), *Cancer* **47,** 146.

Van Etten, R. L., and M. S. Saini (1978), *Clin. Chem.* **24,** 1525.

Vihko, P., M. Konturri, and L. K. Korhonen (1978a), *Clin. Chem.* **24,** 466.

Vihko, P., Sanjati, L. Peltnonen, and R. Vihko (1978b), *Clin. Chem.* **25,** 1915.

Wajsman, Z., T. M. Chu, D. Bross, J. Saroff, and G. P. Murphy (1978), *J. Urol.* **119,** 244.

Wajsman, Z., T. M. Chu, J. Saroff, N. Slack, and G. P. Murphy (1979), *Urol.* **13,** 8.

Wang, M. C., L. Valenzuela, G. P. Murphy, and T. M. Chu (1979), *Invest. Urol.* **17,** 159.

Yam, L. T. (1974), *Am. J. Med.* **56,** 604.

Yarrison, G., B. F. Mertens, and J. C. Mathies (1976), *Am. J. Clin. Path.* **66,** 667.

9

Breast Cancer Markers

Thomas S. Edgington and Robert M. Nakamura

*Department of Molecular Immunology, Research Institute of
Scripps Clinic, La Jolla, California*

1. Introduction

There has been considerable interest in the identification of markers for neoplasms of the human breast. Investigation has included the search for not only discrete molecular markers, but also tumor-specific antigens recognized by the tumor-bearing host and a variety of immune responses of the host that may be associated with carcinoma of the breast. In spite of a substantial body of study, it is fair to say that there is no generally accepted, well-validated, and highly effective single marker or set of markers for the diagnosis, monitoring, or therapy of breast carcinoma on the basis of assay of serum or other body fluids. Histopathological examination remains at the core of definitive diagnosis and prognosis.

Clinical studies have explored the use of oncodevelopmental antigens, differentiation products, and tumor-associated markers. A few candidate tumor-specific antigens have recently been described. These offer potential not only to elucidate basic events in the cell biology of mammary neoplasia, but if established as valid tumor-specific antigens they should also permit analysis of the specificity of the host response in this form of neoplasia. Such immune responses may add a new dimension to the diagnosis and monitoring of tumors. Other byproducts of establishing markers (whether tumor-specific antigens, tumor-associated antigens, or oncodevelopmental antigens) include the potential to image tumors in vivo with labeled purified antibody or hybridoma antibodies. This has been explored in experimental settings and in prototype clinical studies. Treatment of neoplasia of the human breast could also be facilitated by derivative approaches in the future. To facilitate orderly consideration of tumor cell markers in this review, they are taxonomically considered within six classes: (1) candidate tumor-specific antigens; (2) oncodevelopmental markers; (3) differentiation markers; (4) other tumor-associated markers; (5) immune response markers; and (6) genetic markers.

2. Structure of the Breast

The breast is composed of an anatomically restricted and functionally specialized mammary fat pad and its glandular elements. The mammary fat pad plays a specialized role in which it induces, under appropriate genetic and endocrine influences, growth of the epithelial elements of the mammary gland from the cutaneous surface. This structure is virtually nonexistent during fetal development, appearing later as a specialized exocrine gland closely related to sweat glands. Arising at the nipple are from 6 to 15 major ducts, with each major duct in turn supplying a lobe of the breast. These major ducts branch repeatedly until reduced in size to a network of small ducts each of which supplies one of the *terminal ductal lobular units* (Wellings et al., 1975). These latter ducts, termed the *extralobular terminal ducts,* are lined by columnar epithelial cells and they branch to form the *intralobular terminal duct.* This latter duct is lined by cuboidal epithelium and it represents the central and intrinsic stem of each *lobule.* The intralobular terminal duct branches in a racemose fashion giving rise to a large number of blind ductules lined by cuboidal epithelium.

The epithelium of the entire terminal ductular lobular unit is hormone-sensitive and subject to induction in the process of lactation. Following growth of the mammary gland during puberty, it is maintained in a maturated state during adulthood of the female. Regression and atrophy follows; and a number of dysplastic events are common, probably as a byproduct of endocrine stimulation. Neoplasia is a relatively infrequent event in the female breast if one considers the frequency of about 300 cases per million subjects per year; however, it does represent one of the three most frequent forms of human cancer and a disease of great concern.

3. Diseases of the Breast

A simplified, but nonetheless reasonable hypothesis for the origins and relationships of benign and neoplastic diseases of the mammary gland is illustrated in Fig. 1 and is outlined in greater detail by Wellings (1980). A considerable body of data has been accumulated to support the association of intraductal and intralobular hyperplasia with the occurrence of focal car-

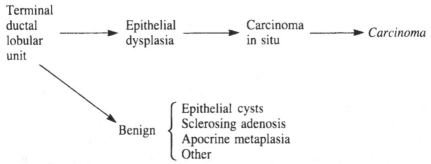

Fig. 1. Proposed sequence of events in progression from normal mammary gland to carcinoma according to Wellings (1980).

cinoma in situ. These observations, though unable to unequivocally establish a causal relationship per se, suggest that the early in situ neoplastic lesion could arise either: (i) in parallel with the hyperplastic lesions or (ii) sequentially from the hyperplastic lesions. A series of cytologic changes in the mammary epithelium, beginning with cytologically normal cells and culminating in neoplastic cells, has been proposed. A progressive increase of epithelial atypia can be observed and transitions to legitimate carcinoma in situ can be illustrated in some tissues. This and other data have suggested a series that is proposed by Wellings (1980).

This neoplastic evolution as proposed embodies a *minimum* of two steps: (1) the transition from normal to preneoplastic epithelium, equated with cytologically atypical cells; and (2) the transition from preneoplastic cells to fully invasive neoplastic cells via non-invasive carcinoma in situ (Fig. 1). This has been extensively investigated in murine mammary carcinomas by DeOme and Medina (1969), Cardiff et al. (1977), and Medina (1978). Indeed, whether two or more steps may be required, it is interesting that the progression from normal mammary epithelium to frank invasive breast carcinoma has been estimated to require as long as 10–20 years in the human.

It should be noted that there is evidence that the atypical or putative preneoplastic lesions need not progress inexorably to neoplasia, but may regress. Thus, when any consideration of markers is raised, it is essential to determine whether the marker is specific for the invasive carcinoma, carcinoma in situ, or whether it may be expressed by some preneoplastic cells. If the marker reflects key events in the biology of the cell in its progression to the neoplastic state, it may appear before other features such as histopathology or cytology permit unequivocal identification of neoplastic cells. Markers for the various states of progression from normal to early neoplastic lesions could prove to be invaluable aids in analysis of the biology of the human breast and its diseases; and selective application might be of aid in clinical diagnosis or management.

Any consideration of markers for carcinoma of the breast cannot proceed without some mention of the most common benign disease, fibrocystic disease (mammary dysplasia, chronic cystic mastitis). This common disease or group of closely related diseases (Haagensen, 1971), appears to represent a hormonally influenced polymorphic imbalance of the growth of the female mammary gland. Both stromal and epithelial elements may be influenced to a variable degree. There is considerable evidence to suggest an increased incidence of carcinoma in breasts with fibrocystic disease, particularly the more florid or hyperplastic forms of the disease (Charteris, 1930; Foote and Stewart, 1945; and Fisher and Paulson, 1978, to mention a few). Since more than 50% of normal breasts are involved to some degree by at least mild forms of fibrocystic disease (Frantz et al., 1951; Wellings et al., 1975) it is difficult, if not impossible, to imply any form of requisite progression. Reliable markers for distinguishing the polymorphic features of fibrocystic disease in its various forms from preneoplastic lesions, carcinoma in situ, and invasive carcinoma would be a major advance. Analysis of the biology of the breast, the relationships of the different types of benign lesions, and more critical examination of the various forms of benign but putative preneoplastic lesions as attempted by Wellings (1980) and many others would greatly benefit from the development of a variety of objective differentiation markers for the mammary epithelium and of markers for steps in the progression from normal epithelium to the neoplastic cell.

4. Oncodevelopmental Markers

Under this category of tumor markers are considered those that are most prominently expressed during embryonic fetal development and thus present at higher concentration in tissues or body fluids during intrauterine development. Classical examples of this group of markers are alphafetoprotein and carcinoembryonic antigen (CEA). In consideration of breast carcinoma, CEA has been of some interest, whereas alphafetoprotein was absent in a study of 91 carcinomas of the breast (Edgington and Nakamura, unpublished observations). The isoferritins are a more specialized example. Oncodevelopmental markers are not intrinsically tumor-specific, but may be present at higher concentrations in tumor cells than in the normally differentiated cells of the breast. This can be thought of as a biochemical mirror of the characteristic cytologic and functional features of tumor cells, which suggest "dedifferentiation" with recapitulation of more embryonic cytology.

4.1. Beta Oncofetal Antigen (BOFA)

This antigen originally described as an oncodevelopmental marker by Fritsche and Mach (1975), was identified with heteroantisera raised against fractions of colon carcinoma extracts. The antigen was observed to have a beta-electrophoretic mobility and was referred to as beta oncofetal antigen or BOFA. The antigen was isolated by aqueous extraction, ion exchange, chromatography of the ultracentrifugal supernatant, and molecular exclusion chromatography. The antisera reacted with an apparently identical molecule in extracts of carcinomas of the breast, colon, lung, liver, pancreas, and also melanomas. It was also observed to react with extracts from a variety of tissues of 16-week gestation from the human fetus, suggesting an oncodevelopmental characteristic. BOFA was estimated to have a molecular weight of 70,000–90,000, and it was also demonstrated to be pronase-sensitive, suggesting that it is a protein. A buoyant density of 1.30–1.32 g/mL suggests a modest carbohydrate content. BOFA was also demonstrated in the plasma of normal adults as well as the plasma of fetuses and of cancer patients. Attempts to apply BOFA assays of serum to diagnosis of cancer were quite unsuccessful. Goldenberg et al. (1978) subsequently reported the characteristics of BOFA and provided independent evidence that this molecule could also be found at *high* concentration in some normal tissues, e.g., spleen. These observations cast considerable doubt on the oncodevelopmental classification of BOFA. The plasma concentrations of BOFA in cancer patients or in fetuses was not significantly higher than in normal individuals, supporting the identity of BOFA as a normal tissue protein rather than an oncodevelopmental molecule.

4.2. Ferritin and Isoferritins

Ferritin is a cellular iron-storage protein that is found in most mammalian tissues. In many tissues ferritin exists in multiple molecular forms, referred to as isoferritins, differing in structure and metabolism. The differing isoferritin forms result from different proportions of acid and basic subunits. The patterns of isoferritins differ between tissues; however, in addition to the normal spectrum of isoferritins most effectively analyzed by isoelectric focusing or other electrophoretic methods, forms at variance with those typical for a given tissue have been observed in human and animal tumor cells. These observations have led to a number of studies of isoferritins in human tumors. Because of the association of certain more acidic isoferritins in both fetal tissue and tumors they have been considered to be oncodevelopmental isoforms (see Drysdale and Singer, 1974).

Much of the surge of interest in isoferritins in breast cancer resulted from a study by Marcus and Zinberg (1974) in which they described an antiserum to breast tumors that reacted strongly with neoplastic mammary epithelial cells, but not with the normal breast. The responsible antigen, at first considered a candidate tumor specific antigen, was subsequently purified. In this study the authors employed affinity chromatography using the responsible antibody, followed by molecular exclusion chromatography and ion exchange chromatography. It is now known that this molecule was identical to an antigen detected in human fetal serum (Burtin et al., 1960) which had been referred to by the same laboratory in a subsequent study as α 2-H protein (Buffe et al., 1972). This molecule was identified as an isoferritin by immunochemical criteria as well as by binding of iron. Marcus and Zinberg (1974) observed acidic isoforms that were not observed in extracts of normal liver; and these were refered to as "carcinofetal" ferritins. Similar acidic isoferritins were observed in placenta and HeLa cells at about the same time by Drysdale and Singer (1974).

Employing a radioimmunoassay of serum, Marcus and Zinberg (1975) described increased ferritin levels in 41% of women with mammary carcinomas and 67% of women with locally recurring or metastatic mammary carcinoma (Table 1). The increases were not specific for breast carcinoma, and were observed also in certain forms of hepatic and gastrointestinal inflammatory disease. Shortly thereafter, Jacobs et al., (1976) confirmed the increased incidence of elevated serum ferritin in 229 women with early breast carcinoma; however, the assays that were utilized did not distinguish between normal and the more acidic isoferritin associated with breast tumors. In fact it is quite doubtful that the assays even assessed the increment owing to the acid isoforms since the isoforms also differ immunochemically. Assay of serum ferritin, although statistically increased, was not comparable to the profound increases observed in acute leukemias where elevations of 25-fold or more have been described by Parry et al. (1975).

Table 1

Serum Ferritin in Patients with Carcinoma of the Breast[a]

Diagnosis	Ferritin, ng/mL		
	Mean	Range	Elevated, %
Normal women(117)	34	10–146	
Normal men(57)	93	10–193	
Breast cancer			
Preoperative(38)	199	10–1394	41
Recurrent(97)	621	10–5875	67
Benign diseases			
Hepatic(42)	364	10–3232	43
GI(31)	106	10–786	13

[a]From Marcus and Zinberg, 1975.

The various isoferritins appear to differ immunochemically as a result of differences between the isoform subunits, or perhaps conformational antigens engendered by different assembly of the subunits in the various isoforms. This influences the quantitation by immunologic assays. As a result, accurate quantitative measurement of ferritin in tissues or serum with a single radioimmunoassay is not entirely valid since it is influenced by the relative proportion of acidic and basic isoferritin subunits and their assembly into the ferritin complex. In an attempt to resolve these problems, Drysdale et al. (1977) resolved ferritin into H and HL subunits and suggested that there is a third or L subunit that is derived from the HL subunit. In an attempt to provide more precise assays of acidic isoferritin, Jones et al. (1980) developed assays for both adult splenic ferritin and for acidic isoferritin. The latter was purified from HeLa cells. They explored the usefulness of assays for acidic isoferritin in parallel with assays relatively specific for splenic ferritins. The study encompassed sera from 1000 patients, including normal controls and individuals with solid cancers and leukemia. They studied 149 patients with benign breast disease, 146 with early breast carcinoma, and 148 with advanced breast carcinoma (Table 2). The median concentration of splenic ferritin was higher in individuals with advanced breast cancer and about half of these also had detectable levels of acidic isoferritin in the serum. The acidic isoferritin was not detected in the majority of normal sera (less than 2 ng/mL), though levels as high as 53 ng/mL were observed in sera from some patients with malignant tumors. The acidic isoferritin/splenic ferritin ratio was, however, consistently very low; and the results were not encouraging in regard to use of the acid isoferritin assay for diagnostic or prognostic application in breast cancer.

4.3. Carcinoembryonic Antigen (CEA)

Carcinoembryonic antigen, a model oncodevelopmental molecule, was first identified and isolated in the search for tumor specific antigens. Gold and Freedman (1965) demonstrated this glycoprotein by immunizing rab-

Table 2
Serum Ferritin and Acidic Isoferritin in Association with Carcinoma of the Breast[a]

Study group	Number	Ferritin, ng/mL	Acidic ferritin, ng/mL	Increased acidic ferritin, %
Normal controls	100	33 (1–260)	<2–3.5	7
Benign breast disease	149	44 (4–322)	<2–15.0	14
Breast carcinoma, early	146	48 (3–1313)	<2–17.0	25
Breast carcinoma, advanced	148	132 (6–8360)	<2–53.0	49

[a]From Jones et al., 1980.

bits rendered tolerant to normal colonic epithelium with extracts of human colonic carcinomas. This resulted in an antibody response to a glycoprotein that was subsequently recognized to be an oncodevelopmental molecule rather than a tumor-specific antigen. CEA is, however, not entirely homogeneous. It varies in degree of glycosylation, isoelectric point, and selected other characteristics when isolated from different tissues (reviewed by Plow and Edgington, 1978). It has been suggested by some investigators, e.g., Accinni et al. (1974), that CEA in breast carcinomas may differ from that of gastrointestinal origin.

CEA received wide attention as a potential diagnostic or prognostic tumor marker and has been observed at elevated concentrations in the serum of individuals with a wide variety of malignant tumors in addition to colon carcinomas (Chu and Nemoto, 1973; Concannon et al., 1973; Steward et al., 1974; and others). Serum or plasma CEA is currently not recommended for diagnosis, but has found utility as a prognostic indicator or in assessing the recurrence of tumors. The existence of metastases is also indicated by the absence of a decline of serum or plasma CEA to baseline levels following removal of primary tumors, including carcinomas of the breast. CEA or related glycoprotein species occur in breast carcinoma tissue, as demonstrated by Wahren et al. (1978) using immunohistochemical analyses.

In assessing the use of plasma CEA in breast carcinoma, Chu and Nemoto (1973) studied 136 patients with breast carcinoma for 2 years and found elevations of CEA in 68% of 83 of these patients who had metastases. The frequency of elevated plasma CEA varied and correlated with the site of metastases; e.g., marked elevations of CEA were observed most characteristically in association with hepatic metastases. In these studies, it did not appear that serial CEA determinations could adequately distinguish between tumor regression or progression. However, Steward et al. (1974) subsequently suggested that elevations of plasma CEA in association with primary mammary carcinoma were infrequent and when observed were relatively mild, requiring the use of a threshold of 2.5 ng/mL (Table 3). In their study, only 27% of 22 patients had elevated CEA. In contrast, 79% of patients with metastatic disease had elevated CEA. However, 6% of patients with benign cystic disease also had CEA elevations greater that 2.5 ng/mL. In contrast to Chu and Nemoto (1973), Steward et al. (1974) suggested a trend of serial CEA values that correlated with the response to treatment, i.e., declining values reflecting a decrease in tumor burden.

The use of plasma or serum CEA assays in the monitoring of mammary carcinoma and in providing prognostic information has continued to receive considerable attention. The high frequency of elevations of plasma CEA has been observed as well by Wang et al. (1975) (69% > 2.5 ng/mL), Tormey et al. (1975) (74% > 5.0 ng/mL), and by Wahren et al.

Table 3
CEA as a Marker for Breast Carcinoma[a]

	CEA	
Diagnosis	Mean, ng/mL	>2.5 ng/mL, %
Benign breast disease(17)	0.8	6
Breast carcinoma		
Stage A	1.1	20
Stage B	1.9	14
Stage C	4.8	60
Stage D	9.8	79

[a]From Steward et al., 1974.

(1978) in which 70% of patients with primary breast cancer had levels above 2.5 ng/mL. The concentration of CEA in association with mammary carcinoma may be lower than in patients with equivalent colonic tumor burden. The detection also may differ with assays. Thus, a very low incidence of positive serum assays were observed (14%) with a colonic CEA species (CEA-S) assay (Edgington et al., 1975). In those tumors that produce significant concentrations of CEA, serial monitoring may provide estimates of relative change in tumor burden.

Some studies have been encouraging in regard to the use of serial CEA determinations, including the recent study by Lamerz et al. (1980). They observed that of 1462 patients without metastases following mastectomy, 91% had normal serum CEA levels. In contrast, of 633 patients with metastases, only 45.7% had normal serum CEA following mastectomy. Thus, 54% of patients with metastatic breast cancer had significant serum CEA elevations after mastectomy; and the increases were most significant with metastases to the skin, lung, bone, and liver, or with multiple organ involvement. They also observed a correlation between decreasing levels of CEA and remission, and between persistent or fluctuating levels with stationary disease. Rising serum CEA antedated the clinical response by some weeks to months. This group also used CEA derived from breast cancers in an attempt to improve the specificity of detection of this form of neoplasia. However, this did not appear to influence the results.

Myers et al. (1980) have conducted a thorough analysis of the use of CEA assays in patients with carcinoma of the breast. They observed that the usefulness of CEA depended on the stage of breast carcinoma and that analysis of CEA provides independent information that when coupled with other criteria can be of use. They observed that 73% of all patients with metastatic breast cancer and CEA, if > 4 ng/mL, had significantly shorter survivals (when analysed at 18 months) than patients with < 4 ng/mL CEA. The reader is referred to this paper for further details of the application of CEA to prognosis.

5. Differentiation Markers

Differentiation markers are discrete molecular entities that are a normal product of the mature or differentiated cell type from with the tumor is derived. The mammary gland contains three epithelial cell types, namely myoepithelial cells, alveolar epithelial cells, and ductal epithelium. The exact origins are debated, but most carcinomas probably arise from the latter. Differentiation markers are not tumor-specific, but can be of potential utility in identifying the histogenetic origin of a tumor, or assessing the potential degree of differentiation of the tumor. If released into the body fluids, they have potential utility in diagnostic, prognostic, or monitoring modalities. Two types of markers can be considered. The first are soluble products of certain modes of differentiation, e.g., lactation. The second are relatively fixed cellular markers that may identify the cell and its pathway of differentiation. It is within this conceptual approach that attention has been addressed to the use of casein, a milk protein. Although primarily an induced differentiation product of the lactating breast, increases in serum levels could be derived from neoplastic mammary epithelial cells that produce small amounts of casein, and as a consequence of their invasive properties are anatomically displaced so as to preclude secretion of the casein into the normal mammary gland lumen. Similarly, other differentiation products of lactation may be observed in some tumors and they might prove useful. These include alpha-lactalbumin, which has received some clinical evaluation. Studies of cellular differentiation have most recently addressed the proteins of the milk fat globule, markers of the apical plasmalemma of mammary epithelium recovered from the functional lactating breast cell. Other differentiation products include the estrogen and progesterone receptors and secretory products such as cyst fluid proteins.

5.1. Hormone Receptors

Hormone receptors, specifically those for estrogen and for progesterone, have been the topic of extensive investigation. They are not specific for the epithelium of the mammary gland, but are clinically useful. They are comprehensively reviewed by McGuire (1978, 1979) and by Thompson and Lippman (1979). The presence or absence of receptors is now often used to select the appropriate therapy.

5.2. Casein

The synthesis of kappa-casein by the mammary epithelium progressively increases during pregnancy (Zangerle et al., 1976). There is a significant difference between mean serum levels of kappa-casein in the 4th to 10th weeks of pregnancy compared to the 30th to 40th weeks of pregnancy. The mean serum kappa-casein level increases during lactation and is found to reach a maximum on the fourth day following delivery. The possibility that mammary carcinomas may produce casein was suggested by Turkington and Riddle (1969) from observations of a "casein-like fluid" in a rat mammary carcinoma cultivated in vitro. Young et al. (1976) made similar observations and extended their review to human breast carcinomas in culture (Engel and Young, 1978). In the latter review only 9 cultures had been tested and three were positive for casein. Normal production of casein by the mammary epithelium is dependent on prolactin stimulation (Little, 1972). Whether additional cultures would have synthesized casein upon appropriate prolactin stimulation or a more optimal nutritional environment is open to question. However, it appears that casein may be an *elective* marker. By this is meant that not all tumors may express this gene product.

In an evaluation of the potential for kappa-casein as a diagnostic marker, it is reasonable to consider that this cellular product would escape into the lymph from invasive carcinoma cells producing kappa-casein. A radioimmunoassay for kappa-casein was developed and evaluated as an index of mammary function and as a tumor marker by Zangerle et al. (1976, 1978). They also demonstrated by immunofluorescence that human breast cancer tissue cells may contain casein (Zangerle et al., 1976). Hendrick and Franchimont (1974) reported previously from the same laboratory that a significant number of patients with breast cancer had elevated levels of circulating casein.

Woods et al. (1977) similarly measured kappa-casein concentrations on patients with breast diseases and observed that 55.6% of patients with metastatic breast cancer and 39.6% of patients with localized breast cancer (with or without tumor in regional lymph nodes) had elevated kappa-casein concentration greater than 50 ng/mL. They observed that 15.2% patients with benign breast disease also had elevated serum kappa-casein, whereas in normal controls only 4.7% were increased above 60 ng/mL. All 62 samples from lactating women had kappa-casein levels from 135 to 1700 ng/mL.

The value of serum kappa-casein as a screening test for breast cancer is limited by the high percentage (15.2%) of positive values in patients in histologically proven benign breast disease and a high number of negative results in patients subsequently found to be diagnosed as breast cancer.

5.3. Alpha-lactalbumin

Alpha-lactalbumin is a differentiation marker that is not specific for the breast, but is frequently produced by tumor cells (Engel and Young, 1978). It is a protein that is important for the conversion of glucose to lactose in the formation of milk and it serves to modify the lactose synthetase reaction (Fitzgerald et al., 1970). The protein is synthesized by differentiated breast epithelial cells, and the concentration of alpha-lactalbumin increases during lactation and falls with involution (Walker, 1979). Alpha-lactalbumin has been demonstrated to be present in the cytosol of human breast carcinomas by radioimmunoassay (Woods et al., 1979), and may be a reasonably promising marker of breast cell differentiation. Walker (1979) demonstrated with an immunoperoxidase method that alpha-lactalbumin could be cytologically localized to tumor cells in 51 of 100 human breast carcinomas. There was no requisite relationship between synthesis of alpha-lactalbumin and histologic differentiation and the absence or presence of lymph node metastasis.

With use of a sensitive radioimmunoassay procedure, Kleinberg et al. (1979) have found that alpha-lactalbumin was detectable in 8 of 25 normal men and 18 of 44 normal women. Significantly higher levels of alpha-lactalbumin were found in 17 of 19 women during pregnancy who were not actively lactating.

However, the reported finding of alpha-lactalbumin in the blood of both men and women has been shown to result from a commonly occurring cross reaction. Laurence (1978) identified antibodies to bovine alpha-lactalbumin that is present in about half of the plasma samples tested (Woods et al., 1979). The latter workers developed a modified assay to negate this interference and noted that alpha-lactalbumin could be detected in the plasma of healthy premenopausal women but not in the plasma of normal postmenopausal women.

Schultz and Ebner (1977) developed a radioimmunoassay with sensitivity to 0.1 ng/mL sample, and demonstrated that 25% of the sera of patients with breast cancer had significant levels of alpha-lactalbumin prior to surgery with disappearance following resection of the tumor. Woods et al. (1979) noted a significant increase in plasma alpha-lactalbumin in one-quarter of postmenopausal patients with disseminated breast cancer. More extensive clinical trials of alpha-lactalbumin assay promises to be of interest.

5.4. Mammary Gland Cyst Fluid Protein

Haagensen et al. described in 1977 a new marker protein, a differentiation product of the mammary and salivary ductal epithelium that is found in high concentration in the fluid from gross cystic disease of the human breast. In this disease, considered by Haagensen (1971) as distinct from fibrocystic disease, aspiration of cyst fluid can be performed. This fluid has been analyzed in detail by Haagensen et al. (1979a), with the identification of four major proteins. One of 15,000 mw by SDS-polyacrylamide gel electrophoresis appeared to be specific for cyst fluid and was not present in plasma by simple immunologic analyses. It was found in human milk, saliva, and by radioimmunoassay. The concentrations of this glycoprotein, designated GCDFP-15, was 7–81 ng/mL. It should be noted that Neville has suggested (personal communication) that this may readily aggregate and occur as polymers. This protein may be the same as EMGP-70 (Imam et al., 1981); however, this remains to be formally established.

Of normal control women, 85% had plasma levels of GCDFP-15 below 50 ng/mL (Haagensen, 1977a) whereas 42% of patients with gross cystic disease of the breast had levels of GCDFP-15 greater than 50 ng/mL plasma (Table 4). Among breast carcinoma patients, the frequency of elevation differed with the stage of disease. Elevations above 50 ng/mL plasma varied from 24% in localized carcinoma to 41% with extensive axillary lymph node involvement and 54% in patients with clinically evident metastases. Elevations above 150 ng/mL were highly significant, being observed in only 30% of patients with clear evidence of metastases. This was most pronounced in osseous metastases.

In two studies using parallel analyses of CEA and GCDFP-15 in plasma (Haagensen et al., 1978, 1980), 216 patients under treatment for metastatic breast carcinoma were studied. One hundred eleven (51%) had abnormally elevated plasma levels of CEA and/or of GCDFP-15. Abnormal plasma levels of CEA were present in 73 patients whereas abnormal GCDFP levels present in 67. Twenty nine of the patients had increased plasma levels of both markers, whereas 44 had increased CEA only and 38 had increased GCDFP-15 only. These two markers thus varied independently of each other in 74% of the patients. Abnormal plasma levels of one

Table 4
Gross Cyst Disease Fluid Protein and Breast Disease[a]

| Diagnosis | Number | GCDFP-15 | |
		>50 ng/mL, %	>150 ng/mL, %
Normal	145	14	0
Gross cystic disease	90	28	0
Benign breast disease	186	16	0
Breast carcinoma			
Stages A and B	154	24	0
Metastatic disease	138	54	30

[a]From Haagensen et al., 1977.

or both markers were present in 74% of the patients with bone metastases, 53% of patients with visceral metastases, but only 26% with soft tissue metastases. It was further suggested that CEA plus GCDFP-15 assays might prove clinically useful in monitoring responsiveness to therapy. An increased concentration of either was indicative of disease progression, and a decreasing plasma level indicative of regression.

In one study (Haagensen et al., 1980), the utility of the dual CEA plus GCDFP-15 assays in evaluating progression and response to therapy of patients with metastases to bone was emphasized. Responses to therapy are most difficult to evaluate in this group. Serial determination of plasma CEA and GCDFP-15 suggested that more objective indication of disease progression and regression could be achieved than with the currently standard X-ray and bone scans.

5.5. Milk Fat Globule Proteins

As a source of mammary epithelial plasmalemma, the milk fat globule (Keenan et al., 1970) has attracted considerable recent attention. These particles of lipid surrounded by membrane are derived from the apical plasma membrane of lactating mammary acinar epithelium (Patton and Keenan, 1975). This is a complex cellular membrane containing surface differentiation antigens (Ceriani et al., 1977) demonstrable by immuno-fluorescence in mammary epithelial cells. One of these referred to as Epithelial Membrane Glycoprotein (EMGP-70) has recently been isolated and characterized (Imam et al., 1981). Using immunohistochemical reactions, this protein has been demonstrated only in the apical plasma membrane of epithelial cells lining the ducts of both normal and lactating breasts. When poorly differentiated epithelium of breast carcinomas were examined, this glycoprotein, or an antigenically related material, was observed in the cytoplasm rather than at the membrane. The pattern of distribution and cytologic distribution differed from normal and represents a potentially useful marker that merits further study.

Antisera to human mammary epithelial antigens (HME Ags) have been prepared by extraction of milk fat globule membranes, immunization, and absorption of the resultant antisera (Ceriani et al., 1977, 1980). When examined by immunofluorescence, HME Ags were demonstrable on the surface of normal viable human mammary epithelium, as indicated by the surface staining pattern, release of these antigens by proteolysis of the cell surface, and the loss of surface reactions after proteolysis. These antigens were retained in human breast cancer cell lines, e.g., HS578T, though not observed in the benign myoepithelial analogs, e.g., HS578 Bst. In some neoplastic breast cell lines, 10–30% of cells were negative by flow cytofluorimetric assay (Ceriani et al., 1980). The possibility of selective deletion of HME Ags in association with neoplasia was examined by radioimmunoassay and in a single reported study Ceriani et al. (1980) observed slightly lower values in two carcinoma cell lines compared to isolated normal mammary epithelium. In view of the limited number of observations a more detailed study would be desirable.

Milk fat globule membranes have been separated into four major proteins of 150,000, 75,000, 60,000, and 48,000 mw. The latter two are PAS positive glycoproteins (Ceriani et al., 1977). Antibodies specific for the 150,000, 75,000, and 48,000 mw antigens have been produced and used to show the presence and specificity of each for mammary epithelium and presence on a breast carcinoma cell line. Shed HME Ags have been demonstrated in the serum of nude mice bearing human breast carcinoma; and specificity was indicated by appropriate controls (Ceriani et al., 1980). In addition, these same investigators have demonstrated the feasibility of in vivo imaging of radiolabeled antibodies to HME Ags on passageable human breast carcinomas in nude mice. The number of specificities as well as quality of available reagents is currently being expanded by use of hybridoma technology.

Currently a variety of monoclonal antibodies to milk fat globulin membrane proteins are being produced and characterized using hybridoma technology. Quite different patterns of reactivity with normal, lactating dysplastic, and neoplastic mammary tissues are being observed. Reports of these reagents are anticipated in the near future.

6. Other Tumor-Associated Molecules

This relatively unrestricted group of markers encompasses those that are not clearly tumor-specific antigens, markers of the differentiation of cells, mammary gland oncodevelopmental markers, or those of the immune response. Such diverse entities as ectopic hormone production, synthesis of β_2-microglobulin, and increased urinary polyamines are representative. Other markers, such as tissue polypeptide antigen (TPA), appear to be a marker of proliferating cells, and may reflect more rapid turnover characteristic of the tumor cell.

6.1. Thomsen-Freidenreich (T) Antigen

The T antigen, first recognized a half century ago on the erythrocyte surface, is now established as a structural precursor of the human erythrocyte blood group MN carbohydrate (Springer and Desai, 1975). As illustrated in Fig. 2, omission of the two ultimate sialic acid residues, or enzymatic removal from the MN structure, results in expression of the T antigen. If the β galactose is omitted during synthesis, the more primitive Tn is expressed. The MN carbohydrate structures and carrier protein occur not

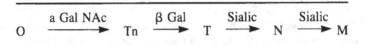

Fig. 2. Structural schematic of the MN carbohydrate radical with the basis of T and Tn antigen expression.

only on erythrocytes, but also on cells of the apocrine glands, such as the salivary gland, as well as the kidney and liver. However, of more interest to the current topic is the incomplete synthesis of this carbohydrate by neoplasms of the breast, colon, and lung with resultant expression of T and very rarely Tn (Springer et al., 1975b, 1976). Enzymatic desialation of the MN structure has been observed in association with bacterial and viral infections, and this also results in expression of the T antigen on cells such as erythrocytes and other cells.

Virtually all adults have humoral anti-T antibodies at relatively high titer. Thus the antibody response is not tumor-associated. In a study of 15 carcinomas of the breast, Springer et al. (1975b) observed T antigen expression by all 15 using human serum anti-T antibody as the analytic reagent. Howard and colleagues (1979, 1980) have confirmed the T antigen expression of breast carcinoma cells using immunocytologic methods, again using human anti-T antibody. They demonstrated that in a small number of benign and malignant breast lesions they could distinguish the malignant from benign mammary epithelial cells by reference to the positive binding of anti-T antibodies by the neoplastic cell (Howard and Taylor, 1979). Subsequently, Howard and Batsakis (1980) utilized a long-known specificity of peanut agglutinin for the T antigen, but coupled it with immunoperoxidase staining, to demonstrate a differential cytologic distribution of binding of peanut agglutinin between benign and neoplastic mammary epithelial cells. The difference between the two reactions and the observed binding of peanut agglutinin to benign cells probably represents the less specific binding of peanut agglutinin; i.e., binding to other β-D-galactose $(1 \rightarrow 3)$-N-acetyl-D-galactosamine containing structures. Similarly, Springer et al. (1980), demonstrated T antigen specificity in all metastatic breast carcinomas and certain other carcinomas that they examined. It was, however, absent from four melanomas and a few other tumors.

Delayed cutaneous hypersensitivity skin reactions to purified T antigen has been observed in breast carcinoma patients, as well as in vitro evidence of cellular immunity to T antigen (Table 5). In this study by Springer et al. (1980) over 85% of ductal breast carcinoma patients and 77% of all breast carcinoma patients gave positive skin tests as compared to about 6% of patients with benign breast disease when tested with purified T antigen. It was also observed (Table 6) that serum anti-T antibody titers were sig-

Table 5
Cellular Immune Responses to Thomsen-Freidenreich (T) Antigen in Patients
with Carcinoma of the Breast[a]

Diagnosis	Leukocyte migration inhibition			Delayed cutaneous hypersensitivity		
	No.	Positive	% Positive	No.	Positive	% Positive
Normal	25	1	4	33	0	0
Benign breast disease	84	11	13	74	4	5
Breast carcinoma	69	25	30	78	60	77

[a]Data from Springer et al., 1980.

Table 6
Humoral Antibody to Thomsen-Freidenreich Antigen
in Patients with Breast Carcinoma[a]

Diagnosis	Number	Decreased anti-T antibody, %
Controls	570	3.6
Breast carcinoma	189	21

[a]From Springer et al., 1980.

nificantly depressed in 21% of 189 individuals with carcinoma of the breast compared to 5% of 270 patients with benign breast disease or 3.6% of 470 other controls (Springer et al., 1976). They interpreted this as in vivo absorption of antibody or induction of immune suppression of this response. This was confirmed by observing increases of anti-T antibody titers following surgical resection of localized carcinomas.

For T antigen, unlike most other markers, we have a well-characterized molecular structure with evidence of systematic expression by breast carcinoma cells as well as other tumors. However, this is clearly not a tumor-specific antigen since it can be expressed under a variety of circumstances, other than neoplasia, including desialation by infectious agents. There is natural immunity to the incomplete carbohydrate structure representative of T, immune tolerance clearly not being established. Nevertheless, potential exists for exploitation in diagnosis, prognosis, and possibly in monitoring of patients with appropriate analytic methods.

6.2. Chorionic Gonadotropin

Human chorionic gonadotropin (HCG) is a product of normal placental metabolism. Ectopic hormone production has been described by a variety of neoplasms; and among these HCG has probably been the most widely observed and certainly the most widely studied. Development of specific radioimmunoassays for HCG as well as subsequent analyses for the alpha and beta chains of HCG have facilitated the detailed analysis of HCG production by tumors including breast carcinomas. Braunstein et al. (1973) utilized a radioimmunoassay specific for HCG, i.e., to the beta chain, and capable of distinguishing HCG from human luteinizing hormone. When the sera of 828 patients with nontesticular tumors were analyzed, HCG was elevated in 4 of 33 patients with breast carcinoma. HCG has since been observed to be elevated in the serum of approximately half of patients with metastatic breast carcinoma and about one-third of patients preoperatively by Tormey et al. (1977). These investigators suggested that elevations of HCG were observed prior to clinical evidence of the recurrence of breast carcinoma. In addition, changes in serum concentrations appeared to reflect therapeutic response or failure. Metastasis to the liver was most frequently associated with elevations of HCG, notably 63% of patients were elevated. These and other data indicate that a relatively high proportion of breast carcinomas are capable of ectopic synthesis of HCG.

The synthesis of this molecule by breast carcinomas appears to reflect aberrant gene expression. In favor of this are the observations of Weintraub et al. (1975) and Rosen and Weintraub (1974) that ectopic HCG synthesis may in some circumstances be associated with an abnormal product. For example, synthesis of only the alpha chain of HCG has been demonstrated. Since only the beta chain is specific for HCG and the alpha chain is nearly identical among four related hormones, analyses of HCG have increasingly adopted reagents specific for the beta chain.

6.3. Calcitonin

The ectopic production of calcitonin has been observed by several types of tumors besides the classical association with Type C cell tumors of the thyroid. Production by breast carcinomas was described by Coombes et al. (1974, 1975). Serum calcitonin, measured by immunoassay, was observed in 22 of 28 patients that they studied with metastatic breast carcinoma. In contrast, only 1 of 13 patients with clinically localized breast carcinoma had elevated serum calcitonin. Elevations of calcitonin have also been observed in association with oat-cell carcinomas of the lung, carcinoid tumors, and pheochromocytomas, thus there is little diagnostic specificity for the origin of the tumor.

6.4. β_2-Microglobulin

β_2-Microglobulin is an 11,800 mw single polypeptide chain molecule that exhibits structural homology with the constant region of immunoglobulin light chain. It appears to represent an evolutionary precursor of light chain, as proposed by Poulik and colleagues (1973, 1975). It is a co-associated chain in cell surface histocompatibility antigens in humans, and is found normally in low concentration in biological fluids.

Three studies have initially demonstrated and subsequently confirmed that β_2-microglobulin frequently occurs in serum at elevated concentrations in patients with advanced tumors (Evrin and Wibell, 1973; Kindt and van Vaerenbergh, 1976; and Poulik, 1979). In the study by Evrin and Wibell, 216 patients were assayed for serum β_2-microglobulin. Because the level of this protein is known to increase with impaired renal function, correction is necessary. Only individuals with serum creatinine in the lower half of the normal range were used in this study. A normal control range was 0.8–2.4 μg/mL serum. Most individuals with serum β_2-microglobulin values of > 3 μg/mL had malignancies, though there were some patients with immunologically mediated diseases and other immunologic disorders in this range. The potential use of β_2-microglobulin as a marker to monitor growth or response to therapy has been considered. Unfortunately, it has provided neither sufficient sensitivity nor the specificity for the clinical stages to aid in initial diagnosis.

Papaioannou et al. (1979) have assessed the potential utility of this marker in 135 patients with breast cancer. Using a solid-phase radioimmunoassay, they observed that there was a significant elevation of β_2-microglobulin associated with advanced metastatic breast cancer. Utilizing an upper normal limit of 2.4 μg/mL, breast cancer patients with Stage I disease had a 30% incidence of elevated β_2-microglobulin; whereas in Stage IV breast cancer β_2-microglobulin was elevated in 50% of patients. Diagnostic application required age-related correction of normal control values since a gradual rise in serum β_2-microglobulin is observed with age. The ratio of serum β_2-microglobulin to creatinine clearance can be used as an index of age-dependent loss of renal function. Whereas Stage I breast cancer patients had a ratio less or equal to 3.1, Stage IV breast cancer patients had ratios of 6.4 or greater. This contrasted with most controls, who did not exceed the ratio of 2.4. They propose that a β_2-microglobulin/creatinine ratio of greater than 3.8 was highly indicative of metastatic breast carcinoma.

6.5. Tissue Polypeptide Antigen

Tissue polypeptide antigen or TPA was described and characterized by Bjorklund and Bjorklund (1957, 1973). TPA is composed of a single polypeptide chain containing predominantly aspartic acid, glutamic acid, and leucine with a mw of 20,000. It appears to be a structural component of cell membranes, apparently localized primarily within the endoplasmic reticulum. TPA was first assayed by passive hemagglutination by the Bjorklunds (1973). More recently Holyoke and Chu (1979) have also conducted clinical evaluations. TPA is not specific for given tissues, nor per-

Table 7
Serum Tissue Polypeptide Antigen in Breast Carcinoma

Diagnosis	CEA >2.4 ng/mL, %	TPA >0.09 U/mL, %
Normal (40)	7.5	12
Benign breast disease (26)	0	27
Localized breast carcinomac (19)	21	53
Metastatic breast carcinoma (67)	61	70

ᵃFrom Nemoto et al., 1979.

haps for the neoplastic cell *per se*. It may reflect increased proliferative rates of cells. It appears at elevated concentrations in the serum in association with a variety of neoplasms including carcinoma of the breast. Nemoto et al. (1979), described the use of dual assays for serum TPA and plasma CEA in 108 patients with breast carcinoma, 26 individuals with benign breast disease, and 40 normal women (Table 7). TPA was elevated above 0.09 U/mL in 10 of 19 patients with primary localized breast carcinoma, whereas plasma CEA levels were elevated in only 5. A significant increase of both was observed in 67 patients with metastatic breast cancer, i.e., 70% by TPA and 67% by CEA.

TPA was increased in 12% of healthy control females and CEA in 8% (Nemoto et al., 1979); but 27% of women with benign breast disease also had increased levels of serum TPA whereas no elevation of plasma CEA was observed. TPA was most frequently increased in individuals with visceral metastases; and only a limited correlation was observed between the clinical course of the tumor and levels of TPA. Schlegel et al. (1981) have recently compared 18 commonly used laboratory tests for a significant association with carcinoma of the breast and for discrimination between actively progressive disease and patients without evidence of residual tumor. Only CEA and TPA gave some discrimination, but it was inadequate. However, they suggest that the product of TPA times CEA is significant. Ninety-four percent of patients with a product value less than 450 had no evidence of progressive disease, whereas at products greater than 450, 47% had active disease and this increased to 96% at products greater than 1200.

6.6. Urinary Polyamines

The polyamines putrescine, spermidine, and spermine are excreted in the urine; however, they are found at increased concentration in association with rapid proliferation of cells. Spermidine and spermine appear to be requisites for maximal DNA synthesis, and they appear to increase intracellularly in an orderly sequential fashion as cells progress from the

G_o state to the mitotic phase of the cell cycle. These three polyamines appear to derive from decarboxylation of ornithine. An additional polyamine of interest is cadaverine. This is produced from lysine by an independent metabolic pathway. The presence of abnormally increased levels of polyamines in a variety of tumor cells, and in the blood and urine of a variety of tumor-bearing patients was observed by De Vita (1971) and by Russell (1971). Only more recently has this been re-examined in the urine of breast cancer patients (Tormey et al., 1975; Waalkes et al., 1975).

Tormey et al. (1975, 1980) assayed the concentration of these polyamines in urine using an amino acid analyzer. He observed that half of the patients with metastatic carcinoma of the breast had elevations of one or more individual polyamines; moreover, they were elevated in 38.5% of pre-operative patients with breast cancer. About a third of patients 5–24 weeks after mastectomy, but with evidence of tumor in regional lymph nodes, had elevated urinary polyamines. They suggest that from sequential sampling of patients with metastatic breast cancer the levels of urinary polyamines correlate with the clinical progression of the disease. Urinary polyamines increased in individuals refractory to therapy. The disease-free period during the post-operative was also somewhat shorter for individuals who had elevated urinary polyamines. These studies suggest application primarily as a prognostic parameter or in assessing changes in tumor burden.

6.7. Assay of Multiple Tumor Markers

This is addressed in part in the various sections above. Franchimont et al., (1977) performed a study using assays of five different tumor markers by radioimmunoassay, namely CEA, alphafetoprotein, human chorionic gonadotrophin (HCG), beta chain HCG, and kappa-casein. The five antigens were only detected within precise limits or were undetectable in 935 healthy subjects. In 145 cases of breast cancer prior to therapy and in absence of metastases, at least one antigen was observed to be elevated in 69% of the cases. The alphafetoprotein was never found to be positive in these cases, whereas the kappa-casein was often elevated in the early clinical stages of breast cancer. The inappropriateness of alpha-fetoprotein is suggested by the inability to demonstrate it by radioimmunoassay in breast carcinoma cytosol (Edgington and Nakamura, unpublished). In metastatic breast carcinoma, the incidence of elevated concentrations of at least one antigen was 80% of the 25 cases. Surgical removal of the breast carcinoma reduced the incidence to 34%. Persistent elevations correlated with recurrence and metastatic spread. In 55 patients with benign breast diseases, elevations of at least one marker was observed in only 5.5%.

In the sera of 935 normal nonpregnant and nonlactating women, CEA, AFP, HCG, beta chain HCG, and kappa-casein were often undetectable in serum and never greater than 10, 20, 1, 1.5, and 25 ng/mL, respectively.

7. Candidate Tumor-Specific Markers

This class of markers is represented by the elusive tumor-specific antigens, molecules that should exist from a wide variety of data derived from study of syngeneic tumor transplantation in animals and a few studies in man. These have not yet been identified as such for human breast carcinoma or other human or animal tumors. The following is a review of the search and some candidate molecules (Tables 8 and 9).

In 1972, Gentile and Flickinger described a putative breast cancer antigen (BCA) in saline extracts of each of 15 carcinomas of the breast (Table 8). These antigens appeared to be of less than 80,000 mw from interpretation of the published elution profiles on Sephadex G-200 chromatography. They were detected by an innovative approach of producing immune complexes by mixing the isolated serum immunoglobulin from breast carcinoma patients with saline extracts of their own tumors. The resultant immune complex fraction was isolated and heat dissociated to yield a putative specific antibody fraction by gel filtration. Positive reactions were obtained with sera from all of 15 breast carcinoma patients when analyzed by hemagglutination assay using extracts of autologous or homologous breast carcinomas, but not with extracts of control tissues. Antibodies appeared to be present only in breast carcinoma patients and were not observed in the serum of patients with other forms of neoplasia. The antigen was not further isolated and characterized. Kuo et al. (1973) described isolation of a glycoprotein from membrane preparations derived from human carcinomas of the breast. This glycoprotein, referred to as BCGP, differed from CEA in molecular weight but cross-reacted with CEA derived from colonic tumors. They suggested that this glycoprotein might account for positive CEA assay results with breast carcinoma. It now seems most likely that this glycoprotein is similar if not identical to the normal cross-reacting glycoprotein (NCA) described by Mach and Pusztaszeri (1972) and von Kleist et al. (1972). Leung et al. (1979) demonstrated that NCA is not present at detectable concentration in carcinomas of the breast.

Subsequently, Humphrey et al. (1974) and Boehm et al. (1974) described humoral antibody responses of breast cancer patients by agar gel diffusion using a concentrated aqueous extract of breast carcinomas. When analyzed by complement fixation, a higher frequency of positive reactions were observed for both controls and breast carcinoma sera. By immunodiffusion the sera of 0–0.9% of women without breast carcinoma gave positive reactions, 46% of breast cancer sera, 34% of sera from fibrocystic disease, and 25% of women with fibroadenomas had antibody to breast carcinoma antigen. These antibodies were not observed in most patients with advanced metastatic carcinoma suggestive of in vivo absorption or suppression of synthesis. The specificity is called into question by the reactions of sera from these patients with extracts of ovarian carcinoma, a sarcoma, and a melanoma. Serum from patients with benign breast disease exhibited similar patterns that were not tumor-specific. Some resolution of the question has been suggested by Lee et al. (1978). Attempts at purification of the antigens using gel chromatography, salt precipitation, and hydrophobic chromatography indicated the presence of two different antigens. One was suggested to be specific for breast carcinoma tumor tissue, whereas the second appeared to be nontissue-specific. The investigators (Humphrey et al., 1979) have subsequently reported the apparent identity of these two antigens as an IgG Fc fragment and an IgG Fab fragment and have suggested that the antibodies thought to be anti-tumor are apparently autoantibodies to immunoglobulin. The significance, fine antigenic specificity, and origin of this response will require further analysis. Insufficient numbers of patients have been studied to substantiate their suggestions of different prognosis for patients with differing immune responses to these immunoglobulin fragments.

Hollinshead et al. (1974) utilized delayed cutaneous hypersensitivity (DCH) to demonstrate sensitization of three of eight breast carcinoma patients to autologous tumor cell membranes. Positive reactions were elicited in all eight when a solubilized fraction prepared by sonication was used. It is notable that half of the patients who were tested with an equivalent sonic solubilized fraction of noncancerous breast tissue also responded. It was suggested that reactivity might not be restricted to tumor or autologous tissue since some patients also gave positive DCH responses with equivalent extracts of allogeneic benign breast. However, in view of the possibility of multiple immune responses these observations could reflect different specificities. When the sonicated and solubilized breast cancer membranes were subjected to polyacrylamide gel electrophoresis, one group of bands (2a) that were recovered and used in skin testing appeared to be associated with tissue-nonspecific reactivity, whereas, a second group of bands (2b) appeared to elicit positive DCH in most breast cancer patients, but did not elicit DCH responses from controls with benign breast diseases. Similarly, patients with other cancers did not respond to the region 2b fractions.

A variety of studies have suggested the existence of a breast carcinoma-specific, or at least a tumor-associated, antigen capable of eliciting immune reactions in vitro. The studies of DCH described by Alford et al. (1973) are complemented by the report of Segall et al. (1972), describing a high frequency of positive leukocyte migration inhibition assay results with extracts of breast carcinomas. This has also been observed by other groups (Cochran et al., 1972, 1974; Wolberg and Golzer, 1971;

Table 8

Candidate Tumor-Specific Markers 1972–1974

Assays	Immune response	Characteristics	References
Hemagglutination	Serum antibody from breast carcinomas	1. Antigens present in all (15) breast carcinomas 2. Antigens not present in normal tissues 3. Antibodies present only in breast carcinoma patients 4. Antigens 80,000 mw not further characterized	Gentile and Flickinger, 1972
Gel diffusion immunofluorescence	Heterologous	1. Glycoprotein isolated BCGP 2. Cross reacts with CEA 3. Probably NCA	Kuo et al., 1973
Gel diffusion (ID) immunoelectro-phoresis	Normal and breast carcinoma serum antibody	1. 0–0.9% antibody incidence in controls (ID) 2. 46% breast carcinoma sera antibody positive 3. 25% sera positive associated with fibroadenomas 4. 34% sera positive in fibrocystic disease 5. Antibody absent in advanced breast carcinoma 6. Not specific, reacts with other carcinomas 7. Probably at least two antigens, one may be breast carcinoma specific/associated	Humphrey et al., 1974 Boehm et al., 1974

Delayed cutaneous hypersensitivity; in vitro lymphocyte response	Host cellular response	1. Tumor cell membranes intact and sonicated 2. A polyacrylamide gel electrophoresis fraction 2b. elicited responses only in breast cancer patients.	Hollinshead et al., 1974
In vitro lymphocyte response	Host cellular response	1. $3M$ KCl extract of MCF-7 cells 2. Appeared specific for breast carcinoma patients 3. Antigens not present in normal or benign tissue	McCoy et al., 1974 Dean et al., 1975 Dean et al., 1977
Radioimmunoassay	Heterologous	$3M$ KCl extract of tumors	Accinni et al., 1974
Radioimmunoassay	Antibody isolated by affinity for immobilized malignant pleural effusion	1. Antigens present in pleural effusions produced by metastatic breast carcinoma; 2. Antibody or antigen capable of inhibition in 52% of breast carcinoma sera, 16% of sera from other malignancies, and 5% of normal sera	Gorsky et al., 1976

Table 9
Candidate Tumor-Specific Markers: 1974–1980

Assays	Immune response	Characteristics	References
Blocking tube leukocyte adherence test	Host cellular immune response	1. Serum antigen(s) 80,000–150,000 mw 2. Urine antigen(s) 40,000 mw 3. Antigenically related to HLA	Lopez and Thomson, 1977
Indirect immuno-fluorescence on viable tumor cells BOT-2	Serum antibody from breast carcinoma patients	Antibody induced capping and shedding of surface antigen from BOT-2 cells	Nordquist et al., 1977
Immunoperoxi-dase on human breast carcinomas	Rabbit anti-MMTV; Rabbit anti-MMTV gp 52	Cross reaction between a tryptic peptide of MMTV pg52 and some breast carcinoma cells; no characterization of human tumor antigen molecule	Mesa-Tejada et al., 1979 Ohno et al., 1979 Spiegelman, et al.

Method	Antibody	Antigen	Reference
Indirect immunofluorescence	Heterologous antiserum to acid soluble extract of breast carcinoma	Antigen is organelle or membrane-associated, but is solubilized in acid buffer	Loisillier et al., 1978
Indirect immunofluorescence	Sera antibody from breast ca. patients	Solubilized by 3M KCl; approximately 20,000 mw	Holton et al., 1978
Immunodiffusion; electroimmunodiffusion	Heterologous antiserum to isolated MTGP	20,000 mw glycoprotein (MTGP) 37–58% carbohydrate Pi, density, and sedimentation velocity varies with tumor	Leung et al., 1978 Leung et al., 1979 Leung et al., 1981a
Radioimmunoassay; immunohistochemical methods		Breast carcinoma specific; 53,000 mw membrane MTGP	Leung and Edgington, 1980a,b, 1981b
Immunoperoxidase on human breast cancer	Human hybridoma antibody	Antigens are uncharacterized	Schlom et al., 1980

Andersen et al., 1970; Black et al., 1974; McCoy et al., 1974; Dean et al., 1975, 1977). Although all of these studies suggested the existence of one or more tumor-associated antigens recognized by the host, and thus from one point of view, tumor-specific antigens, there has been no discrete identification or characterization of specific molecular entities. In vitro cellular immune responses were demonstrated by McCoy et al. (1974) and Dean et al. (1975, 1977) to 3M KCl extracts of breast carcinomas, and a correlation to the stage of disease was noted. In addition there appeared to be a reasonably high degree of specificity for breast carcinoma. It also appeared that normal or benign breast tissue did not possess the relevant antigens.

In a brief report, Accinni et al. (1974) suggested the presence in 3M KCl extracts of breast carcinomas of not only a carcinoembryonic antigen (CEA)-like molecule (which might not be identical to colonic CEA), but also the presence of a breast tumor-associated antigen independent of CEA. This germinal observation requires substantiation and considerably more analysis.

Gorsky et al. (1976) developed a solid-phase radioimmunoassay for detection of breast cancer-associated antigen in the serum and body fluids (Table 8). The antibodies were isolated from serum by affinity for breast carcinoma pleural fluids immobilized in polyacrylamide gel. A very small fraction of the eluted antibodies, after radioiodination, were observed to again bind to immobilized pleural fluid. Binding was inhibited by the presence of breast cancer sera (52%) and sera from patients with other malignancies (16%). Only about 5% sera of normal women also inhibited the binding of the antibody. The antigens with which these antibodies react are under investigation by these workers. At this point it is not known whether the antigens that were detected are present only in breast carcinomas or could be present in other types of neoplastic cells or normal cells. The absence of the relevant antibody in normal sera indicates that the antigens are not T antigen.

The blocking-tube leukocyte adherence inhibition assay was used by Lopez and Thomson (1977) to detect and isolate an antigen present in serum and in urine of individuals with carcinoma of the breast (Table 9). The serum antigen appeared to have a molecular weight in the range of 80,000–150,000 and a buoyant density similar to high density plasma lipoprotein (1.063–1.21 g/mL). This feature raises questions regarding a lipid or lipoprotein antigen. In the urine the tumor-specific antigen appeared to be of circa 40,000 mw, suggesting either cleavage of the larger serum antigen or a different, but antigenically homologous, antigen. The serum antigen appeared to possess antigenic determinants related to HLA using xenoantisera. It should be noted that HLA antigens also have been demonstrated to associate with plasma high density lipoprotein. These observations also raised questions as to the presence in these patients of a modified HLA, or simply sensitization to common framework epitopes of the HLA molecule. Purification and structural analysis of these candidate tumor-specific antigens is clearly essential to resolving structural relationships and their biological significance.

In 1977, Nordquist et al. described the presence of serum antibodies in breast cancer patients. These antibodies were observed by indirect immunofluorescence to react with viable cells in suspension. The line BOT-2 was derived from a human breast carcinoma. Antibodies were not only demonstrated to bind to the surface of BOT-2 cells, but they could be observed to patch, cap, and shed by following the fate of the fluorescein-labeled second antibody on the surface of the cells. The possibility that this mechanism might induce shedding of antigen–antibody complexes containing cell surface tumor-specific antigen and antibody and as such represent the source of immune complexes in breast cancer patients might be considered. The mechanism of induced transposition of breast tumor specific antigens from the surface of the cell to the extracellular space and ultimately the plasma has been thought of as a primary property of the tumor-specific or tumor-associated antigen. This may not be the case, since many plasmalemma molecules are not shed to a significant degree. This possibility of immune shedding is worth considering. As of the present, the characteristics of the antigens shed from BOT-2 have not been described.

Two-candidate tumor-associated antigens are briefly described. The first (Loisillier et al., 1978) evolved from the preparation of heterologous antiserum raised by immunization with a low pH extract of insoluble pellets from human mammary carcinomas. After extensive absorption, the antiserum gave a single precipitin line in gel diffusion against the immunizing material. They first observed that the antiserum reacted only with human mammary carcinoma cells by immunofluorescence. The antiserum did not react with normal mammary gland epithelium nor with cells of benign mammary lesions. Although originally described as unreactive with other tumors, more recent observations suggest that it may react with some carcinomas of the colon and some normal tissues to a lesser degree (personal communication).

At approximately the same time, Holton et al. (1978) using indirect immunofluorescence and serum from breast carcinoma patients observed reactions with a human mammary carcinoma cell line (SW527). Using $3M$ KCl extracts, these workers have provided initial evidence for the isolation of a molecule of approximately 20,000 mw that appears to neutralize homologous antitumor cell antibodies.

7.1. MMTV-Related Antigen

A substantial and provocative advance in identification of what may be a tumor-specific antigen of human breast carcinomas has been provided by Spiegelman and his colleagues (Mesa-Tejada et al., 1978; Ohno et al.,

1979). Based on earlier observations of a reputed slight homology between the RNAs of human and murine mammary tumor particles using assays of low stringency, they suspected the possibility of an immunochemical cross-reaction between proteins of the murine mammary tumor virus particles and constituents of human mammary carcinomas. The possibility of this was not entirely hypothetical since humoral antibodies to constituents of murine mammary tumor virus (MMTV) had been described in the serum of a number of breast cancer patients by Charney and Moore (1971) and others (Muller and Grossmann, 1972, 1973; Holder et al., 1976; Bowen et al., 1976). In addition, cellular immune response assays as exemplified by leukocyte migration inhibition (Black et al., 1976) describe responses to gp52, the major surface glycoprotein of MMTV in breast cancer patients. Yang et al. (1977) have also described a possible cross reaction between MMTV and the human breast carcinoma derived cell line MCF-7. Using the IgG from a rabbit immunized with MMTV that had been isolated from the milk of Paris RIII mice, immunohistochemical reactions with cells of human breast tumors were reported by Mesa-Tejada et al. (1978). They observed reactions with various histological types of human breast carcinomas in 39% of 131 cases. No reactions were observed with 119 benign breast lesions, 18 normal breast tissues and only with 1 of 99 carcinomas from other tissue sites. In Table 10 the results of this group are summarized. It is notable that the reactions were not uniform in that only a minor portion of cells were positive by this assay. Whether this is a problem of sensitivity of the assay and the inability to detect a few molecules of antigen that are indeed present in the remaining neoplastic cells is not known. If this MMTV cross-reacting antigen is truly a focal and elective marker not expressed by most neoplastic cells of the mammary epithelium, then it may not play an essential role in the biology or immunobiology intrinsic of the neoplastic cell. In addition, in vitro imaging with radiolabeled antibody and attempts at immunotherapy may be precluded from the outset.

The specificity of the MMTV cross-reaction observed by Spiegelman and associates was demonstrated through blocking of the reaction by prior

Table 10
MMTV-Related Antigen in Breast Carcinoma Tissue[a]

Patient group	Number	% Positive
Benign breast lesions	137	0
Breast carcinoma	447	47.4
Other malignancies	107	0
Cystosarcoma, breast	8	0

[a]Assay by immunoperoxidase staining of breast biopsies with anti-MMTV gp 52.

absorption of the anti-MMTV antiserum with MMTV isolated from three sources. The reaction was also neutralized by gp52 from two different strains isolated by two independent methods. A variety of tissues including human milk were observed not to block the reactions. The specificity of the reaction was further extended by demonstrating that the gp52 polypeptide chain rather than the carbohydrate radicals were responsible for the specificity (Ohno et al., 1979). Deglycosylated gp52 was equally effective in neutralizing the anti-MMTV reaction with human cells, whereas the isolated polysaccharides were ineffectual. More recent studies have further defined a single tryptic peptide as possessing the cross-reacting antigenic epitope. To date, there is no characterization of the molecule in human breast carcinoma cells that bears this cross-reacting epitope. With the available information and analytic approaches, it is reasonable to anticipate information regarding the biochemical characteristics of the human tumor specific molecule in the near future.

It should be noted in respect of the above observations that most antisera to MMTV, or to MMTV structural proteins such as gp52, have not reacted with human mammary carcinomas in other laboratories. If indeed there is such a cross-reaction with heterologous antisera, it must be rare and only fortuitously encountered. Cardiff has observed reactions similar to those described by Mesa-Tejada et al. (1978) using their antiserum (personal communication).

A critical question has been introduced recently by Dion et al. (1980). They have identified and isolated a human milk protein that is structurally and antigenically related to MMTV gp52 (referred to by this group as gp55). Immunoprecipitation analyses indicated the presence of an antigenically cross-reacting protein of about 58,000 mw, about three kilodaltons larger than the MMTV protein. In an extensive structural analysis they demonstrated that both contained amino terminal serine. Further homology was demonstrated by tryptic peptide mapping. Although Mesa-Tejada (1978) did not observe inhibition of their rabbit anti-MMTV or anti-MMTV gp52 by human milk assaying reactivity of their antisera by immunoperoxidase with human breast carcinomas, the studies of Dion et al. (1980) suggest the need for critical re-examination of this point. The possibility that the MMTV gp52 cross-reacting molecule observed in some human neoplastic mammary epithelial cells might represent a differentiation product present in only low concentration in human breast milk cannot be safely dismissed without further study.

7.2. Mammary Tumor-Specific Glycoprotein (MTGP)

In 1978, Leung et al. described a new trace glycoprotein in human breast carcinomas that has since appeared to be tumor-specific with a reasonably high degree of confidence. A variety of immobilized antibodies to normal tissues, blood group antigens, and known oncodevelopmental antigens, such as CEA, were used to deplete the cytosol glycoprotein fractions of human breast carcinomas. What remained was fractionated by size. Following immunization, a single rabbit produced antibodies to one fraction containing what is now designated Mammary Tumor-Specific Glycoprotein (MTGP). Following absorption with a wide battery of tumors and nonneoplastic tissues, a single precipitin formed in agar gel diffusion against very high concentrations of glycoprotein from all of 6 breast carcinomas, but no other tumor or normal tissue that was analyzed. Using a quantitative electroimmundiffusion assay, molecules were isolated from the cytosol fractions of human ductal carcinomas of the breast and were characterized by isoelectric point, sedimentation velocity, carbohydrate composition, buoyant density in cesium chloride, diffusion constant, estimated molecular weight, and amino acid composition (Table 11). Though bearing common antigenic determinants that appeared to exhibit antigenic identity by gel diffusion, the physicochemical properties and composition were quite discrete and homogeneous for a single tumor, but differed for different tumors. Although cytosol MTGP was of approximately the same size (19,000–19,800 mw) significant differences were observed in sedimentation velocity, isoelectric point, and buoyant density, as well as carbohydrate composition between Type I and Type II tumors. Further, the MTGP of Type II tumors lacked tyrosine whereas that from Type I tumors possessed a single tyrosine residue with a reciprocal difference in arginine. This antigen was demonstrated by immunohistochemical techniques to be present in the cytoplasm cytosol preparations from biopsies of breast carcinomas, but could not be identified in benign breast cells. It was expressed

Table 11
Properties of Cytosol and Membrane Forms of MTGP[a]

Characteristic	Cytosol MTGP	Membrane MTGP
Solubility	Water	Ionic detergent
$D^0_{20,w}$[b]	$9.1 \times 10^{-7} cm^2/s$	$5.6 \times 10^{-7} cm^2/s$
$S^0_{20,w}$	2.50	2.90
Density[c], ρ	$1.48 g/cm^3$	$1.32 g/cm^3$
Molecular weight		
Svedberg equation	19,800	52,800
SDS polyacrylamide gel	41,000	64,000
Carbohydrate	58%	
Electrophoretic mobility	a_1	a_2
Isoelectric point	5.35	6.10

[a]Both forms derived from Type I tumors.
[b]From molecular exclusion chromatography
[c]From buoyant density in cesium chloride

both in the cytoplasm of fixed breast carcinoma cells in culture or in biopsies of tumors by immunohistochemical methods as well as at the surface of viable cells (Leung et al., 1978).

The frequency of association of this 19,000–20,000 mw glycoprotein (MTGP 20) with breast carcinomas was examined and it was found in each of seven metastatic breast tumors in which 1g of tissue was assayed. MTGP 20 was not demonstrated in 76 normal tissue samples or tumors other than of breast origin. It was present in 79.5% of histologically confirmed biopsies of ductal carcinomas of the breast or 76.2% of 101 breast carcinomas of all types that were examined (Leung et al., 1979). The presence or concentration of MTGP 20 did not significantly correlate with the presence or concentration of CEA or estrogen receptor. It was also independent of a variety of histological features. It was suggested that MTGP 20 represented an independent marker that only reflected the neoplastic nature of the mammary epithelial cells.

Subsequently, Leung and Edgington (1980a) identified a second form of MTGP in the plasmalemma of breast carcinoma cells. This very insoluble form of the molecule required ionic detergent such as SDS for solubilization, being refractory to solubilization by a variety of non-ionic detergents. This MTGP segregated in parallel with markers for plasmalemma and was recovered at high yield in the isolated plasma membrane fraction. Subsequent studies (Leung et al., 1981a) have more carefully delineated the physicochemical heterogeneity of both types of MTGP molecules in different breast carcinomas. Using fifteen cell lines of breast carcinoma origin and tumor tissue, MTGP was identified in all (Leung and Edgington, 1980b). However, there was a marked variation in concentration, some cells contained only membrane MTGP with no MTGP 20. Though each was homogeneous by physicochemical characteristics in individual cell lines and their derivative clones over some years, discrete and consistent differences were observed in the MTGP molecules between different cell lines. This permitted grouping breast carcinomas into four MTGP types. These could be distinguished by the combined isoelectric point and buoyant density of the cytosol MTGP 20 and membrane form of the molecule. These studies further suggest the existence of common tumor-specific antigenic determinants as well as structural variation that could accommodate hypothesized "variable" or individual tumor-specific structures on tumor-specific antigens.

Radioimmunoassay suggests the absence of MTGP, or at least the tumor-specific antigenic determinants, from a variety of tissues, both neoplastic and benign. In some cases, the level of confidence for the absence of MTGP in these tissues has been extended to less than 100 pg for 5 mg of tissue or tumor glycoprotein or less than one molecule of MTGP per tissue culture cell plasmalemma. Although variable in concentration, the highest of cell lines (734-B, the parent culture from which MCF-7 was derived) had approximately 10,000 molecules of MTGP per plasmalemma. Most tumor cells had considerably less. This membrane form of MTGP has recently been isolated to near homogeneity (Leung et al., 1981b). The membrane molecule from one tumor had a mw of 52,800 estimated from Svedberg equation using sedimentation velocity, density, and diffusion constant (Table 10). Preliminary studies have suggested the existence of humoral antibody responses specific for the plasmalemma form of the molecule, but this remains to be formally established.

7.3. Human Monoclonal Antibody-Defined Markers

Schlom et al. (1980) have recently reported a new approach to the identification of immunobiologically relevant tumor-specific antigens of breast carcinomas. Cells from lymph nodes derived at the time of mastectomy of 13 breast carcinoma patients were fused with murine myeloma cells to produce human–mouse hybrid cells, some of which synthesize human monoclonal antibodies. Of 52 hybridoma cultures synthesizing human immunoglobulin, four hybridoma antibodies were identified that react with tumor cells by immunoperoxidase reactions with sections of human breast carcinomas. Three of these did not react with normal mammary epithelium. They reacted with both primary and metastatic cells, but gave different patterns of reactivity with breast carcinoma cells. One appeared to discriminate between mammary carcinoma cells and benign cells from 55 of 59 tumors. With this approach, reasonably unlimited quantities of antibodies may become available for isolation of the responsible antigen to which the tumor-bearing host has made the immune response. A wide variety of studies of the host immune response to breast carcinomas as well as characterization of the candidate tumor-specific antigen are clearly possible.

8. Immune Response Markers

Immune responses will only be briefly addressed, since this topic is both complex in its own right and difficult to satisfactorily resolve at this time. Two general types of immune responses may however be of significance in respect to the basic biology of the neoplastic cell, elucidation of the interaction between the host and neoplasms of the mammary gland, and in potential clinical application such as to provide markers for the diagnosis, prognosis, or for potential immunotherapy. The first of these, and clearly the most elusive, are the immune responses to tumor-specific or tumor-associated molecules. The second is immune responses to potentially tumor-associated markers of oncogenic agents that have been hypothesized and could be implicated in the biology of these tumors. Current information regarding the host immune response to tumor-specific antigens is limited owing to the lack of established tumor-specific antigens of breast cancer as well as other tumors. In the absence of well-established molecular entities, the immune phenomena described remain debatable. A number of studies purport to demonstrate immune responses to autologous or homologous breast cancer. On the other hand, considerable interest and a body of data are available in regard to immune responses to structural proteins of the murine mammary tumor virus.

8.1. Humoral Immune Responses to MMTV

The most extensive studies have been those to MMTV. A number of investigators have reported the presence of antibody to MMTV in the serum of humans, and in elevated titer or frequency in the sera of patients with breast carcinoma. Charney and Moore (1971) observed neutralization of infectivity of MMTV by human sera. The specificity of the reaction was not further confirmed, and the number of sera examined in this initial study were too low to permit interpretation. Muller and Grossmann (1972) observed reactions of some breast cancer sera with MMTV-rich murine mammary tumor tissue sections. Specificity was in part demonstrated through absorption; however, this does not firmly establish specificity since neutralization may have occurred as a result from contaminants of the MMTV preparation or from relatively nonspecific interactions with the carbohydrate of MMTV. In a subsequent report, Muller et al. (1976) demonstrated that antibodies described in women with fibrocystic disease or breast cancer were directed to intracytoplasmic type A particles of MMTV. Immunofluorescence demonstrated that the human antibodies were bound only by tumors producing such type A particle clusters visible by light microscopy. The reaction was blocked by rabbit antisera to type A intracytoplasmic particles and much less of antisera to type B particles. It is notable that this group has not observed a diagnostically useful correlation of this anti-MMTV with breast carcinoma, and antibodies were frequently associated with benign breast disease and were also observed in a significant number of normal women.

Zangerle et al. (1977) attempted without success to demonstrate antibodies to structural proteins of MMTV in 100 sera from controls, patients with benign breast disease, or breast cancer patients. Witkin et al. (1979) addressed the problem that apparent neutralization of MMTV by certain human sera might reflect antibody independent, but complement-mediated, reactions. They have provided evidence that the type B retrovirus MMTV is not disrupted by normal human serum via the alternative complement pathway, demonstrating that specific antibody was required for lysis of the viral particle. They developed an assay based on the release of reverse transcriptase from the disrupted virions; and this was used to assay antibodies to MMTV in human sera. Greater virolytic activity was detected in the sera of patients with breast disease or colorectal cancer than in sera from healthy individuals. Based on this apparent confirmation of the presence of anti-MMTV antibody, they also developed an en zyme-linked immunoassay (Witkin et al., 1980) that detected antibodies both to the internal viral protein p28 as well as to viral envelope components gp52 and gp34. A statistically higher frequency of IgG binding to MMTV was observed in the sera of breast cancer patients, 26% of which were positive. Ten percent of sera from benign breast disease and 8% of normal sera were also positive. Their reactions were blocked with rabbit antisera to MMTV gp34 and less well with anti gp52.

8.2. Cellular Immune Responses to MMTV

The possibility of the presence of cellular immune reactivity to MMTV or some related viral product has been suggested with an increased incidence of such reactions in breast cancer patients. In an initial study, Black et al. (1974) observed positive leukocyte migration inhibition, an indicator of cellular immunity, in a third of breast cancer patients using milk from RIII mice as a source of MMTV antigen. In contrast, MMTV-free murine milk did not induce such responses. It was of interest to note that a high percentage of individuals who responded by this assay to breast cancer tissue also responded to the MMTV positive milk. These investigators subsequently suggested that diminished LMI responses correlated with more advanced disease and tumor progression (Black et al., 1975). This group, Black et al. (1976), further demonstrated some specificity for the major viral envelope glycoprotein gp55. The correlation between putative cellular immune responses in vitro to autologous or homologous breast cancer tissue and the structural protein of MMTV have been considered by Zachrau et al. (1978), who concluded that reactivity was primarily to the major glycoprotein gp55 (or gp52 in other laboratories). This correlated well with reactivity to autologous or homologous breast tissue. These workers also observed a high correlation with reactivity to MCF-7 extracts. These studies represent a body of evidence linking a putative cross-reactivity between constituents of neoplastic mammary epithelium and constituents of MMTV.

9. Genetic Markers

9.1. Cytogenetic Markers

Whereas the genetics of murine mammary tumor virus susceptibility and the incidence of mammary tumors has been extensively characterized, only limited reports of genetic markers of human breast carcinoma cells or susceptibility are available. The existence of a cytogenetic marker in common for a number of human breast carcinoma cells has been reported (Cruciger et al., 1976; Barker et al., 1977; Cailleau et al., 1979). This group first observed that seven long-term breast carcinoma lines had a common abberation upon G-banding chromosome analysis. Each had a translocation of the q or long arm of chromosome 1. This was extended to an additional six lines on further analysis. The possibility of contamination of the cultures by one of the cell lines is always a serious consideration; however, this group has subsequently demonstrated that sixteen of seventeen breast carcinoma lines that were characterized had independent genetic signatures by analysis at 17 enzyme loci (Siciliano et al., 1979). The relationship of the $1q$ chromosomal translocation to other properties of the breast carcinoma cell lines, e.g., estrogen receptor or tumorigenicity, has yet to be established through offering interesting possibilites.

9.2. GPT Linked Marker

Data has long been available to suggest an increased risk of breast cancer in the immediate family, particularly if the onset of the relative was at a young age, the disease was bilateral or if more than one member of the family had breast cancer (Anderson, 1972, 1974; Maclin, 1959). The possibility that this could be genetic predisposition or increased risk rather than environmental has been examined by King et al. (1980) in 11 high risk families. Of four models of genetic transmission or environmental influence that were tested, the data most closely approximated that expected from autosomal dominant transmission of risk. Twenty genetic markers were analyzed and linkage analyses were consistent with a dominant allele closely linked to the glutamate-pyruvate transaminase (GPT) gene in six families. The remaining five families provided weak evidence against linkage. Within the six families with suggestion of linkage of breast cancer risk to GPT the probability was 80 to 1 in favor of linkage ($p=0.04$). It is possible that this linkage may occur only in some families, and that in other families there is no genetic basis for the elevated risk or that if genetically based, the allele(s) is not linked to any of the tested gene products.

10. Comment

A variety of markers that have exhibited biological or clinical correlation with breast cancer have been considered. These reflect a variety of approaches to the study of the biology of the malignant breast cancer cell, as well as the application to diagnosis of carcinoma of the breast and its prognosis. No single marker other than CEA is in wide clinical use. Perhaps as the apparent relationship between murine mammary tumor virus and human breast carcinoma-associated antigens are clarified and true tumor specific antigens are identified, a new era of understanding of the neoplastic cell of the mammary gland will emerge as well as a far greater potential for application of discrete and biologically meaningful markers in this form of neoplasia.

Acknowledgments

The dedicated assistance of Alycia Bittick in the preparation of this manuscript is readily acknowledged. This is publication number 2461 from the Immunology Department. Portions of this work were supported by grants CA-28166 and CA-16600 from the National Cancer Institute.

References

Accinni, R., A. Bartorelli, R. Ferrara, C. Biancardi (1977), *Experientia* **33,** 88.
Alford, C., A. C. Hollinshead, and R. B. Herberman (1973), *Ann. Surg.* **178,** 20.
Anderson, V., O. Bjerrum, G. Bendixen, T. Schiodt, and I. Dissing (1970), *Inter. J. Cancer* **5,** 357.
Anderson, D. E. (1972), *J. Natl. Cancer Inst.* **48,** 1029.
Anderson, D. E. (1974), *Cancer* **43,** 1090.
Barker, P. E., Q. V. J. Cruciger, R. Cailleau, and H. J. Siciliano (1977), *J. Cell Biol.* **75,** 379.
Bjorklund, B., and V. Bjorklund (1957), *Inter. Arch. Allerg. Immunol.* **10,** 153.
Bjorklund, B., V. Bjorklund, B. Wiklund, R. Lundstrom, P. H. Ekdahl, L. Hagbard, I. Kaijser, G. Eklund and B. Luning (1973), in *Immunological Techniques for Detection of Cancer,* Bonniers, Stockholm, 133–187.
Black, M. M., H. P. Leis, B. Shore, and R. E. Zachrau, (1974), *Cancer* **33,** 952.
Black, M. M., D. H. Moore, B. Shore, R. E. Zachrau, and H. P. Leis, (1974), *Cancer Res.* **34,** 1054.
Black, M. M., R. E. Zachrau, A. S. Dion, B. Shore, D. L. Fine, H. P. Leis, and C. J. Williams (1976), *Cancer Res.* **36,** 4137.
Black, M. M., R. G. Zachrau, B. Shore, D. H. Moore, and H. P. Leis (1975), *Cancer* **35,** 121.
Boehm, O. R., B. J. Boehm, and L. J. Humphrey (1974), *Clin. Exptl. Immunol.,* **16,** 31.
Bowen, J. M., L. Dmochowski, M. F. Miller, E. S. Priori, G. Seman, M. L. Dodson, and K. Maruyama (1976), *Cancer Res.* **36,** 759.
Buffe, D., C. Rimbaut, C. Fuccaro, and P. Burtin (1972), *Ann Inst. Pasteur* **123,** 29.
Burtin, P., S. von Kleist, and D. Buffe (1960), *Bull. Soc. Chim. Biol.* **49,** 1389.
Cailleau, R., M. Olive, and Q. Cruciger (1979), *In Vitro* **14,** 911.
Cardiff, R. D., S. R. Weelings, and L. J. Faulkin (1977), *Cancer* **39,** 2734.
Ceriani, R. L., M. Sasalei, J. A. Peterson, and E. W. Blank (1980), in *Cell Biology of Breast Cancer,* McGrath, C. H., M. J. Brennan, and M. A. Rich, Eds., Academic Press, New York, p. 33.

Ceriani, R. L., K. Thompson, J. A. Peterson, and S. Abraham (1977), *Proc. Natl. Acad. Sci. (USA)* **74**, 582.

Charney, J, and D. H. Moore (1971), *Nature* **229**, 627.

Charteris, A. A. (1930), *J. Pathol. Bacteriol.* **33**, 101.

Chu, T. M. (1979), in *Immunodiagnosis of Cancer*, R. B. Herberman and K. R. McIntire, eds., Marcel Dekker, New York, p. 513.

Chu, T. M., and T. Nemoto (1973), *J. Natl. Cancer Inst.* **51**, 1119.

Cochran, A. J., W. G. S. Spilg, R. M. Mackie, and C. E. Thomas (1972), *Brit. Med. J.* **4**, 67.

Cochran, A. J., R. M. Grant, W. G. Spilg, R. M. Mackie, C. E. Ross, D. E. Hoyle, and J. M. Russell (1974), *Inter. J. Cancer* **14**, 19.

Concannon, J. P., M. H. Dalbow, and J. C. Frich (1973), *Radiology* **108**, 191.

Cruciger, A. V. J., S. Pathak, and R. Cailleau (1976), *Cytogenet. Cell Genet.* **17**, 231.

Cunningham-Rundles, S., W. F. Feller, C. Cunningham-Rundles, B. Dupont, H. Wanebo, R. O'Reilly, and R. A. Goode (1976), *Cell Immunol.* **25**, 322.

Dean, J. J., J. S. Silva, J. L. McCoy, C. M. Leonard, H. Middleton, G. B. Cannon, and R. B. Herberman (1975), *J. Natl. Cancer Inst.* **54**, 1295.

Dean, J. H., J. L. McCoy, G. B. Cannon, C. M. Leonard, E. Perlin, A. Kreutner, R. K. Oldham, and R. B. Herberman (1977), *J. Natl. Cancer Inst.* **58**, 549.

DeOme, K. B., and D. Medina (1969), *Cancer* 1255.

DeVita, V. T. (1971), *Cancer Chemo. Rept.* **2**, 23.

Dion, A. S., D. C. Farwell, A. A. Pomenti, and A. J. Girardi (1979), *Proc. Natl. Acad. Sci USA* **77**, 1301.

Drysdale, J. W., T. G. Adelman, P. Arosio, D. Casareale, P. Fitzpatrick, J. T. Hazard, and M. Yokota (1977), *Semin. Hematol.* **14**, 71.

Drysdale, J. W., and R. M. Singer (1974), *Cancer Res.* **34**, 3352.

Edgington, T. S., R. W. Astarita, and E. F. Plow (1975), *New Eng. J. Med.* **293**, 103.

Edynak, E. M., M. P. Lardis, and M. Vrana (1971), *Cancer* **28**, 1457.

Engel, L. W., and N. A. Young (1978), *Cancer Res.* **38**, 4327.

Ervin, P. E., and L. Wibell (1973), *Clin. Chimica Acta* **43**, 183.

Fisher, E. R., and J. D. Paulson (1978), in *Cancer Campaign*, Grundmann, E., and L. Beck, eds., vol. 1, Fischer Verlag, Stuttgart and New York, pp. 65–80.

Fitzgerald, D. K., V. Brodbeck, I. Kiyosawa, R. Marval, B. Colvin, and K. E. Ebner (1970), *J. Biol. Chem.* **245**, 2103.

Foote, F. W., and F. W. Stewart (1945), *Ann. Surg.* **121**, 197.

Franchimont, P., P. F. Zangerle, J. C. Hendrick, A. Reuter, C. Colin (1977), *Cancer* **39**, 2806.

Frantz, V. K., J. W. Pickren, G. W. Melcher, and M. Auchincloss, Jr. (1951), *Cancer* **4**, 762.

Fritsche, R., and J. P. Mach (1975), *Nature* **258**, 734.

Gentile, J. M., and J. T. Flickinger (1972), *Surg. Gyn. Ob.* **135**, 69.

Gold, P., and S. O. Freedman, *J. Exptl. Med.* **121**, 439.

Goldenberg, D. M., T. F. Garner, K. D. Pant, and J. R. van Nagell, Jr. (1978), *Cancer Res.* **38**, 1246.

Gorsky, Y., F. Vanky, and D. Sulitzeanu (1976), *Proc. Natl. Acad. Sci. USA,* **73,** 2101.

Haagensen, C. D. (1971), in *Diseases of the Breast,* 2nd Ed., Saunders, Philadelphia, Chapter 7, 155.

Haagensen, D. W., W. F. Barry, T. A. McCook, J. Giannola, S. Ammirata, and S. A. Wells (1980), *Ann. Surg.* **191,** 599.

Haagensen, D. W., S. J. Kister, J. Panick, J. Giannola, H. J. Hansen, and S. A. Wells (1978), *Cancer* **42,** 1646.

Haagensen, D. E., G. Mazoujian, W. G. Dilley, C. E. Pedersen, S. J. Kister, and S. A. Wells (1979b), *J. Natl. Cancer Inst.* **62,** 239.

Haagensen, D. E., G. Mazoujian, W. D. Holder, S. J. Kister, and S. A. Wells (1977), *Ann. Surg.* **185,** 279.

Hendrick, J. C., and P. Franchimont (1974), *Eur. J. Cancer* **10,** 725.

Holder, W. D., Jr., G. W. Peer, D. P. Bolognesi, and S. A. Wells (1976), *Surg. Forum* **27,** 102.

Hollinshead, A. C., W. T. Jaffurs, L. K. Alpert, J. E. Harris, and R. B. Herberman (1974), *Cancer Res.* **34,** 2961.

Holton, O. D., J. W. Fett, E. M. Alderman, and R. E. Lovins (1978), *Fed. Proc.* **37,** 1485.

Howard, D. R., and C. R. Taylor (1979), *Cancer* **43,** 2279.

Howard, D. R., and J. G. Batsakis (1980), *Science* **210,** 201.

Humphrey, L. J., N. C. Estes, P. A. Morse, W. R. Jewell, R. A. Boudet, and M. J. K. Hudson (1974), *Cancer* **34,** 1516.

Humphrey, L. J., P. J. Volenec, N. C. Estes, and F. J. Volenec (1979), *J. Surg. Oncol.,* **11,** 141.

Imam, A., D. J. R. Laurence, and A. M. Neville (1981), *Biochem. J.,* in press.

Imam, A., and Z. A. Tokes (1981), *J. Histochem. Cytochem.,* in press.

Jacobs, A., B. Jones, C. Ricketts, R. D. Bulbrook, and D. Y. Wang (1976), *Brit. J. Cancer* **34,** 286.

Jones, B. M., M. Worwood, and A. Jacobs (1980), *Clin. Chimica Acta* **106,** 203.

Keenan, T. W., D. J. Moore, D. E. Olson, W. N. Yunghans, and S. Patton (1970), *J. Cell Biol.* **44,** 80.

Kindt, R., and P. M. Van Vaerenbergh (1976), *Acta Clin. Belgium* **31,** Suppl., 8, 33.

King, M. C., R. C. P. Go, R. C. Elston, H. T. Lynch, and N. L. Petrakis (1980), *Science* **208,** 406.

Kleinberg, D. L., J. Todd, and M. L. Groves (1977), *J. Clin. Endo. Metab.* **45,** 1238.

Kuo, T., Rosai, J., and T. W. Tillack, (1973), *Int. J. Cancer* **12,** 532.

Lamerz, R., A. Leonhardt, H. Ehrhart, and H. V. Lieven (1979), *Oncodev. Biol. Med.* **1,** 123.

Laurence, D. J. R. (1978), *Invest. Cell Pathol.* **1,** 5.

Lee, C. K., L. Humphrey, and A. B. Rawitch (1978), *Fed. Proc.* **37,** 1485.

Leung, J. P., E. F. Plow, R. M. Nakamura, and T. S. Edgington (1978), *J. Immunol.* **121,** 1287.

Leung, J. P., G. M. Bordin, R. M. Nakamura, D. H. DeHeer, and T. S. Edgington (1979), *Cancer Res.* **39,** 2057.

Leung, J. P., and T. S. Edgington (1980a), *Cancer Res.* **40,** 316.

Leung, J. P., and T. S. Edgington (1980b), *Cancer Res.* **40,** 662.

Leung, J. P., W. Nelson-Rees, G. C. Moore, R. Cailleau, and T. S. Edgington (1981a), *Int. J. Cancer*, in press.

Leung, J. P., G. E. Moore, and T. S. Edgington (1981b), *Fed. Proc.* **40**, 1118.

Little, M. (1972), *Acta Endocr. Suppl.* **159**, 41.

Loisillier, F., D. Metivier, and P. Burtin (1978), *Compt. Rend. Acad. Sci. Paris* **287**, 1169.

Lopez, M. J., and D. M. P. Thomson (1977), *Int. J. Cancer* **20**, 834.

Mach, J. P., and G. Pusztaszeri (1972), *Immunochem.* **9**, 1031.

Maclin, M. T. (1959), *J. Natl. Cancer Inst.* **22**, 927.

Marcus, D. M., and N. Zinberg (1974), *Arch. Biochem. Biphys.* **162**, 493.

Marcus, D. M., and N. Zinberg (1975), *J. Natl. Cancer Inst.* **55**, 791.

McCoy, J. L., L. F. Jerome, J. H. Dean, G. B. Cannon, T. C. Alford, T. Doering, and R. B. Herberman (1974), *J. Natl. Cancer Inst.* **53**, 11.

McGuire, W. L. (ed.) (1978), *Hormones, Receptors and Breast Cancer*, Raven Press, New York.

McGuire, W. L. (1979), *Adv. Int. Med.* **24**, 127.

Mesa-Tejada, R., I. Keydar, M. Ramanarayanan, T. Ohno, C. Fenoglio, and S. Spiegelman (1978), *Proc. Natl. Acad. Sci. USA* **75**, 1529.

Muller, M., and Grossmann, H. (1972), *Nature* **237**, 116.

Muller, M., S. Zotter, C. Kemmer (1976), *J. Natl. Cancer Inst.* **56**, 295.

Myers, R. E., J. A. Sutherland, J. W. Meakin, D. G. Malkin, J. A. Kellen, and A. Malkin (1980), *Protides Biol. Fluids*, 285.

Nemoto, T., R. Constantine, and T. M. Chu (1979), *J. Natl. Cancer Inst.* **63**, 1347.

Nordquist, R. E. J. H. Anglin, and M. P. Lerner (1977), *Science* **197**, 366.

Ohno, T., R. Mesa-Tejada, I. Keydar, M. Ramanarayanan, J. Bausch, and S. Spiegelman (1979), *Proc. Natl. Acad. Sci USA* **76**, 2460.

Papaioannou, D., P. Geggie, and J. Klassen (1979), *Clin. Chimica Acta* **99**, 37.

Parry, D. H., M. Worwood, and A. Jacobs (1975), *Brit. Med. J.*, **i**, 245.

Patton, S., and T. W. Kennan (1975), *Biochim. Biophys. Acta* **415**, 273.

Plow, E. F., and T. S. Edgington (1978), in *Immunodiagnosis of Cancer*, R. B. Herberman, and K. R. McIntire, eds., Marcel Dekker, New York, pp. 181–239.

Poulik, M. D. (1979), in *Compendium of Assays for Immunodiagnosis of Human Cancer*, Herberman, R. B., ed., Elsevier, New York, p. 107.

Poulik, M. D., and A. D. Bloom (1973), *J. Immunol.* **110**, 1430.

Poulik, M. D., and R. A. Reisfeld (1975), in *Contemporary Topics in Molecular Immunology*, Inman, F. P., and W. J. Mandy, eds., vol. 4, Plenum, New York, pp. 157–204.

Russell, D. H. (1971), *Nature* **233**, 144.

Schlom, J., D. Wunderlich, and Y. A. Teramoto (1980), *Proc. Natl. Acad. Sci. USA* **77**, 6841.

Schultz, G. S., and K. E. Ebner (1977), *Cancer Res.* **37**, 4489.

Segall, A., O. Weiler, J. Genin, J. Lacour, and F. Lacour (1972), *Int. J. Cancer* **9**, 417.

Slemmer, G. (1980), in *Breast Cancer: New Concepts in Etiology and Control*, McGrath, C. M., M. J. Brennan, and M. A. Rich, eds., Academic Press, p. 93.

Springer, G. F., and P. R. Desai (1975a), *Carbohyd. Res.* **40**, 183.

Springer, G. F., P. R. Desai, and I. Banatwala (1975b), *J. Natl. Cancer Inst.* **54,** 335.

Springer, G. F., P. R. Desai, and E. F. Scanlon (1976), *Cancer* **37,** 169.

Springer, G. F., M. S. Murthy, R. Desai, and E. F. Scanlon (1980), *Cancer* **45,** 2949.

Steward, A. M., D. Nixon, N. Zamcheck, and A. Aisenberg (1974), *Cancer* **33,** 1246.

Thompson, E. B., and M. E. Lippman (1979), *Steroid Receptors and the Management of Cancer.* Vol. 1, CRC Press, Boca Raton.

Tormey, D. C., T. P. Waalkes, D. Ahmann, C. W. Gehrke, R. W. Zumwalt, J. Snyder, and H. Hansen (1975), *Cancer* **35,** 1095.

Tormey, D. C., T. P. Waalkes, K. C. Kuo, C. W. Gehrke (1980), *Cancer* **46,** 741.

Turkington, R. W., and M. Riddle (1969), *Endocrinol.* **84,** 1213.

von Kleist, S., G. Chavanel, and P. Burtin (1972), *Proc. Natl. Acad. Sci. USA* **64,** 161.

Waalkes, T. P., C. W. Gehrke, D. C. Tormey (1975), *Cancer Chemo. Rept.* **59,** 1103.

Wahren, B., E. Lidbrink, A. Wallgren, P. Eneroth, and J. Zajicek (1978), *Cancer* **42,** 1870.

Walker, R. (1979), *J. Pathol.* **129,** 37.

Wang, D. Y., R. D. Bulbrook, J. L. Hayward, J. C. Hendrick, and P. Franchimont (1975), *Eur. J. Cancer* **11,** 615.

Witkin, S. S., R. A. Egeli, N. H. Sarkar, R. A. Good, and N. K. Day (1979), *Proc. Natl. Acad. Sci USA* **76,** 2984.

Witkin, S. S., N. H. Sarkar, R. A. Good, and N. R. Day (1980), *J. Immunol. Methods* **32,** 85.

Wolberg, W. H., and M. L. Goelzer (1971), *Nature* **229,** 632.

Woods, K. L., D. H. Cove, and A. Howell (1977), *Lancet* **II,** 14.

Woods, K. L., D. H. Cove, D. M. Morrison, and D. A. Heath (1979), *Eur. J. Cancer* **15,** 47.

Yang, N. S., H. D. Soule, and C. M. McGrath (1977), *J. Natl. Cancer Inst.* **59,** 1357.

Young, S., L. S. C. Pang, and I. Goldsmith (1976), *J. Clin. Path. Suppl.* **7,** 94.

Zachrau, R. E., M. M. Black, A. S. Dion, B. Shore, C. J. Williams, and H. P. Leis (1978), *Cancer Res.* **38,** 4314.

Zangerle, P. F., C. M. Carlberg-Bacq., C. Colin, P. Franchimont, L. Gosselin, S. Kozma, and P. M. Osterrieth (1977), *Cancer Res.* **37,** 4326.

Zangerle, P. F., J. C. Hendrick, A. Thiron, and P. Franchimont (1976), in *Cancer Related Antigens,* Franchimont, P., ed., Elsevier, New York p. 61.

Zangerle, P. F., A. Thiron, J. C. Hendrick, and P. Franchimont (1978), in *Laboratory Testing for Cancer,* vol. 22, Karger, Switzerland, p. 141.

10

Ovarian and Uterine Cancer Markers

Markku Seppälä

Department of Obstetrics and Gynecology,
University Central Hospital, Helsinki, Finland

Laboratory tests have long been an integral part of the diagnosis and management of gynecological cancer. Cytology permits easy detection of premalignant and early malignant lesions of the cervix, and as a result new cases are now diagnosed earlier and can be more successfully managed. Research on biochemical tumor markers is directed to the same goal. The classic example is choriocarcinoma, which can be diagnosed and monitored by measurement of chorionic gonadotropin. But many gynecologic tumors are still fatal. Thus, ovarian cancer has defied all attempts at early diagnosis, and treatment of advanced cases remains unsatisfactory.

Potential markers for gynecologic cancer include oncodevelopmental antigens, enzymes, hormones, and other proteins. This review summarizes the current state of knowledge on tumor markers for the management of trophoblastic and nontrophoblastic gynecologic cancer.

1. Oncodevelopmental Antigens

1.1. Alphafetoprotein

1.1.1. Trophoblastic Disease

Alphafetoprotein (AFP) is synthesized by the fetal liver, yolk sac, and the gastrointestinal tract (Gitlin et al., 1972). AFP reappears in most cases of primary liver cancer and yolk sac tumors, and very occasionally in gastric cancer (see Abelev, 1974). Considering the embryonic sites of AFP production one would not expect AFP secretion by trophoblastic tumors; serum AFP levels are usually not elevated in patients with choriocarcinoma (Seppälä et al., 1972), but may be in some patients with hydatidiform mole (Seppälä and Ruoslahti, 1974). Vesicular fluid from hydatidiform moles may also contain AFP at high concentrations (Grudzinskas et al., 1977). However, measurement of serum AFP does not contribute to the management of patients with gestational trophoblastic disease.

1.1.2. Nontrophoblastic Tumors

Nontrophoblastic gynecologic neoplasms rarely secrete AFP in increased amounts detectable in serum. In a study of 92 patients with nontrophoblastic gynecologic neoplasms, of which 53 were ovarian cancers, Seppälä and coworkers (1975) found an elevated serum AFP level in only one patient (ovarian carcinoma with liver metastases).

Germ cell tumors may secrete AFP (Abelev et al., 1967; Ballas, 1972; Talerman and Haije, 1974). Germ cell tumors differentiate along either embryonic or extraembryonic pathways (Teilum, 1965), or along both; dysgerminomas proliferate without differentiation. Extraembryonic differentiation may yield yolk sac or trophoblastic tissue, the former secreting AFP and the latter chorionic gonadotropin (HCG). Embryonic differentiation yields teratomas that usually do not secrete AFP. Many germ cell tumors have mixed components and virtually all teratocarcinomas are mixed tumors (see Fox, 1980). Cells that secrete AFP or HCG may be unrecognized by routine histopathology unless specific immunohistochemical staining is used. In pure yolk sac tumors, AFP can be identified in cells lining the endodermal sinuses as well as in intra- and extracytoplasmic PAS-positive hyaline globules (Teilum et al., 1974).

In patients with yolk sac tumors, circulating AFP levels reflect the activity of the tumor. The normal half-life of AFP is 4–5 days (Seppälä and Ruoslahti, 1972), and postoperative estimation of half-life permits early determination of the completeness of surgical removal.

The use of radiolabeled anti-AFP antibodies has been exploited for in vivo localization of AFP-producing tumors (e.g., a Sertoli-Leydig cell tumor of both ovaries) (Goldenberg et al., 1980b). For example, a "second-look" operation was performed on a patient with a yolk sac tumor who had a rising AFP level despite chemotherapy. Small nodules of yolk sac tumor were removed from the peritoneal cavity, but this had no effect on the serum AFP level. Radioimmunodetection was attempted in order to localize tumor deposits. Scanning revealed an accumulation of radioactivity in the peritoneal cavity and retroperitoneal space, but the liver and the lungs were free of apparent tumor tissue. The absence of remote metastases was confirmed at a third operation, and by later autopsy. Previous experimental (Primus et al., 1973; Mach et al., 1974) and clinical studies (Goldenberg et al., 1978; Dykes et al., 1980; Goldenberg et al., 1980) indicate that radioactive antibody scanning can show tumor deposits. Although, unlike CEA, AFP is not a cell surface marker, the local antigen concentration appears to be sufficient for successful radiolocalization (Goldenberg et al., 1980b).

AFP from yolk sac tumors differs from fetal serum AFP in that a greater proportion of it does not bind to concanavalin A (Ruoslahti et al., 1978). In the patient with yolk sac tumor described above, 40–60% of circulating AFP did not bind con A, suggesting yolk sac origin, and reflecting differences in glycosylation between AFP from fetal liver and yolk sac (Ruoslahti and Seppälä, 1979). The difference does not, however, affect the immunoreactivity of AFP (Ruoslahti et al., 1978).

In summary, AFP is an excellent marker for yolk sac tumors. Demonstration of AFP can be used for histopathological classification, localization of metastases in the body, and for monitoring of treatment. Pregnancy-related disorders and liver disease may also cause elevated serum AFP levels (Brock, 1977; Seppälä, 1977), but these can be easily recognized and cause no major problems in differential diagnosis.

1.2. Carcinoembryonic Antigen

1.2.1. Trophoblastic Tumors

CEA levels are usually normal in patients with trophoblastic tumors (Seppälä et al., 1976).

1.2.2. Nontrophoblastic Tumors

CEA has been demonstrated in premalignant lesions and malignant tumors of the female reproductive system (Lindgren et al., 1979; Marchand et al., 1975; Goldenberg et al., 1976; Rutanen et al., 1978) as well as in mucinous cyst fluid (van Nagell et al., 1975b), ascitic fluid (Seppälä et al., 1975), and serum of such patients (Khoo and Mackay, 1973; Seppälä et al., 1975; van Nagell et al., 1975a; DiSaia et al., 1975). CEA from gynecological cancers appears to be immunologically identical with colon cancer CEA (Seppälä et al., 1975), but CEA from some ovarian cancers has been reported to have a higher molecular weight (Pletsch and Goldenberg, 1974).

1.2.2.1. Expression of CEA in Premalignant Lesions and Invasive Cancer. CEA has been identified in tissue from early premalignant lesions. Using immunoperoxidase staining for epithelial lesions of the uterine cervix, Lindgren and coworkers (1979) found that normal epithelium was CEA-negative, whereas 25% of early dysplasias were CEA-positive, principally in the keratinized surface layers. The incidence of CEA-positivity increased from premalignant to malignant lesions (Fig. 1). Increased CEA levels may reflect malignant potential in premalignant lesions.

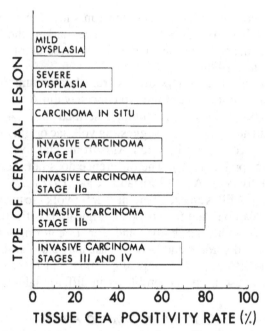

Fig. 1. CEA-positivity rate in tissue of premalignant and malignant squamous cell lesions of the uterine cervix. Data from Lindgren et al., 1979.

1.2.2.2. The Relationship of CEA to Prognosis of Patients with Gynecologic Cancer. In patients with ovarian cancer, elevated serum CEA levels are associated with a poor prognosis (Levin et al., 1976). This has been ascribed to the greater volume of such tumors rather than any inherent aggressiveness of CEA-positive lesions. Studies by Lindgren et al. (1979) have demonstrated that the invasive properties of squamous cell carcinoma of the cervix are not related to the presence or absence of CEA, since patients with CEA-positive and CEA-negative lesions had similar 10-year survival rates within tumors of the same clinical stage (Figs. 2 and 3).

1.2.2.3. CEA in Histopathological Classification of Gynecologic Tumors. Immunoperoxidase staining for CEA in tissue may improve the histopathologic classification of certain tumors of uterus and ovary. For example, the histological variability of endocervical and endometrial adenocarcinomas has created problems of differential diagnosis, in part because specimens obtained by endocervical curettage of the endocervix may contain endometrial tissue. Recent studies suggest that diagnosis can be improved by the demonstration of CEA in tissue (Fig. 4). Thus, in a study by Wahlström et al. (1979), tissue from 131 of 163 patients (80%) with endocervical adenocarcinoma, but only 11 of 137 patients (8%) with endometrial adenocarcinoma, was CEA-positive. The commonest exceptions were endocervical mesonephroid adenocarcin-

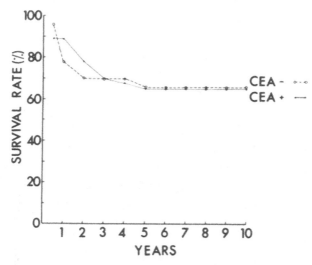

Fig. 2. Survival rates for patients with CEA-positive and CEA-negative state I–II$_A$ cervical cancer treated by radical surgery. Reproduced by permission from Lindgren et al. (1979), *Int. J. Cancer* **23,** 448.

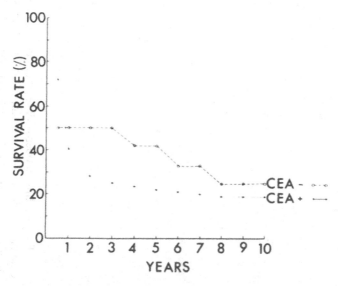

Fig. 3. Survival rates for patients with CEA-positive and CEA-negative with advanced cervical cancer (Stages II$_B$–III) treated by radiotherapy. Reproduced by permission from Lindgren et al. (1979), *Int. J. Cancer* **23,** 448.

omas (which were CEA-negative) and endometrial adenosquamous carcinomas (which were CEA-positive). After exclusion of these on simple morphological criteria, 86 of 107 endocervical adenocarcinomas (80%) were CEA-positive, and all endometrial adenocarcinomas were CEA-

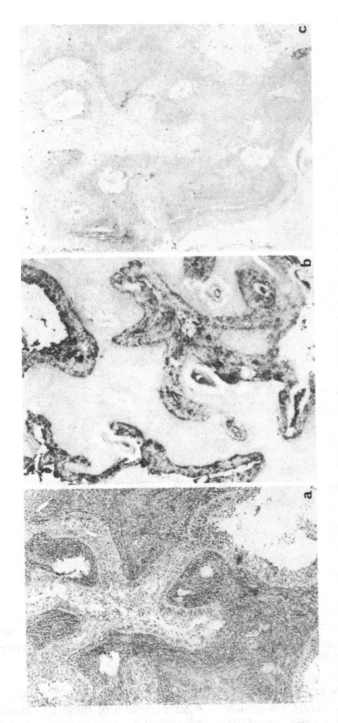

Fig. 4. Immunoperoxidase staining of CEA in endocervical adenocarcinoma. (a) Hematoxylin–eosin; (b) anti-CEA antiserum; (c) anti-CEA antiserum absorbed with purified CEA. By courtesy of Dr. T. Wahlström, Helsinki.

negative. Although the qualitative interpretation of immunoperoxidase slides is unambiguous when appropriate controls are included, the difference between positive and negative results must also be quantitative because the immunoperoxidase test can only detect CEA concentrations of 3–5 μg/g or greater in formalin-fixed specimens (Goldenberg et al., 1976). However, not all workers agree that a clear distinction can be made. In a smaller series of endocervical adenocarcinomas, van Nagell et al. (1979) reported a lower frequency (36%) of CEA-positivity. The usefulness of CEA-staining has also been questioned on the basis of the relative incidence of endometrial and endocervical adenocarcinomas (Dufour and Stock, 1980). Since endometrial adenocarcinoma is over 20 times more common than endocervical adenocarcinoma, endometrial adenocarcinoma would contribute more CEA-positives than would endocervical adenocarcinomas in a random sample of adenocarcinomas. However, if tumors with squamous elements are rigorously excluded, 99% of CEA-negative adenocarcinomas would be endometrial. This information can be of great diagnostic value.

Immunohistochemical staining of CEA may also be useful in some ovarian tumors. A study of tissue CEA content of 82 ovarian epithelial neoplasms showed that mucinous tumors contain more CEA than serous tumors (Heald et al., 1979). There was only partial correspondence between the degree of malignancy of mucinous tumors, as assessed histologically, and their content of CEA. From these studies it was postulated that examination of tissue CEA might sharpen the morphological distinction of these neoplasms and thus allow for a more precise grading of their degree of malignancy (Heald et al., 1979).

1.2.2.4. Circulating CEA Levels. Elevated serum CEA levels have been noted in 13–80% of patients with gynecologic cancer. The highest frequency is seen with endocervical cancer, and lower frequencies in endometrial adenocarcinoma. Elevated levels are also commoner and more striking in patients with advanced disease (Seppälä et al., 1975; Kjörstad and Orjaseter, 1977; Rutanen et al., 1978), though they are occasionally seen even in patients with benign mucinous cystadenoma (Fig. 5). The great variation in the reported frequencies of elevated serum CEA levels results from variability in cutoff levels and on differences in assay protocols and reagents. All workers agree, however, that in gynecologic cancer elevated CEA levels are not as high as in colorectal cancer. Most studies show that circulating CEA levels correlate with the spread of disease (Seppälä et al., 1975; DiSaia et al., 1975; Rutanen et al., 1978). Elevated levels have been reported in early stages, e.g., carcinoma *in situ* (Khoo and Mackay, 1976), but most would agree that this is uncommon (Stone et al., 1977; Seppälä et al., 1975; Kjörstad and Orjaseter, 1977; Rutanen et al., 1978).

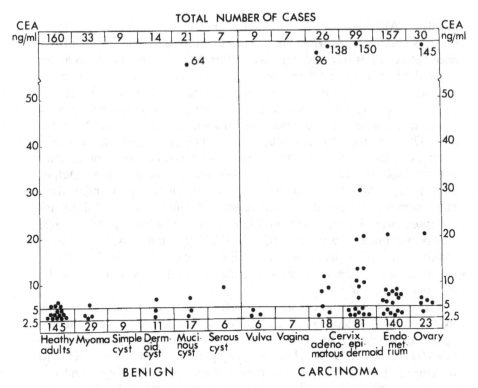

Fig. 5. Serum CEA concentration in 160 apparently healthy adults and 412 patients with gynecologic tumors before treatment. Reproduced by permission from Rutanen et al. (1978), *Cancer* **42**, 581.

In gynecologic cancer, immunoperoxidase staining of tumor tissue is more sensitive than measurement of serum CEA levels for the identification of CEA-positive tumors. Thus, when tumors are CEA-positive, the serum level may be either normal or elevated, but when the tumor is CEA-negative, the serum CEA level is usually normal (Fig. 6). Exceptions to the latter have been observed among patients with advanced disease, liver disease, infectious disease, and in heavy smokers. Some studies (Khoo and Mackay, 1974) suggest that, in gynecologic cancer, reelevation of serum CEA level precedes clinical symptoms and clinical tumor by an average of 10.8 weeks. However, this does not improve prognosis since little can be done following radical surgery and full radiotherapy. Persistence or decrease of elevated CEA levels may also be used to determine the completeness of surgery.

1.2.2.5. Radioimmunodetection of Gynecologic Tumors by Anti-CEA Antibodies and External Photoscanning. Although the first attempt to identify human neoplasms with radiolabeled anti-CEA was unsuccessful (Reif et al., 1974), subsequent studies have been more promising. Goldenberg et al. (1978) described 18 patients with various cancers

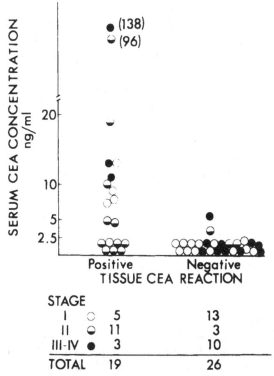

Fig. 6. Serum CEA concentration and tissue CEA staining in 45 cancer patients classified according to clinical stage. Reproduced by permission from Rutanen et al. (1978), *Cancer* **42**, 581.

in whom all but 6 out of 38 tumor deposits were revealed using a subtraction technique. The studies were expanded to include ovarian cancer. ^{131}I-labeled goat immunoglobulin G (IgG) against CEA was administered to patients with ovarian cancer (average dose 1.0 mCi; 180–250 μg IgG protein). The primary cancer was localized in all 13 patients and the metastases in 6 out of 9 cases (van Nagell et al., 1980). More conventional diagnostic techniques such as computer-assisted tomography, ultrasonography, and angiography were less efficient. However, lesions smaller than 2 cm in diameter could not be detected. Tumors containing a CEA concentration above 115 ng/g could be localized with radioactive anti-CEA antibodies, and these included a benign neoplasm (van Nagell et al., 1980). Thus, primary and secondary ovarian cancers could be detected in 100 and 67% of cases, respectively. Although these preliminary results are promising, CEA is not a specific marker for ovarian cancer but merely serves as a target for immunolocalization.

The same principle applies to all tumors or tissues containing more CEA than the surrounding tissue. In studies on colonic cancer, radioactivity in the tumor has been 1.5–5.3 times higher than in the adjacent tissue (Mach et al., 1979), and successful radioimmunodetection has been achieved even in the presence of high circulating CEA concentrations (Goldenberg et al., 1978; Dykes et al., 1980). It is obvious that both specificity and purity of anti-CEA antibody are prerequisites, and demand the use of affinity-purified antibodies. Nonetheless, the method has great potential value in the immunodetection of cancer (van Nagell et al., 1980; Dykes et al., 1980; Mach et al., 1980).

1.3. Chorionic Gonadotropin and Subunits of Glycoprotein Hormones

1.3.1. Trophoblastic Tumors

Chorionic gonadotropin is synthesized by the placental syncytiotrophoblast and trophoblastic tumors (Midgley and Pierce, 1962). Of all tumor markers, HCG is the most fully investigated with regard to physiocochemical properties, physiology, and clinical application. The estimated secretion rate of HCG by one trophoblastic cell for a 10-day old human placenta is 1.4×10^{-2} IU/day (Braunstein et al., 1973a), and the estimated production rate of HCG by malignant trophoblast in vivo is 5×10^{-5} IU/cell/day (Bagshawe, 1969) and in vitro 5×10^{-6}–10^{-7} IU/cell/day (Kohler and Bridson, 1971). Evidence from in vitro and in vivo studies indicates that the amount of HCG produced is proportional to the number of viable tumor cells (Bagshawe, 1969; Lewis et al., 1969).

In addition to HCG the normal placenta also contains subunits of HCG, the free alpha subunit being in excess of the beta subunit (Vaitukaitis, 1974). In choriocarcinoma the proportion of free alpha secretion is less than in normal pregnancy (Vaitukaitis and Ebersole, 1976; Rutanen, 1978), and it has been suggested that free alpha secretion is related to an unfavorable prognosis.

Treatment of patients with choriocarcinoma relies heavily on information about circulating HCG levels (Hertz et al., 1961). HCG becomes detectable in blood when as few as 10^4–10^5 tumor cells are present in the body (Bagshawe, 1975), whereas 10^9–10^{12} cells are required before tumor becomes demonstrable by other clinical measures. The measurement of serum HCG levels by radioimmunoassay (Vaitukaitis et al., 1972) has become vital for the patient because effective treatment can be offered. The prognosis of these patients has improved to near 100% survival rate following improvements in early diagnosis and treatment.

1.3.2. HCG in Nontrophoblastic Gynecologic Cancer

Studies using radioimmunoassays specific to the HCG beta subunit have revealed the presence of HCG-like immunoreactivity in a number of nontrophoblastic tumors, including gynecologic cancer (Braunstein et al., 1973b). Although the clinical significance of HCG measurement is now

Table 1
Elevated Serum Levels of HCG
in Gynecological Cancer
before Treatment[a]

Site	Elevated/total	%
Vulva	2/8	25
Vagina	2/6	33
Cervix	23/111	21
Endometrium	17/125	14
Ovary	5/26	19
All patients	49/276	18

[a]From Rutanen and Seppälä, 1978.

generally accepted for the management of choriocarcinoma and germ cell tumors (Bagshawe, 1979), its application to nontrophoblastic gynecologic cancer is less apparent. Rutanen and Seppälä (1978) examined the circulating levels of HCG by radioimmunoassay specific to HCG beta subunit in 380 patients with nontrophoblastic gynecologic disease. HCG-like immunoradioactivity was found in 49 of 276 cancer patients (18%) (Table 1) and in 15 of 104 patients (14%) with nonmalignant conditions. In malignant disease, HCG values were higher than in nonmalignant conditions. No difference was observed between the mean age of HCG-positive and HCG-negative cancer patients, but HCG-positive patients in the nonmalignant group were older. The frequency of HCG-positives was not related to clinical stage (Tables 2 and 3) or histological differentiation (Tables 4

Table 2
Elevated Serum Levels of HCG
in Cervical Cancer
before Treatment[a]

Clinical stage[b]	Elevated/total	%
0	2/6	33
I_A	1/4	25
I_B	13/45	29
II_A	1/21	5
II_B	3/11	27
III	3/20	15
IV	0/4	0
All patients	23/111	21

[a]From Rutanen and Seppälä, 1978.
[b]FIGO classification. Figures for adenocarcinoma of the cervix were 4/23 (17%).

Table 3
Elevated Serum Levels of HCG
in Endometrial Cancer
before Treatment[a]

Clinical stage[b]	Elevated/total	%
I	14/104	13
II	3/13	23
III	0/6	0
IV	0/2	0
All patients	17/125	14

[a]From Rutanen and Seppälä, 1978.
[b]FIGO classification.

Table 4
Elevated Serum Levels of HCG in Relation to Histological Degree of Differentiation of
Cervical Cancer[a]

Degree of differentiation	Elevated/total	%	HCG concentration, mIU/mL (mean ± SEM)
High	3/12	25	16.2 ± 3.3
Medium	7/28	25	16.6 ± 3.4
Low	5/34	22	14.6 ± 3.0
Not stated	5/34	15	13.9 ± 2.8
Total	23/111	21	

[a]From Rutanen and Seppälä, 1978.

Table 5
Elevated Serum Levels of HCG in Relation to Histological Differentiation of Endometrial
Cancer[a]

Degree of differentiation	Elevated/total	%	HCG concentration, mIU/mL (mean ± SEM)
High	7/39	18	25.7 ± 10.9
Medium	2/51	4	9.4
Low	5/19	26	11.4 ± 0.8
Not stated	3/16	19	9.6 ± 1.3
Total	17/125	14	

[a]From Rutanen and Seppälä, 1978.

and 5). After radical surgery 12 of 17 HCG-positive cancer patients became HCG-negative (71%), while 5 remained HCG-positive. Remarkably enough, 49 initially negative patients transiently became HCG-positive after radical surgery, which included oophorectomy, and 42 remained negative. It was also observed that high concentrations of the crude pituitary HFSH/HLH* reference preparation LER 907 cross-reacted in the HCG assay. These and other results (Chen et al., 1976) suggest the possible existence of a pituitary HCG-like substance, and HCG-like immunoreactivity has recently been demonstrated in many normal tissues (Braunstein et al., 1979). Oophorectomy is included in the radical surgery for gynecologic cancer, and this may cause supraphysiological HLH levels to interfere with the HCG assay unless the cutoff level is set above the level of HLH crossreaction.

The above observations raise questions regarding the value of HCG measurement in the demonstration of residual HCG-producing cells in patients with nontrophoblastic neoplasms.

Eutopic and ectopic secretion of subunits of pituitary and placental glycoprotein hormones have been shown both in vivo and in vitro (Vaitukaitis, 1973; Rosen and Weintraub, 1974; Hussa, 1977), and free alpha subunits are detectable in the serum of pregnant and postmenopausal women (Franchimont et al., 1972). HeLa cells also release HCG and free alpha subunit in culture (Lieblich et al., 1976), but patients with cancer of the cervix do not have elevated levels of alpha subunit. Rutanen (1978) examined serum samples from 101 patients with nontrophoblastic gynecologic cancer including cervical cancer (43 cases), endometrial cancer (40 cases), ovarian cancer (11 cases), carcinoma of the vulva (3 cases), and of the vagina (4 cases), and found that the levels of alpha subunit were no different from those of controls in corresponding age groups.

1.4. Pregnancy-Specific Beta-1-Glycoprotein (SP1)

1.4.1. Trophoblastic Tumors

Pregnancy specific beta-l-glycoprotein (Bohn, 1971) has been identified by immunofluorescence methods in normal human placenta and choriocarcinoma (Tatarinov et al., 1976; Horne et al., 1976), and also in the serum of patients with malignant trophoblastic disease (Tatarinov et al., 1974). Subsequent studies using highly sensitive radioimmunoassays have shown that SP1 is detectable in the serum of virtually all patients with untreated choriocarcinoma, and the levels approximately parallel those of HCG (Fig. 7). Isolated secretion of SP1 (without HCG) has been observed in some patients with choriocarcinoma (Searle et al., 1978; Seppälä et al., 1978). The significance of this observation was examined by Rutanen

*Human follicle-stimulating hormone/human luteinizing hormone (HFSH/HLH).

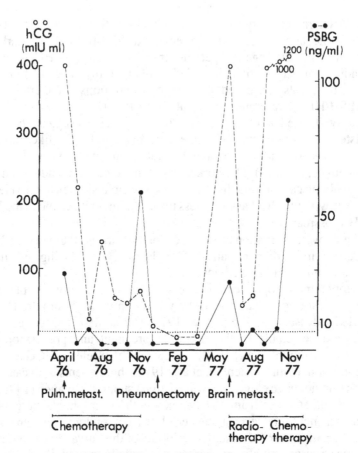

Fig. 7. Serum SPl (PSBG) and HCG levels in a choriocarcinoma patient who developed clinical metastases in spite of extensive chemotherapy. Reproduced by permission from Seppälä et al. (1978), *Int. J. Cancer* **21**, 265.

and Seppälä (1980) in a series of 17 patients with choriocarcinoma (Fig. 8), 7 patients with hydatidiform mole, and patients with rheumatoid arthritis, liver disease, infections, and apparently healthy nonpregnant women. Immunoreactive SPl was identified in 1 out of 20 patients with rheumatoid arthritis (3.7 μg/L), 1 out of 20 patients with liver disease (4.8 μg/L), and in none of the 29 patients with infectious disease. Four out of 85 healthy nonpregnant women (4.7%) had apparent serum levels up to 2.2 μg/L. In choriocarcinoma, trophoblastic activity was assumed when over 5 U/L were found in serum. SPl was elevated (over 4.8 μg/L) in 80 out of 129 HCG-positive samples (62%), but SPl was also found in 27 out of 238 HCG-negative samples (11%) from choriocarcinoma patients. After 3 months remission, judged by the absence of demonstrable HCG, SPl was found in 11 out of 112 HCG-negative samples (10%), and after 12 months

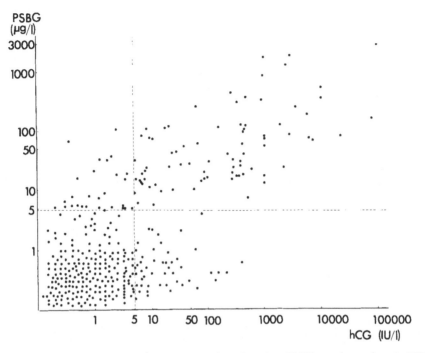

Fig. 8. Serum SPl concentrations plotted against HCG concentrations in 367 serum samples obtained from 17 patients with choriocarcinoma before, during, and after chemotherapy. Six to 47 samples came from each patient. Reproduced by permission from Rutanen and Seppälä (1980), *J. Clin. Endocrinol. Metab.* **50**, 57.

remission SPl was found in 6 out of 42 HCG-negative samples (17%). Peaks of SPl and/or HCG were sometimes observed in asymptomatic patients, and chemotherapy was given only to those patients in whom HCG was found. The significance of isolated SPl peaks is not clear, and further chemotherapy has not been recommended on the basis of such elevations in asymptomatic HCG-negative patients (Fig. 9).

1.4.2. Nontrophoblastic Tumors

SPl-like activity has been detected in various types of nontrophoblastic malignant neoplasms (Tatarinov and Sokolov, 1977; Bagshawe et al., 1978), but this has not been confirmed in all studies (Engvall and Yonemoto, 1979). Wurz (1979) reported elevated serum SPl levels in some patients with ovarian cancer, but the levels in the tumor itself were lower than those in serum. It is difficult to assess from these results whether the elevated serum SPl level was secondary to the tumor, though this was suggested by the fact that the levels fell after radical surgery. Crowther et al. (1979) examined 37 patients with ovarian cancer and found

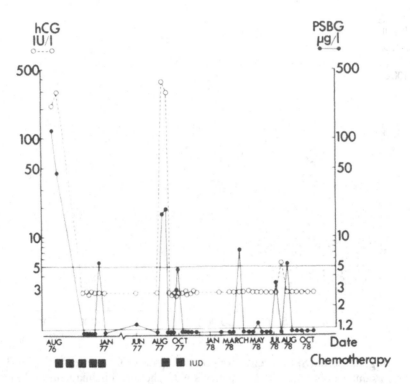

Fig. 9. Serum SPl and HCG levels in a patient with choriocarcinoma. Small elevations above the cut-off level were considered to be nonspecific and did not warrant chemotherapy.

elevated SPl levels (up to 15.5 μg/L) in 5 cases. The author has also seen transient minor elevations of serum SPl level in patients with invasive epidermoid cancer of the cervix, but the origin and significance of such peaks is not clear. SPl has been identified in teratocarcinomas of the testis (Tatarinov et al., 1977; Johnson et al., 1977) and it is possible that some ovarian teratocarcinomas may produce SPl. Apart from germ cell tumors it is likely that estimation of circulating SPl levels will not be useful for monitoring of patients with nontrophoblastic gynecologic cancer.

It has not as yet been ascertained whether normal human serum is completely devoid of SPl. Searle et al. (1978) reported a low level of circulating SPl in 13% of healthy adults, and Rutanen and Seppälä (1980) found similar levels in 5% of apparently healthy women and patients with nonneoplastic disease. Rosen and coworkers (1979) have observed immunoreactive SPl production by human fibroblast cultures, and this material has been shown to have the same molecular weight as placental SPl. There is a certain noise level (a few μg/L) in the sensitive part of any radio-immunoassay and, therefore, some of the low values observed by radioimmunoassay may result from a nonspecific effect. Hence, the cutoff level must be chosen so that it excludes the values that may arise from non-specific variation in the assay "blank" when SPl measurement is used in clinical studies.

1.5. Placental Protein 5 (PP5)

PP5 is a unique protein isolated from the human placenta (Bohn, 1972). PP5 is a glycoprotein containing 20% carbohydrate. It has a molecular weight of 36,000 and appears to inhibit the action of trypsin and plasmin (Bohn and Winckler, 1977). PP5 also forms complexes with heparin (Salem et al., 1980).

1.5.1. Trophoblastic Tumors

PP5 has been localized by the immunoperoxidase technique in the syncytiotrophoblast of normal human placenta and hydatidiform mole (Seppälä et al., 1979). In normal pregnancy, PP5 becomes detectable in maternal serum at 8–10 weeks gestation (Seppälä et al., 1979). The levels increase as the pregnancy progresses and plateau in the third trimester (Obiekwe et al., 1979). PP5 has been found in the serum and tissue of patients with hydatidiform mole, whereas it is undetectable in the serum and tumor of patients with chroriocarcinoma (Seppälä et al., 1979). Even patients with high circulating levels of HCG are PP5-negative (Lee et al., 1981). Thus there is a considerable difference between normal and malignant trophoblast in the concentration of PP5, and it is possible that the low concentration of PP5 (protease inhibitor) is associated with the invasiveness of malignant trophoblast.

1.5.2. PP5 in Nontrophoblastic Tumors

The author has studied PP5 levels in 12 patients with invasive squamous cell carcinoma of the cervix and 17 patients with adenocarcinoma of the endometrium, and none of these patients had a PP5 level elevated above the 1.2 μg/L detection limit. Small elevations (up to 2.5 μg/L) of PP5 were occasionally seen in a patient with an AFP-producing ovarian yolk sac tumor, and in some patients with nonneoplastic liver disease, but these lay near the minimum detection limits of the assay and may represent nonspecific "noise."

2. Enzymes

Abnormal enzyme activity is well-recognized in many cancers (for a review, see Schwartz, 1973). Deficiency or altered specificity of enzymes results in accumulation of incomplete or abnormal glycoproteins. Barlow and Dillard (1972) reported increased serum levels of fucosyl glycoprotein in a high percentage of patients with advanced ovarian cancer. Battacharya and Barlow (1979) found elevated levels of galactosyl transferase and sialyl transferase in all ovarian tumors, whereas the levels of β-N-acetyl-glucosaminide fucosyl transferase and β-galactoside fucosyl transferase activity were high in some ovarian tumors only. On the other hand, a deficiency of α-L-fucosidase was found in the serum of patients with epithelial ovarian cancers and α-L-fucosidase deficiency may be a genetic marker for patients with epithelial ovarian cancers (see Battacharya and Barlow, 1979). Another enzyme that is deficient in ovarian tumors is phosphodiesterase, but the circulating activity of the same enzyme may be paradoxically increased (Schwartz, 1973). Chatterjee and colleagues (1978) and Battacharya and Barlow (1979) reported elevated serum levels of galactosyltransferase in all 30 patients with ovarian adenocarcinoma compared with age- and blood group-matched controls, and N-acetyl glucosaminyl transferase 1 and 2 were elevated in most of the same patients. Sialyl transferase concentration was high in all tumor tissues, while elevated serum levels were seen in only 20% of patients. Elevated leucine aminopeptidase levels have been reported in patients with ovarian cancer (Blum and Sirota, 1977). A plasminogen-activating enzyme identical to urokinase is released by ovaian carcinoma in tissue culture (Astedt and Holmberg, 1976).

Carcino-placental alkaline phosphatase, Regan isoenzyme, is frequently elevated in the serum of patients with ovarian cancer (Stolbach et al., 1969). Fishman and coworkers (1975a,b) studied 833 cancer patients and f ound elevated levels of Regan isoenzyme in 43% of patients with ovarian adenocarcinoma, and increasing enzyme levels were generally correlated with advancing disease. By contrast, Cadeau and coworkers (1974) found that patients with early stages of cervical cancer had higher levels of heat stable alkaline phosphatase than patients in later stages. The D-phenotype of placental alkaline phosphatase, Nagao isoenzyme, has been recovered in 82% of ascitic fluids from ovarian cancer patients (Inglis et al., 1973). Though these observations add to our knowledge of the biology of cancer, the assessment of clinical utility for diagnosis or monitoring of cancer awaits more detailed studies.

3. Other Antigens

3.1. Ovarian Cancer-Associated Antigens OCAA and OCAA-1

Bhattacharya and Barlow (1973) described two tumor-associated antigens, OCAA and OCAA-1, in serous and mucinous cystadenocarcinomas of the ovary that were not detectable in the normal ovary. OCAA was present in 26 of 37 serous and 7 of 7 mucinous cystadenocarcinomas, but not in benign serous or mucinous cystadenomas or normal ovaries. OCAA-1 was identified in 90% of all malignant ovarian and other gynecologic neoplasms as well as in some colon, breast, pancreatic, and other malignant tumors. OCAA has not been found by immunodiffusion techniques in normal human serum.

3.2. Ovarian Cancer Antigens OvC-1–OvC-6

Imamura and coworkers (1978) isolated six antigens OvC-1, 2, 3, 4, 5, and 6 from human ovarian cancer that were not detected in normal ovary. OvC-4 was identified as CEA and OvC-5 was the normal crossreacting antigen, NCA (von Kleist et al., 1972). OvC-3 was the same as pregnancy-associated macroglobulin (see Stigbrand, Chapter 12), while OvC-6 was an individual specific antigen detectable in the immunizing tumor only. OvC-1 and OvC-2 were unrelated to any well-defined tumor antigen. OvC-1 was present in 48 of 93 epithelial cancers of the ovary, but also in some cervical, breast, gastric, and pancreatic cancers, and in normal kidney and lung. OvC-1 was also present in cord serum and pregnancy sera and in the placenta and amniotic fluid. OvC-2 was confined to ovarian cancers (8/93) and was not detected in other types of tumors or normal adult tissues. OvC-2 was also found in the placenta, amniotic fluid, and fetal intestine.

3.3. Miscellaneous Markers

Ovarian cancer-associated antigens have also been reported by several other investigators, and some of them may overlap with each other. Burton and coworkers (1976) isolated a thermostable glycoprotein antigen in 70% of human ovarian cancers and cysts. Knauf and Urbach (1974) described a perchloric acid soluble antigen in 70% of patients with ovarian cancer. About 50% of ovarian cancers contain embryonic prealbumin (EPA) (Tatarinov and Kalashnikov, 1977), and Bagshawe and coworkers (1980) isolated an ovarian tumor associated antigen (OTAG) in ascitic fluids of patients with ovarian cystadenocarcinomas. Hamazaki and Hotta (1975) found a fucose-rich glycoprotein (FRGP) in ovarian cyst fluid, and Bara et al. (1977) described an antigen that was common to human mucinous cyst fluid and gastric mucosa.

A collaborative study (Bagshawe et al., 1979) on ovarian cancer antigens was arranged by Sizaret of the International Agency for Cancer in which various ovarian cancer-associated antigens and antisera were compared by Axelsen. Testing of over 30 antigens and antisera revealed that a number were not pure or monospecific. Studies by fused rocket immunoelectrophoresis, crossed immunoelectrophoresis, and tandem crossed immunoelectrophoresis revealed CEA-like immunoreactivity in OCAA-5 of Bhattacharya and Barlow (1973), OCAA-2 of Lamerz et al. (1979)

OvC-3 of Knauf and Urbach (1974), and OvC-4 of Imamura et al. (1978). OCAA of Bhattacharya and Barlow (1973) was shown to be unique, whereas their OCAA-3 and OCAA-4 corresponded to the M4-antigen of Bara et al. (1977). M1-antigen of the latter workers, EPA, FRGP, and OTAG were unique proteins. Many of the above tumor-associated antigens are candidates for diagnosis and monitoring of cancer patients, but prospective clinical trials are required to decide whether any of them will be useful.

A tumor antigen for human cervical squamous cell carcinoma (TA-4) was isolated by Kato and Torigoe (1977). The antigen has a molecular weight of 48,000 and is destroyed by treatment with perchloric acid. The antigen has not been detected in normal women or patients with other carcinomas, whereas 27 of 35 patients with squamous cell carcinoma showed detectable serum antigen levels. All patients with advanced disease had detectable levels in serum. A rough correlation with disease progress has been reported (Kato et al., 1979). However, a detailed comparison of this protein with other well-established tumor markers is not available.

4. Summary

A number of tumor-associated substances have been isolated from malignant gynecologic neoplasms, but few, if any, are strictly organ specific. Research on these markers will increase understanding and management of gynecologic cancer in several ways:

1. Tumor-associated antigens may aid in histopathological classification of certain tumors (AFP in yolk sac tumors, CEA in endocervical vs endometrial adenocarcinomas).

2. Demonstration of an antigen in tissue by immunohistochemical methods may help to identify those patients in whom measurement of circulating levels of the same antigen may reveal early recurrence (CEA in cancers of the uterine cervix or ovary).

3. Response to surgery of elevated marker levels may indicate completeness of removal (CEA, AFP, HCG).

4. Elevation of the serum tumor marker level can occur before symptoms appear or other methods indicate a recurrence. This will become increasingly important when more effective means of treatment are available (HCG in choriocarcinoma, AFP in yolk sac tumors).

5. Some lesions considered as premalignant express tumor-related substances (CEA). It remains to be seen whether cells containing tumor markers are those with malignant potential.

6. The presence or relative absence of certain substances in tumors adds to our knowledge of tumor biology. The concentration of a pro-

tease inhibitor (PP5) is lower in choriocarcinoma than in normal placenta, and it is possible that absence of protease inhibitor is related to the invasive properties of choriocarcinoma.

7. Radioimmunodetection of tumors in vivo by radiolabeled IgG and subsequent photoscanning presents a challenging new approach to the localization of tumors and their metastases.

Acknowledgments

The author thanks Professor Tim Chard and Ms. Eileen Rubenstein for valuable suggestions and preparation of this manuscript. Original studies and preparation of this chapter were supported by grants from the Research Council for Medical Sciences, Academy of Finland, the Finnish Cancer Society, and the UK Medical Research Council.

References

Abelev, G. I. (1974), *Transplant. Rev.* **20**, 3.
Abelev, G. I., I. V. Assercritova, N. A. Kraevsky, S. D. Perova, and N. I. Perevodchikova (1967), *Int. J. Cancer* **2**, 551.
Astedt, B., and L. Holmberg (1976), *Nature* **261**, 595.
Bagshawe, K. D. (1969), in *Choriocarcinoma: The Clinical Biology of the Trophoblast and Its Tumours* (K. D. Bagshawe, ed.), Edward Arnold, London, 153 pp.
Bagshawe, K. D. (1975), in *Medical Oncology: Medical Aspects of Malignant Disease* (K. D. Bagshawe, ed.), Blackwell, London, 453 pp.
Bagshawe, K. D. (1979), in *Alpha-fetoprotein in Clinical Medicine* (Weitzel, H. K., and J. Schneider, eds.), Thieme, Stuggart.
Bagshawe, K. D., R. M. Lequin, P. H. Sizaret, and Yu. S. Tatarinov (1978), *Eur. J. Cancer* **14**, 1331.
Bagshawe, K. D., J. N. Gennings, and F. Searle (Organizers) (1979), in *International Workshop on Ovarian Tumour-Associated Antigens*, carried out under auspices of P. H. Sizaret and N. H. Axelsen, London, to be published.
Bagshawe, K. D., M. Wass, and F. Searle (1980), *Arch. Gynecol.* **229**, 303.
Ballas, M. (1972), *Am. J. Clin. Path.* **57**, 511.
Bara, J., A. Malarewicz, F. Loisillier, and P. Burtin (1977), *Brit. J. Cancer* **36**, 49.
Barlow, J. J., and P. H. Dillard (1972), *Obstet. Gynecol.* **39**, 727.
Bhattacharya, M., and J. J. Barlow (1973), *Cancer* **31**, 588.
Bhattacharya, M., and J. J. Barlow (1979), *Int. Adv. Surg. Oncol.* **2**, 155.
Blum, M., and P. Sirota (1977), *Isr. J. Med. Sci.* **13**, 875.
Bohn, H. (1971), *Arch. Gynäk.* **210**, 440.
Bohn, H. (1972), *Arch. Gynäk.* **220**, 105.
Bohn, H., and Winckler (1977). *Arch. Gynäk.* **233**, 1979.

Braunstein, G. D., J. M. Grodin, J. L. Vaitukaitis, and G. T. Ross (1973a), *Am. J. Obstet. Gynecol.* **115**, 447.

Braunstein, G. D., J. L. Vaitukaitis, P. P. Carbone, and G. T. Ross (1973b), *Ann. Intern. Med.* **78**, 39.

Braunstein, G. D., V. Kamdar, J. Rasor, N. Swaminathan, and M. E. Wade (1979), *J. Clin. Endocrinol. Metab.* **49**, 917.

Brock, D. J. H. (1977), *Eur. J. Clin. Invest.* **7**, 465.

Burton, R. M., N. J. Hope, and L. M. Lubbers (1976), *Am. J. Obstet. Gynecol.* **125**, 472.

Cadeau, B. J., M. E. Blackstein, and A. Malkin (1974), *Cancer Res.* **34**, 729.

Chatterjee, S. K., M. Bhattacharya, and J. J. Barlow (1978), *Proc. Am. Assoc. Cancer Res.* **19**, 165 (Abstr.).

Chen, H.-C., G. D. Hodgen, S. Matsuura, L. J. Lin, E. Gross, L. E. Reichert, Jr., S. Birken, R. E. Canfield, and G. T. Ross (1976), *Proc. Natl. Acad. Sci. USA* **73**, 2885.

Crowther, M. E., J. G. Grundzinskas, T. A. Poulton, and Y. B. Gordon (1979), *Obstet. Gynecol.* **43**, 59.

DiSaia, P., B. J. Haverback, B. J. Dyce, and C. P. Morrow (1975), *Am. J. Obstet. Gynecol.* **121**, 159.

Dufour, D. R., and R. J. Stock (1980), *Lancet* **1**, 596.

Dykes, P. W., K. R. Hine, A. R. Bradwell, J. C. Blackburn, T. A. Reeder, Z. Drolc, and S. N. Booth (1980), *Brit. Med. J.* **1**, 220.

Engvall, E., and R. H. Yonemoto (1979), *Int. J. Cancer* **23**, 759.

Fishman, W. H., N. R. Inglis, J. L. Vaitukaitis, and L. L. Stolbach (1975a), *J. Natl. Cancer Inst. Monogr. Ser.* **42**, 63.

Fishman, W. H., S. Raam, and L. L. Stolbach (1975b), *Semin. Oncol.* **2**, 211.

Fox, H. (1980), in *Biology of Ovarian Neoplasia* (Murphy, E. D., and W. G. Beamer, eds.), *UICC Technical Report Series* **50**, 22.

Franchimont, P., U. Gaspard, A. Reuter, and G. Heynen (1972), *Clin. Endocrinol.* **1**, 315.

Gitlin, D., A. Perricelli, and G. M. Gitlin (1972), *Cancer* **32**, 979.

Goldenberg, D. M., R. M. Sharkey, and F. J. Primus (1976), *J. Natl. Cancer Inst.* **57**, 11.

Goldenberg, D. M., F. DeLand, E. Kim, S. Bennett, F. J. Primus, J. R. van Nagell, Jr., N. Estes, P. DeSimone, and P. Rayburn (1978), *New Engl. J. Med.* **298**, 1384.

Goldenberg, D. M., F. H. DeLand, E. E. Kim, F. J. Primus, S. Bennett, S. Casper, and R. L. Corgan (1979), VIIth Meeting of International Society for Oncodevelopmental Biology and Medicine, Surrey, UK. Abstr. 59a.

Goldenberg, D. M., E. E. Kim, F. H. DeLand, J. R. van Nagell, Jr., and N. Javadpour (1980a), *Science,* **208**, 1284

Goldenberg, D. M., E. E. Kim, F. DeLand, E. Spremulli, M. O. Nelson, J. P. Gockerman, F. J. Primus, R. L. Corgan, and E. Alpert (1980b), *Cancer* **45**, 2500.

Grudzinskas, J. G. (1977), *Lancet* **2**, 1008.

Hamazaki, M. H., and K. Hotta (1975), *Experientia* **31**, 241.

Heald, J., C. H. Buckley, and H. Fox (1979), *J. Clin. Path.* **32**, 918.

Hertz, R., J. Lewis, Jr. and M. B. Lipsett (1961), *Am. J. Obstet. Gynecol.* **83**, 631.

Horne, C. H. W., C. M. Towler, R. G. P. Pugh-Humphreys, A. W. Thomson, and H. Bohn (1976), *Experientia* **32**, 1197.

Hussa, R. O. (1977), *J. Clin. Endocrinol. Metab.* **44**, 1154.

Imamura, N., T. Takahashi, K. P. Lloyd, J. L. Lewis, Jr., and L. J. Old (1978), *Int. J. Cancer* **21**, 570.

Inglis, N. R., S. Kirley, L. L. Stolbach, and W. H. Fishman (1973), *Cancer Res.* **33**, 1657.

Johnson, S. A. N., J. G. Grudzinskas, Y. B. Gordon, and A. T. M. Al-Ani (1977), *Brit. Med. J.* **1**, 951.

Kato, H., and T. Torigoe (1977), *Cancer* **40**, 1621.

Kato, H., P. Miyauchi, H. Morioka, T. Fujino, and T. Torigoe (1979), *Cancer* **43**, 585.

Khoo, S. K., and E. V. MacKay (1973), *Aust. New Zeal. J. Obstet. Gynaecol.* **13**, 1.

Khoo, S. K., and E. V. MacKay (1974), *Cancer* **34**, 542.

Kjorstad, K. E., and H. Orjaseter (1977), *Cancer* **40**, 2956.

Knauf, S., and G. I. Urbach (1974), *Am. J. Obstet. Gynecol.* **119**, 966.

Kohler, P. O., and W. E. Bridson (1971), *J. Clin. Endocrinol. Metab.* **32**, 683.

Lamerz, R., G. Schnabl, G. Stein, H. J. Kumper, and A. Brandt (1979), in *Carcinoembryonic Proteins: Biology, Chemistry, Clinical Application* (Lehmann, F.-G., ed.), Elsevier/North Holland, Amsterdam, vol. 2, p. 509.

Lee, J. N., H. T. Salem, A. T. M. Al-Ani, T. Chard, S. C. Huang, P. C. Ouyang, P. Y. Wei, and M. Seppälä (1981), *Am. J. Obstet. Gynecol.* **139**, 702.

Levin, L., and J. E. McHardy, T. A. Poulton, P. M. Curling, M. J. Kitau, A. M. Neville, and C. N. Hudson (1976), *Brit. J. Cancer* **33**, 363.

Lewis, J. L., Jr., R. C. Davis, and G. T. Ross (1976), *Am. J. Obstet. Gynecol.* **104**, 472.

Lieblich, J. M., B. D. Weintraub, S. W. Rosen, J. Y. Chou, and J. C. Robinson (1976), *Nature* **260**, 530.

Lindgren, J., T. Wahlström, and M. Seppälä (1979), *Int. J. Cancer* **23**, 448.

Mach, J. P., S. Carrel, C. Merenda, B. Sorbat, and J. C. Cerottini (1974), *Nature* **248**, 704.

Mach, J. P., S. Carrell, M. Forni, J. Ritschard, A. Donath, and P. Alberto (1979), VIIth Meeting of International Society for Oncodevelopmental Biology and Medicine, Surrey, UK, Abstract 59c.

Mach, J. P., M. Forni, J. Ritschard, F. Buchegger, S. Carrel, S. Widgren, A. Donath, and P. Alberto (1980), *Oncodevel. Biol. Med.*, **1**, 49.

Midgley, A. R., Jr., and G. B. Pierce, Jr. (1962), *J. Exp. Med.* **115**, 289.

Marchand, A., C. M. Fenoglio, R. Pascal, R. M. Richart, and S. Bennett (1975), *Cancer Res.* **35**, 3807.

Obiekwe, B. C., D. J. Pendlebury, Y. B. Gordon, J. G. Grudzinskas, T. Chard, and H. Bohn (1979), *Clin. Chim. Acta* **95**, 509.

Pletsch, Q. A., and D. M. Goldenberg (1974), *J. Natl. Cancer Inst.* **52**, 1201.

Primus, F. J., R. H. Wang, D. M. Goldenberg, and H. J. Hansen (1973), *Cancer Res.* **33**, 2977.

Reif, A. E., L. E. Curtis, R. Duffield, and I. A. Shauffer (1974), *J. Surg. Oncol.* **6**, 133.

Rosen, S. W., and B. D. Weintraub (1974), *New Engl. J. Med.* **290**, 1441.

Rosen, S. W., J. Kaminska, I. S. Calvert, and S. A. Aaronson (1979), *Am. J. Obstet. Gynecol.* **134**, 834.

Ruoslahti, E., and M. Seppälä (1979), *Adv. Cancer Res.* **29**, 275.

Ruoslahti, E., E. Engvall, A. Pekkala, and M. Seppälä (1978), *Int. J. Cancer* **22**, 515.

Rutanen, E.-M. (1978), *Int. J. Cancer* **22**, 413.

Rutanen, E.-M., and M. Seppälä (1978), *Cancer* **41**, 692.

Rutanen, E.-M., and M. Seppälä (1980), *J. Clin. Endocrinol. Metab.* **50**, 57.

Rutanen, E.-M., J. Lindgren, P. Sipponen, U.-H. Stenman, E. Saksela, and M. Seppälä (1978), *Cancer* **42**, 581.

Salem, H. T., B. C. Obiekwe, A. T. M. Al-Ani, M. Seppälä, and T. Chard (1980), *Clin. Chim. Acta*, **107**, 211.

Schwartz, M. K. (1973), *Clin. Chem.* **19**, 10.

Searle, F., K. D. Bagshawe, B. A. Leake, and J. Dent (1978), *Lancet* **1**, 579.

Seppälä, M. (1977), *Clin. Obstet. Gynecol.* **20**, 737.

Seppälä, M., and E. Ruoslahti (1972), *Am. J. Obstet. Gynecol.* **112**, 208.

Seppälä, M., and E. Ruoslahti (1974), in *Recent Progress in Obstetrics and Gynecology* (Persianinov, L. S., T. V. Chervakova, and J. Presl, eds.), Excerpta Medica, Amsterdam, 449 pp.

Seppälä, M., K. D. Bagshawe, and E. Ruoslahti (1972), *Int. J. Cancer* **10**, 478.

Seppälä, M., H. Pihko, and E. Ruoslahti (1975), *Cancer* **34**, 1377.

Seppälä, M., E.-M. Rutanen, T. Ranta, I. Aho, U. Nieminen, H.-A. Unnerus, and E. Saksela (1976), *Cancer* **38**, 2065.

Seppälä, M., E.-M. Rutanen, M. Heikinheimo, H. Jalanko, and E. Engvall (1978), *Int. J. Cancer* **21**, 265.

Seppälä, M., T. Wahlström, and H. Bohn (1979), *Int. J. Cancer* **25**, 1489.

Stolbach, L. L., W. H. Fishman, and M. J. Krant (1969), *New Engl. Med.* **281**, 757.

Stone, M., K. D. Bagshawe, A. Kardana, F. Searle, and J. Dent (1977), *Brit. J. Obstet. Gynaecol.* **84**, 375.

Talerman, A., and W. G. Haije (1974), *Cancer* **34**, 1722.

Tatarinov, Y. S., and V. V. Kalashnikov (1977), *Nature* **265**, 638.

Tatarinov, Y. S., and A. V. Sokolov (1977), *Int. J. Cancer* **19**, 161.

Tatarinov, Y. S., N. V. Mesenyankina, D. M. Nikoulina, L. A. Novikova, B. O. Toloknov, and D. M. Falaleeva (1974), *Int. J. Cancer* **14**, 548.

Tatarinov, Y. S., D. M. Falaleeva, V. V. Kalashnikov, and B. O. Toloknov (1976), *Nature*, **260**, 263.

Teilum, G. (1965), *Acta Pathol. Microbiol. Scand.* **64**, 407.

Teilum, G., R. Albrechtsen, and B. Norgaard-Pedersen (1974), *Acta Pathol. Microbiol. Scand. A.* **82**, 586.

Vaitukaitis, J. L. (1973), *J. Clin. Endocrinol. Metab.* **37**, 505.

Vaitukaitis, J. L. (1974), *J. Clin. Endocrinol. Metab.* **38**, 755.

Vaitukaitis, J. L., and E. R. Ebersole (1976), *J. Clin. Endocrinol. Metab.* **42**, 1048.

Vaitukaitis, J. L., G. D. Braunstein, and G. T. Ross (1972), *Am. J. Obstet. Gynecol.* **113,** 751.

van Nagell, J. R., Jr., W. R. Meeker, J. C. Parker, Jr., and J. D. Harralson (1975a), *Cancer* **35,** 1372.

van Nagell, J. R., Jr., Q. A. Pletsch, and D. M. Goldenberg (1975b), *Cancer Res.* **35,** 1433.

van Nagell, J. R., Jr., E. S. Donaldson, E. C. Gay, S. Hudson, R. M. Sharkey, F. J. Primus, D. F. Powell, and D. M. Goldenberg (1979), *Cancer* **44,** 944.

van Nagell, J. R., Jr., E. Kim, S. Casper, F. J. Primus, S. Bennett, F. H. DeLand, and D. M. Goldenberg (1980), *Cancer Res.* **40,** 502.

von Kleist, S., G. Chavanel, and P. Burtin (1972), *Proc. Natl. Acad. Sci. USA* **64,** 161.

Wahlström, T., J. Lindgren, M. Korhonen, and M. Seppälä (1979), *Lancet* **2,** 1159.

Wurz, H. (1979), *Arch. Gynäk.* **227,** 1.

11

Testicular Cancer Markers

Paul H. Lange

Department of Urologic Surgery, University of Minnesota College of Health Sciences, Minneapolis, Minnesota

1. Introduction

In perhaps no other human malignancy have the potential value and drawbacks of tumor markers become as evident as they have during the recent experience with serum alphafetoprotein (AFP) and human chorionic gonadotropin (HCG) in testicular cancer. At present, these two markers, when used together, are the best available in clinical oncology.

The details of the use of AFP and HCG have been described extensively (Waldmann and McIntire, 1974; Perlin et al., 1976; Lange and Fraley, 1977; Schultz et al., 1978; Javadpour et al., 1978b; Lange et al., 1976; 1980b) and so will only be summarized here. This article will concentrate on those aspects of AFP and HCG that are still controversial and on those applications that are now being developed. It will also mention other tumor markers that have demonstrated their clinical value more recently. Finally, it will speculate about the future of markers for testicular tumors.

2. Clinical Aspects of Testicular Cancer

Our discussion requires a prefatory review of certain clinical aspects of testicular cancer, a subject we have examined in more detail recently (Fraley et al., 1979). More than 95% of these cancers belong to a heterogenous group called germ-cell tumors because it is widely believed that they arise in primordial germ cells (reviewed by Nochomovitz and Rosai, 1978). Germ-cell tumors are classified either as seminomas, of which there are at least three variants, or as nonseminomatous tumors, which are classified further as embryonal carcinoma, teratoma (mature or immature), or choriocarcinoma. The many histologic types of germ-cell tumors may occur singly or in various combinations, and mixtures of embryonal carcinoma and teratoma are common enough to warrant a separate name, teratocarcinoma.

Except for the rare extragonadal tumors that arise in midline structures (retroperitoneum, mediastinum, pineal gland), germ-cell tumors in men nearly always appear first as an intrascrotal mass; and the definitive diagnosis is made after the primary tumor has been extirpated by radical orchiectomy. Thereafter, the patient is "staged"; tests are performed to determine to what extent, if any, the cancer has spread. Because testicular germ-cell tumors usually metastasize first to the lymph nodes along the great vessels in the retroperitoneum and then to the lungs, other lymph nodes, and viscera, staging tests commonly include full-lung tomography, computed axial tomography or ultrasonography of the abdomen, and, in some hospitals, bipedal lymphangiography. A tumor confined to the testis and spermatic cord is said to be in Stage I, one that has metastasized only to the retroperitoneum in Stage II, and one that has spread outside the retroperitoneum in Stage III. Often it is necessary to specify whether the stage is clinical (based on the results of tests such as lymphangiography) or pathologic (based on histologic examination of the retroperitoneal lymph nodes).

If the primary tumor is pure seminoma, the accepted treatment after orchiectomy is radiation of the retroperitoneal lymph nodes and perhaps of the mediastinum and supraclavicular nodes, depending on the stage of the disease. Cure rates exceed 90% except in patients who present with far-advanced cancer.

If the primary tumor is partly or entirely nonseminomatous cancer, there is considerable debate about the best course of treatment after orchiectomy. In many medical centers, particularly in the United States, patients without evidence of Stage III disease are treated by retroperitoneal lymphadenectomy. Histologic examination of the resected tissue will show that many patients whose tumors appear to be in Stage I actually have metastases; and, in rare instances, that patients thought to have retroperitoneal tumor do not. Thus, lymphadenectomy is the most accurate staging method for nonseminomatous tumors as well as a highly effective treatment method (Fraley et al., 1980). In other medical centers, particularly in Europe, patients without Stage III disease are treated by radiation at doses higher than those used for seminoma.

If the patient presents with Stage III disease, it is generally agreed that he should be treated primarily by chemotherapy, with surgery or radiation if he does not respond completely. Newer drug regimens have been so effective in Stage III that consideration is being given to administering chemotherapy instead of surgery or radiation for Stage II nonseminomatous cancer.

As recently as ten years ago, nonseminomatous testicular cancer was often fatal. Now, however, most patients, even those who present with disseminated disease, are cured. As just mentioned, much of this success is attributable to advances in chemotherapy, but the clinical use of AFP and HCG has been essential also.

3. Incidence and Specificity of AFP and HCG

Markers may be expected to be useful in four ways: diagnosis, staging, monitoring of treatment (especially chemotherapy), and followup. To be of great value, however, a marker must be associated with the particular tumor in many or most instances, and, ideally, it should be specific for that tumor. Elevated levels of one or both or the markers AFP and HCG often accompany nonseminomatous cancer, and, in practice, these markers have proved to be specific.

Although it was known for many years that patients with testicular cancer sometimes had elevated serum levels of AFP, HCG, or both, it was not until sensitive radioimmunoassays became available that it was realized that the substances were prevalent enough to be useful clinically. The necessary limit of sensitivity for an assay is still being debated. Usually, 5–10 ng/mL (5.15–10.3 IU/mL) for AFP and 1–2 ng/mL (5–10 mIU/mL) for HCG are satisfactory (Nørgaard-Pedersen and Raghavan, 1981). However, the markers not only must be measured with sensitive assays to be useful in testicular cancer, they must be measured together. First, approximately 40% of patients with nonseminomatous tumors have elevations of only one marker. Second, during the clinical course, the levels of the two markers do not always parallel each other (Lange et al., 1980b). Investigators who have followed only one marker (usually AFP) generally have been disappointed with their results.

It also was known for many years that elevated levels of AFP or HCG may occur in patients with cancers other than those of the testicle or with certain nonmalignant diseases (Table 1). However, we and others have found that in patients thought or known to have testicular cancer, these markers are, in a practical sense, specific (Waldmann and McIntire, 1974; Perlin et al., 1976; Schultz et al., 1978; Lange et al., 1980b). To my knowledge, there is only one case in which an elevated marker level in a patient with testicular cancer was caused by some other pathologic condition, and it was not a clinical problem. (This patient died at one of our hospitals of cancer of the liver with an elevated AFP level. An embryonal car-

Table 1
Incidence of Elevated AFP or HCG Levels in Human Disease[a]

Cancer	Elevated AFP, %	Elevated HCG, %
Hepatocellular carcinoma	72	21
Nonseminomatous germ-cell testicular cancer	75	60
Pancreatic carcinoma	23	33
Gastric carcinoma	18	23
Colonic carcinoma	5	12
Breast cancer	—	11
Hereditary tyrosinemia	100	—
Ataxia telangiectasia	100	—
Nonmalignant hepatic disease	0.3	
Nongastrointestinal tumor metastatic to liver		
Renal cell carcinoma	0	6
Transitional cell carcinoma	0	8
Benign genitourinary disease	0	0

[a]References: Waldmann and McIntire, 1971; 1974; McIntire et al., 1975; Lange et al., 1976; Grenier et al., 1979; Griffing et al., 1980.

cinoma of the left testicle was an incidental finding at autopsy.) Should such an event occur, I believe that routine clinical evaluation could easily clarify the situation.

It is often stated that no true false-positive marker levels have been recorded in patients with testicular cancer (i.e., elevations found by accurate, sensitive radioimmunoassays in a patient who has no evidence of tumor at the time or soon thereafter). This statement is true, providing that two qualifications are understood.

First, marker levels may be elevated in a tumor-free patient because the substance has not yet been metabolically cleared after removal of the tumor. For example, marker levels may be elevated a few days after orchiectomy in a patient with pathologic Stage I nonseminomatous cancer. This is a more relevant consideration for AFP, which has a half-life of about five days, than for HCG, with its half-life of about 30 h.

Second, one must be certain that the HCG assay is measuring HCG. As discussed elsewhere in this book, the hormone is composed of two dissimilar polypeptide chains, designated alpha and beta. The alpha chain is similar to the alpha subunits of the pituitary glycoprotein hormones, viz. follicle-stimulating hormone (FSH), thyroid-stimulating hormone (TSH), and luteinizing hormone (LH). However, the beta chain of HCG is much less similar to the beta subunits of these other hormones, particularly in its 20 terminal amino acids. Thus, xenogeneic antibodies can be produced against purified HCG beta chains that cross-react very little with physiological concentrations of LH. Most radioimmunoassays for HCG are beta-HCG assays and thus are usually very specific for that hormone and its freely circulating beta chain.

However, cross-reactivity with LH varies considerably among beta-HCG assays, depending on the antibody used. As a result, slight elevations of HCG occasionally are recorded in patients who actually have only an elevated LH level. Although this mistake is made most often with the less-specific commercial beta-HCG assays, in our experience it can also occur with highly specific assays if the serum LH level is especially high. Thus cross-reaction may be a problem if a man has been rendered hypogonadal by chemotherapy or orchiectomy. If necessary, the patient can be given a short course of testosterone to lower the LH level and then retested (Catalona et al., 1979).

4. Markers as Aids in Diagnosis and Staging

4.1. Diagnosis

Knowledge of the prevalence and meaning of elevated marker levels in patients with scrotal masses has lagged behind that of other aspects of markers in testicular cancer, because until recently these assays were performed primarily in referral centers, which often do not see patients until after their orchiectomies. However, as news of the value of AFP and HCG has spread, the assays have become more widely available and more primary-care physicians are sending preorchiectomy blood specimens for analysis. The following conclusions have emerged to date.

First, AFP and HCG are never elevated in patients whose scrotal masses are benign.

Second, marker levels also are normal in all patients with nongerm-cell tumors (e.g., Leydig-cell tumors, lymphoma).

Third, HCG levels, but not AFP levels, may be elevated in patients with pure seminoma. The frequency with which this occurs is still being defined, but it probably is about 10% in Stage I disease and greater in higher stages. More will be said about seminoma and markers later in this article.

Fourth, levels of either or both of the markers may, of course, be elevated before orchiectomy if the patient has nonseminomatous cancer, and the incidence probably increases with increasing stage. About 60% of patients with Stage I disease have elevations of at least one marker before the primary tumor is removed, and in those with Stage III disease, as many as 90% have elevated markers. Whether the increasing frequency reflects only the amount of tumor or some biological difference (e.g., greater likelihood of marker production by a tumor that metastasizes more readily) has not been examined satisfactorily as yet (Lange et al., 1980b).

Fifth, marker assays of percutaneously aspirated fluid from around the testicle, as seen most prominently in hydrocele, is diagnostically useless and medically ill-advised. Transscrotal aspiration carries a risk of contamination of the inguinal lymphatic chain that normally is protected from testicular tumors by anatomical barriers. Further, detectable levels of an HCG-like substance, which does not appear to be LH, are found in testicular fluid in benign conditions (Scardino et al., 1980). This phenomenon is not inconsistent with earlier findings; HCG-like substances have been found in apparently normal testicle (Braunstein et al., 1975).

Therefore, our present knowledge of markers in patients with scrotal masses shows that AFP and HCG are helpful in diagnosis only if the levels are elevated, in which case the patient almost certainly has a testicular tumor. If the AFP level is elevated, he does not have pure seminoma.

4.2. Staging

The addition of marker determinations to other clinical staging methods has been beneficial, although there is still some controversy about the markers' exact role. Retroperitoneal lymphadenectomy remains the only certain method of distinguishing patients with metastases of nonseminomatous cancer from those without.

In determining the stage of disease after orchiectomy, one must take the metabolic clearance rate into account to be certain that any AFP or HCG in the serum is not left over from the removed testicle. Usually, two determinations several days apart suffice (for the formulae, see Lange and Fraley, 1977, or Lange et al., 1980b). If the marker levels are truly elevated, one can be certain that metastatic disease is present, even if there is no clinical evidence of it, because there have been no true false-positives. The distinction between Stages II and III is usually made by full-lung tomography and occasionally by biopsy of the supraclavicular lymph nodes or other lesions or by liver, brain, or bone scans.

If the levels of both markers are normal after orchiectomy, the situation is more complicated. This could, of course, mean Stage I disease. However, in several series in which routine retroperitoneal lymphadenectomy made accurate staging possible, the false-negative rate (normal marker levels in the face of active tumor) in Stage II disease has ranged from 20 to 50%. Many of these false-negatives occur in patients who have only microscopic metastases in a few nodes. The frequency of false-negative markers in untreated Stage III disease is 10–12%, but there usually are clinical signs of the disseminated tumor. More will be said about these cases later in this article.

Newer methods, especially computed tomography, have been used in attempts to improve the accuracy of staging, with some success. However, they suffer from significant false-positive rates. At present, no combination of nonoperative methods, including AFP and HCG assays, is sufficiently accurate in staging nonseminomatous tumors that one can use the results to decide against lymphadenectomy or other treatment of the retroperitoneal nodes.

5. Markers in Treatment Monitoring and Followup

Unquestionably, the greatest value of AFP and HCG determinations in testicular cancer is in the monitoring of patients during chemotherapy and followup after initial treatment (Waldmann and McIntire, 1974; Perlin et al., 1976; Lange et al., 1976; Lange and Fraley, 1977; Scardino et al., 1977; Schultz et al., 1978; Javadpour, 1978; Lange, 1978; Thompson et al., 1979; Lange et al., 1980b). Marker levels have predicted progression or recurrence of disease as much as 6 months earlier than did other methods. Confidence in these markers is now such that an unequivocal elevation is sufficient evidence of tumor for chemotherapy to be started or resumed without pathologic confirmation if that would require major surgery. Likewise, on occasion an elevated marker is the only sign of disease, and here again, treatment can be started with confidence that the patient does have growing tumor.

However, this is not to say that the markers alone can be used to monitor patients. As mentioned, 10–12% of patients with untreated Stage III disease will have normal marker levels. Also, patients with a history of nonseminomatous cancer, clinically evident tumor, and normal marker levels may have adult teratoma, seminoma, or even benign disease, not recurrence of their initial tumor. Consequently, it has been recommended that any patient with a history of nonseminomatous cancer, persistent or growing masses, and normal marker levels should have the nature of the masses confirmed by biopsy before chemotherapy is begun or continued (Lange et al., 1980b). (An exception might be made for those patients whose marker levels have been falsely normal from the beginning.)

Finally, it must be remembered that AFP and HCG production is only one of the biological activities of these cancers and is not essential to their survival. Therefore, a tumor that has ceased to produce detectable amounts of markers is not necessarily dead. It often happens that serum marker levels return to normal during chemotherapy months before the tumor disappears clinically. Obviously, therefore, normal marker levels are not a sign that planned treatment can be discontinued.

6. Markers in Seminoma

In the past, seminoma was considered a very curable tumor, in part because it often is slow to metastasize so that patients present with low-stage disease and in part because of its great sensitivity to radiation. However, with recent advances in chemotherapy, high-stage nonseminomatous cancers often are more curable than are high-stage seminomas.

Regular determinations in serum of AFP and HCG are not always part of the management of seminoma, but efforts to improve the treatment results in these tumors may soon involve marker assays. There are several reasons why this is advisable.

First, patients with apparently pure seminoma in the primary tumor may have nonseminomatous metastases. This was true in a third of the patients in one series of autopsies (Maier et al., 1968). Regular marker determinations often would reveal this so that treatment could be changed appropriately.

Second, patients with apparently pure seminoma occasionally have elevated markers early in the clinical course. If the AFP level is elevated, nonseminomatous cancer always is present somewhere, so this marker may be helpful in diagnosis. An elevated HCG level also may mean nonseminomatous metastases.

However—a third reason why markers can be useful in seminoma —some of these tumors produce HCG. Early pathologic studies showed that some seminomas contain syncytiotrophoblastic cells resembling those in the placenta and in choriocarcinoma (Friedman and Pearlman, 1970). Recent histochemical studies have shown that these cells contain HCG (Javadpour et al., 1978a). Understanding of the significance of HCG in seminoma is far from complete, but our experience suggests that high-stage HCG-producing seminomas do not respond well to classical treatment plans (Lange et al., 1980c). It is our impression that between 10 and 20% of pure seminomas produce HCG.

7. Other Uses of AFP and HCG in Testicular Cancer

Some other aspects of AFP and HCG may become clinically useful in the future. For example, there are two ways in which marker levels may have prognostic value.

First, the initial level of the marker (normal, slightly elevated, or high) may indicate something about the behavior of the tumor. Evaluation of this hypothesis is complicated by the correlation between frequency of elevation and stage of disease and by the difficulties in determining the amount of tumor present. Thus, in our series, 66% of the patients in Stage I, but 93% of those in Stage II or greater, had elevated markers before orchiectomy. It is unclear whether these data are a commentary only on the amount of disease or on its biologic behavior. As newer staging methods make it easier to determine the amount of tumor present, answers may be forthcoming. There is some evidence that AFP/HCG levels are a prognostic indicator independent of tumor size.

Second, the rate of decline of marker levels during treatment, especially chemotherapy, may have prognostic value (Kohn, 1979). For example, it may be that, as a group, patients who respond well to therapy will have faster declines in marker levels (closer to the theoretical decay rates) than do those who respond poorly. Theoretically, this difference would be evident long before there were obvious differences in the clinical response. Thus, one may be able to predict that a patient will respond poorly even if his marker levels return temporarily to normal. The results of our retrospective analysis suggest that this is true and worth further study (P. H. Lange, N. J. Vogelzang, A. Goldman, B. J. Kennedy, E. E. Fraley, submitted).

Newer methods of detecting HCG may become important clinically. For example, because the molecule is excreted intact in the urine, concentrating techniques and more specific assays can increase the sensitivity of HCG determinations as much as 200-fold (Ayala et al., 1978). Although more control and research data are needed before firm conclusions can be drawn, it does appear that this approach can reveal residual disease in some patients with normal serum markers (Javadpour and Chen, 1980). Wider application of this method may change our ideas on the frequency and meaning of marker-negative cases.

It is now apparent that tumors and, indeed, the normal placenta, secrete not only intact HCG, but also free alpha and beta chains and chain fragments (Papapetrou et al., 1980). In gestational trophoblastic tumors, the proportion of the various forms appears to have prognostic significance (Vaitukaitis and Ebersole, 1976). Studies are in progress to determine whether this is true in nonseminomatous testicular cancer also.

Refinements in the use of AFP also can be envisioned. Different species of AFP molecules have been detected by various immunochemical methods and may be related to the tissue source. For example, there are reproducible differences in the amount of marker binding to concanavalin A between AFP from yolk sac and that from fetal liver. Moreover, the percentage of binding differs among various types of human and animal tumors (Smith and Kelleher, 1980). Studies now are exploring AFP in patients with nonseminomatous cancer to see whether there are different molecular species and, if so, whether this is important clinically.

8. Other Markers for Testicular Cancer

Several other substances have been evaluated for possible clinical use in testicular cancer (Table 2). Carcinoembryonic antigen (CEA), human placental lactogen, alpha-1 antitrypsin, and ferritin either are not sufficiently prevalent, specific, or sensitive, or add nothing to the information obtained from AFP and HCG. However, lactic dehydrogenase (LDH), pla-

Table 2
Possible Markers Found in Serum of Patients with
Germ-Cell Testicular Cancer

Marker	Detectable in tumor tissue?	Useful clinically?
AFP	Yes	Yes
HCG	Yes	Yes
HCG-alpha[a,b]	Yes	?
HCG-beta[a]	Yes	?
CEA[a]	Yes	No
LDH	?	?
SP1[b]	Yes	Yes?
PLAP[a,c]	Yes	?
Alpha-1 antitrypsin[a]	Yes	No
Human placental lactogen[d]	Yes	No
Ferritin[a]	Yes	No
Pregnancy protein 5 (PP5)[e]	Yes	No?
Gamma-glutamyl transferase[f]	?	?

[a]Nørgaard-Pedersen and Raghavan (1981).
[b]P. H. Lange and C. H. W. Horne, unpublished data.
[c]Wahren et al., 1979.
[d]Horne and Bremner (1980).
[e]C. H. W. Horne, personal communication.
[f]Fishman et al. (1979).

cental alkaline phosphatase (PLAP), SP1, and F9-like antigens show promise.

There is some evidence that serum LDH or one of its isoenzymes may be useful despite the number of conditions in which it may be elevated (Edler von Eyben, 1978; Cheng et al., 1978). In our studies, the LDH level was elevated in 63% of patients, including some with normal levels of AFP and HCG (Bosl et al., 1981). However, Javadpour and Lippert (1980) believe that LDH is of clinical value primarily in advanced disease. In our hospital, LDH is measured routinely in patients with testicular cancer, and it is our impression that it is useful occasionally in clinical management. However, because it is not specific, special care is needed in defining its clinical role.

Placental alkaline phosphatase is one of a group of fetal isoenzymes that can be distinguished biochemically from one another and from "adult" alkaline phosphatases such as those of the liver and bone (Fishman et al., 1976). Ectopic PLAP was found in a human lung carcinoma (and called Regan isoenzyme) and has since been found in a variety of cancers (Nathanson and Fishman, 1971). Various nonenzymatic methods (including radioimmunoassay) now are available that increase the ease of measurement and perhaps the sensitivity. Serial measurements were made in many patients with cancer, but except perhaps in ovarian carcinoma, PLAP did not appear to be useful. However, Fishman et al., (1979), who used an enzymatic assay, suggested that PLAP might be prevalent enough in patients with seminoma to be useful. Wahren et al. (1979), who used a radioimmunoassay, reported that PLAP is an important marker in seminoma and is elevated more often than is HCG. However, a significant number of patients believed to be free of disease had elevated levels. We used an enzymatic method to measure PLAP and found that 12 of 22 patients with seminoma had elevated levels and that in some patients the marker provided unique clinical information in serial studies (P.H. Lange, J. Millan, E. Ruoslahti, E.E. Fraley, in preparation). Further work on this marker, perhaps with more reliable assays, is needed and studies of other fetal alkaline phosphatases (e.g., chorionic) should be pursued when better assays for them become available. Whether or not PLAP turns out to be useful in seminoma, studies of it and of HCG already have changed the thinking about the histogenesis of this type of tumor.

The pregnancy protein SP1 (from *Schwangerschaftsproteine* No. 1) is produced by the syncytiotrophoblastic cells of the placenta. It is detectable in the serum of pregnant women as early as 7 days after ovulation and reaches 95–315 μg/mL by 36 weeks' gestation. SP1 also is detectable in 80–100% of women with trophoblastic tumors (Horne and Nisbet, 1979). Recently, we found elevated serum SP1 levels in approximately half of a group of men with active testicular cancer. These elevations were associated more often with elevated HCG levels than with elevated AFP levels (as expected) but also occurred in men with normal levels of both of the established markers. More important, serial measurements showed that SP1 occasionally provided clinically valuable information not revealed by AFP and HCG (Lange et al., 1980a). However, SP1 cannot be recommended yet for routine use in testicular cancer since the limits of normal are not adequately defined and more serial studies are needed.

Studies of murine teratocarcinoma models have shown that these tumors have unique oncodevelopmental antigens (reviewed by Jacob, 1977). One such antigen, called F9 after the cell line on which it was discovered, has been detected on cultured human nonseminomatous cancer cells (Holden et al., 1977) and may be present on fresh tissue also (P. H. Lange and D. Solter, unpublished data). Another of these embryonic murine antigens, called stage-specific embryonic antigen No. 1 (SSEA-1), was detected with monoclonal antibody produced by hybridoma techniques (Solter and Knowles, 1978). This antigen has been detected on cell lines of human nonseminomatous testicular cancer (Bronson et al., 1980). One might speculate that these embryonic antigens mark more primitive, and thus more aggressive, tumors, but it is not known whether they can be useful prognostically.

9. Location of Tumors with Oncodevelopmental Markers

Markers may be useful not only as signals of the presence of tiny foci of tumor, but in revealing their location. The idea is to tag antimarker antibody (usually xenogeneic) with a radioactive label and inject it into the tumor-bearing host. Radiodiagnostic methods then are used to locate metastases.

The difficulties are many. For example, high-quality antibody is essential, and this is not easy to obtain. In addition, if xenogeneic antibody is used, the possibility of allergic reactions must be considered. Also, there are technical problems with background "noise," particularly with an oncodevelopmental protein, since it might be present in small amounts on normal tissue. Consequently, a second antibody, usually tagged with a different isotope, must be used simultaneously in a subtraction method.

Despite these problems, Goldenberg and his group have succeeded in radioimmunodetection of animal and human tumors with CEA (Goldenberg et al., 1978; van Nagell et al., 1980) and obtained some evidence that a similar method, with radiolabeled antibody to AFP or HCG, may be useful with human nonseminomatous testicular tumors (Goldenberg et al., 1980a,b).

Radioimmunodetection of teratocarcinomas in mice has been accomplished with the F9-like antigen, SSEA-1 (Ballou et al., 1979). Because SSEA-1 also appears to be expressed in human tumors, efforts to detect teratocarcinomas in man are under way.

10. Tumor Markers in Pathology

Histochemical methods, particularly immunofluorescence or immunoperoxidase, have been used to identify the cells of origin of many markers associated with germ-cell testicular tumors (Table 2).

HCG has been located by several authors (reviewed by Nørgaard-Pedersen and Raghavan, 1981) in syncytiotrophoblastic cells of both seminomas and nonseminomatous tumors. There is some question as to whether other cells stain for HCG. Similar studies of AFP have been more difficult, probably because of the quality of the antibody available, and nonspecific staining has been a problem. More recently, better absorption techniques have improved the antibody preparations, and AFP studies may become easier. AFP has been located primarily in yolk-sac elements, although occasionally other cells, such as embryonal carcinoma, also appear to stain for AFP (Kurman et al., 1977). Seminomas apparently do not stain for AFP. Finally, in preliminary studies, SP1 appeared to be located in cytotrophoblastic cells (Javadpour, 1980). It has been suggested that histochemical analysis may be useful clinically, perhaps in developing a new pathologic classification system for germ-cell testicular tumors (Kurman et al., 1977; Raghavan et al., 1979). However, although there is no doubt that histochemical studies have increased understanding of cell types that produce markers and may aid in the identification of certain cells, so far it has not changed diagnosis or classification significantly. Moreover, the correlation between serum levels and the presence or absence of positive tissue staining is incomplete, with serum levels generally being a more sensitive indicator of marker production. Also, the correlation between tumor-tissue staining and the clinical course has not been investigated. Such studies will continue to be hampered by problems of adequate tissue sampling.

11. The Future

Tumor markers will maintain a prominent place in the research on and management of testicular cancer. Three things are needed: consolidation, innovation, and implementation.

For example, data are available (or could be accumulated quickly) that would define the prognostic value of half-life calculations, the exact meaning of HCG in pure seminoma, and the value of histochemical marker studies. Innovations that are needed include studies of marker subspecies, such as molecular forms of HCG, and better methods of radioimmunodetection with oncodevelopmental markers. Also, new markers (especially developmental antigens) may become available and require study.

Implementation may seem the most obvious, but it may be the most difficult. The cure rate for Stage III nonseminomatous testicular cancer is now 70–80%, and new knowledge must be applied so that we do not lose ground already gained in attempting to cure the others. New information will have to be especially precise, and studies of the role of new markers will be difficult to design.

References

Ayala, A. R., B. C. Nisula, H. C. Chen, G. D. Hodgen, and G. T. Ross (1978), *J. Clin. Endocrinol. Metab.* **47,** 767.

Ballou, B., G. Levine, T. R. Hakala, and D. Solter (1979), *Science* **206,** 844.

Bosl, G. J., P. H. Lange, L. E. Nochomovitz, A. Goldman, E. E. Fraley, J. Rosai, K. Johnson, and B. J. Kennedy (1981), *Cancer* **47,** 572.

Braunstein, G. D., J. Rasor, and M. E. Wade (1975), *New Engl. J. Med.* **293,** 1334.

Bronson, D. L., P. W. Andrews, D. Solter, J. Cervenka, P. H. Lange, and E. E. Fraley (1980), *Cancer Res.* **40**, 2500.

Catalona, W. J., J. L. Vaitukaitis, and W. R. Fair (1979), *J. Urol.* **122**, 126.

Cheng, E., E. Cvitkovic, R. D. Wittes, and R. B. Golbey (1978), *Cancer* **42**, 2162.

Edler von Eyben, F. (1978), *Cancer* **41**, 648.

Fishman, W. H., T. Nishiyama, A. Rule, S. Green, N. R. Inglis, and L. Fishman (1976), in *Onco-Developmental Gene Expression* (Fishman, W. H., and S. Sell, eds.), Academic Press, New York.

Fishman, W. H., P. R. Krishaswamy, L. Fishman, J. L. Millan, and K. R. McIntire (1979), in *Carcino-Embryonic Proteins* (Lehmann, F.-G., ed.), vol. 2, Elsevier/North Holland, Amsterdam.

Fraley, E. E., P. H. Lange, and B. J. Kennedy (1979), *New Engl. J. Med.* **301**, 1370, 1420.

Fraley, E. E., P. H. Lange, R. D. Williams, and S. A. Ortlip (1980), *Cancer* **45**, 1762.

Friedman, M., and A. W. Pearlman (1970), *Cancer* **26**, 46.

Goldenberg, D. M., F. DeLand, E. Kim, S. Bennett, F. J. Primus, and J. R. van Nagell, Jr. (1978), *New Engl. J. Med.* **298**, 1384.

Goldenberg, D. M., E. E. Kim, F. DeLand, E. Spremulli, M. O. Nelson, J. P. Gockerman, F. J. Primus, R. L. Corgan, and E. Alpert (1980a), *Cancer* **45**, 2500.

Goldenberg, D. M., E. E. Kim, F. H. DeLand, J. R. van Nagell, Jr., and N. Javadpour (1980b), *Science* **207**, 1284.

Grenier, A., C. LaBerge, J. P. Valet, J. Morissette, and L. Belanger (1979), in *Carcino-Embryonic Proteins* (Lehmann, F.-G., ed.), vol. 2, Elsevier/North Holland, Amsterdam, p. 425.

Griffing, G., and J. L. Vaitukaitis (1980), in *Cancer Markers: Diagnostic and Developmental Significance* (Sell, S., ed.), Humana, Clifton, New Jersey, p. 16.

Holden, S., O. Bernard, K. Artzt, W. F. Whitmore, Jr., and D. Bennett (1977), *Nature* **270**, 518.

Horne, C. H. W., and R. D. Bremner (1980), in *Cancer Markers: Diagnostic and Developmental Significance* (Sell, S., ed.), Humana, Clifton, New Jersey, p. 225.

Horne, C. H. W., and A. D. Nisbet (1979), *Invest. Cell Pathol.* **2**, 217.

Jacob, F. (1977), *Immunol. Rev.* **33**, 3.

Javadpour, N. (1978), *J. Urol.* **120**, 651.

Javadpour, N. (1980), *J. Urol.* **123**, 514.

Javadpour, N., and H. C. Chen (1980), paper presented at the American Urological Association Meeting, San Francisco.

Javadpour, N., and M. Lippert (1980), paper presented at the American Urological Association Meeting, San Francisco.

Javadpour, N., K. R. McIntire, and T. A. Waldmann (1978a), *Cancer* **42**, 2768.

Javadpour, N., K. R. McIntire, T. A. Waldmann, and S. M. Bergman (1978b), *J. Urol.* **119**, 759.

Kohn, J. (1979), in *Carcino-Embryonic Proteins* (Lehmann, F.-G., ed.), vol. 2, Elsevier/North Holland, Amsterdam, p. 383.

Kurman, R. J., P. T. Scardino, K. R. McIntire, T. A. Waldmann, and N. Javadpour (1977), *Cancer* **40**, 2136.

Lange, P. H. (1978), *Natl. Cancer Inst. Monogr.* **49**, 215.

Lange, P. H., and E. E. Fraley (1977), *Urol. Clin. North Am.* **4**, 393.

Lange, P. H., K. R. McIntire, T. A. Waldmann, T. R. Hakala, and E. E. Fraley (1976), *New Engl. J. Med.* **295**, 1237.

Lange, P. H., R. D. Bremner, C. H. W. Horne, R. L. Vessella, and E. E. Fraley (1980a), *Urology* **15**, 251.

Lange, P. H., K. R. McIntire, and T. A. Waldmann (1980b), in *Testicular Tumors: Management and Treatment* (Einhorn, L. E., ed.), Masson, New York.

Lange, P. H., L. E. Nochomovitz, J. Rosai, E. E. Fraley, B. J. Kennedy, G. J. Bosl, J. Brisbane, W. J. Catalona, J. S. Cochran, R. H. Comisarow, K. B. Kummings, J. B. deKernion, L. H. Einhorn, T. R. Hakala, M. A. S. Jewett, M. R. Moore, P. T. Scardino, and J. M. Streitz (1980c), *J. Urol.*, **124**, 472.

Maier, J. G., M. H. Sulak, and B. T. Mittemeyer (1968), *Am. J. Roentgenol.* **102**, 596.

McIntire, K. R., T. A. Waldmann, C. G. Moertel, and V. L. W. Go (1975), *Cancer Res.* **35**, 991.

Nathanson, L., and W. H. Fishman (1971), *Cancer* **27**, 1388.

Nochomovitz, L. E., and J. Rosai (1978), *Pathol. Annu.* **13** (part 1), 327.

Nørgaard-Pedersen, B., and D. Raghavan (1981), *Onco-develop. Biol. Med.* **1**, 327.

Papapetrou, P. D., N. P. Sakarelou, H. Braouzi, and P. H. Fessas (1980), *Cancer* **45**, 2583.

Perlin, E., J. E. Engeler, Jr., M. Edson, D. Karp, K. R. McIntire, and T. A. Waldmann (1976), *Cancer* **37**, 215.

Raghavan, D., E. Heyderman, and M. J. Peckham (1979), in *Tumor Markers: Impact and Progress* (Boelsma, E., and P. H. Rumke, eds.), Elsevier/North Holland, Amsterdam.

Scardino, P. T., H. D. Cox, T. A. Waldmann, K. R. McIntire, B. Mittemeyer, and N. Javadpour (1977), *J. Urol.* **118**, 994.

Scardino, P. T., T. A. Waldmann, and K. R. McIntire (1980), paper presented at the American Urological Association Meeting, San Francisco.

Schultz, H., A. Sell, B. Nørgaard-Pedersen, and J. Arends (1978), *Cancer* **42**, 2182.

Smith, C. J. P., and P. C. Kelleher (1980), *Biochim. Biophys. Acta* **605**, 1.

Solter, D., and B. B. Knowles (1978), *Proc. Natl. Acad. Sci. USA* **75**, 5565.

Thompson, D.K., and J. E. Haddow (1979), in *Carcino-Embryonic Proteins* (Lehmann, F.-G., ed.), vol. 2, Elsevier/North Holland, Amsterdam, pp. 379–381.

Vaitukaitis, J. L., and E. R. Ebersole (1976), *J. Clin. Endocrinol. Metab.* **42**, 1048.

van Nagell, J. R., Jr., E. Kim, S. Casper, F. J. Primus, S. Bennett, F. H. DeLand, and D. M. Goldenberg (1980), *Cancer Res.* **40**, 502.

Wahren, B., P. Å. Holmgren, and T. Stigbrand (1979), *Int. J. Cancer* **24**, 749.

Waldmann, T. A., and K. R. McIntire (1971), *Lancet* **2**, 1112.

Waldmann, T. A., and K. R. McIntire (1974), *Cancer* **34**, 1510.

12

Placental Proteins as Tumor Markers

Torgny Stigbrand[1,2] and Eva Engvall[2]

[1]Department of Physiological Chemistry, University of Umeå, Umeå, Sweden and [2]La Jolla Cancer Research Foundation, La Jolla, California

1. Introduction

The placenta was long regarded as a simple barrier between mother and fetus. As readily available tissue, it has more recently attracted interest from several biological fields. In research on malignancy, on the mechanisms of transplantation rejection, and even on aging, useful information can be obtained from studies of the growth, development, and rejection of the placenta (Beaconsfield and Ginsburg, 1979).

One of the striking properties of placental tissue is its complexity with regard to cellular components and functional versatility. The cell lineages found in the placenta include trophectoderm, primitive endoderm, and primitive ectoderm. The placenta performs a variety of functions that in the adult are served by a number of different organs such as the alimentary canal, lung, kidney, liver, and endocrine glands. However, the stage of differentiation of placental tissue in these processes compared to that of adult organs is not necessarily the same (Gardner, 1979). The placenta thus has many of the characteristic functions of adult specialized tissues, but at the same time it is also an embryonic tissue with a predestined life cycle of nine months. Moreover, some properties of the placenta are

275

clearly shared with malignant tumors. These include rapid cell division, local infiltration, and invasion. A high level of energy metabolism and a high production of lactate are also characteristics shared by the placenta and many malignant tissues. (For a review, see Beaconsfield and Ginsburg, 1979). Significant differences also exist between the placenta and malignant tissues; placental growth is limited in extent and duration, and true metastasis normally does not occur. In spite of this, the placenta does seem to have a significant degree of autonomy. It can survive and synthesize and release proteins in the absence of a fetus (Petropoulus, 1973), and the cells responsible for this synthesis have already differentiated from the blastocyst before implantation.

A significant similarity of tumors and the placenta (and other fetal tissues) is their frequent expression of fetal proteins. The term ''oncodevelopmental gene products'' has been coined to characterize such substances (Fishman et al., 1968a). The existence of oncodevelopmental gene products suggests that malignancy may result from disturbances in the regulation of the expression of genes normally active in the embryo and the fetus. Oncodevelopmental gene products also provide useful markers for tumor detection.

Most of the placental proteins thought to be of potential use as tumor markers are synthesized by the syncytiotrophoblast. This cell type, which constitutes about 13% of the placental tissue, is in direct contact with the intervillous maternal blood and is separated from the fetal capillaries by a basement membrane. As a consequence of these anatomical arrangements, the products of the syncytiotrophoblast are mainly secreted into the maternal circulation. The concentrations of proteins synthesized by the placenta are generally 100–1000 times higher in the maternal than in the fetal circulation. It should be noted that significant differences in the pattern of protein release exist between the human placenta and the nonhemochordial placentas of some higher animals (Davies and Ryan, 1972). This greatly influences the distribution of placental and fetal proteins in both fetus and mother of various species. The vascular structure of a tumor may similarly be of importance in determining the amount of a given tumor marker that reaches the circulation.

Several of the placental proteins have been found to have analogs in the normal adult, i.e., they share some chemical, immunological, or biological features with proteins from adult tissues. This is particularly true of the hormones and enzymes of the placenta (Table 1).

Several of the placental proteins can serve as markers for monitoring fetal well-being or placental function during pregnancy (Gordon and Chard, 1979). The levels of the various placental proteins generally show parallel changes in maternal circulation. This is not the case with tumors. When originating from a tumor, the placental proteins often show a discordant behavior, suggesting that activation of the corresponding embry-

Table 1
Proteins Synthesized by the Human Placenta

Protein	Abbreviation	mw	References
Human chorionic gonadotropin	HCG	45,000–50,000	Morgan et al., 1973 Vaitukaitis, 1977
Human placental lactogen (human chorionic somatomammotropin)	HPL (HCS)	21,000–23,000	Josimovich, 1977
Human chorionic thyrotropin	HCT	45,000	Hershman and Starnes, 1971
Human chorionic corticotropin	HCCT	5,000	Opsahl and Long, 1951
Human chorionic gonadotropin-releasing hormone	HCGRH	1,000	Gibbons et al., 1975
Schwangerschafts-spezifisches proteine (pregnancy specific β_1-glycoprotein, trophoblast specific β_1-globulin, pregnancy-associated plasma protein C)	SP1 (PSβG, TBG, PAPP-C)	90,000–100,000	Bohn, 1971 Towler et al., 1976 Tatarinov and Masyukevich, 1970 Lin et al., 1976
Pregnancy-associated plasma protein A	PAPP-A	750,000	Lin et al., 1976
Pregnancy-associated plasma protein B	PAPP-B	1,000,000	Lin et al., 1976
Placental alkaline phosphatase (heat-stable alkaline phosphatase)	PLAP (HSAP)	120,000	Boyer, 1961 Fishman and Ghosh, 1967
Cystine aminopeptidase (oxytocinase)	CAP	—	Tuppy and Nesvadba, 1957
Diamine oxidase (histaminase)	DO	190,000	Lin and Kirley, 1976

onic genes can take place selectively, and resulting in synthesis of oncodevelopmental markers in combinations different from that characteristic of the normal placenta.

The aim of the present chapter is to review our current knowledge of the expression and properties of those oncofetal gene products that are normally synthesized by the placenta.

2. Placental Alkaline Phosphatase

Alkaline phosphatases have been studied more than any other group of enzymes. A monograph on alkaline phosphatases (McComb et al., 1979) lists more than 6000 references. In man, alkaline phosphatases with hydrolase and/or transferase activity have been demonstrated in many organs such as the liver, placenta, intestine, bone, and kidney. In spite of their abundant distribution in nature, including bacteria, plants, and animals, the physiological functions of these enzymes remain a mystery. More than a dozen different cellular processes (McComb et al., 1979) have been associated with the enzymatic activity, but no final conclusions about its biological role have been drawn thus far. The alkaline phosphatases are, however, often present in plasma membranes where intense transport through the membranes takes place. This is obviously the case in placenta, intestine, kidney, and liver.

2.1. Isoenzymes and Multiple Forms of Placental Alkaline Phosphatase

In humans, the alkaline phosphatase of placenta is evolutionarily unique (Goldstein and Harris, 1979; Doellgast and Benirschke, 1979) and distinct from that of liver, bone, and kidney, as well as from that of intestine (McKenna et al., 1979; Goldstein et al., 1980). The placental enzyme can be identified by its unusual heat stability (heat-stable alkaline phosphatase) (Posen et al., 1965; Fishman and Ghosh, 1967; Fishman et al., 1968c) and by its immunochemical reactivity (Sussman et al., 1968; Lehman, 1975). On the other hand, placental alkaline phosphatase is genetically polymorphic and displays more allelic variants, as defined electrophoretically, than any other human enzyme studied so far (Boyer, 1961; Robson and Harris, 1965; 1967; Beckman et al., 1966). Six common phenotypes can be recognized electrophoretically (Fig. 1). In addition, several other rare allelic variants have been reported. The structural basis for this polymorphism has not yet been elucidated. Point mutations at the placental phosphatase locus offer one explanation, but there is evidence also that post-translational modifications of the enzyme can occur. These could significantly affect both the surface charge of the molecule and its affinity to

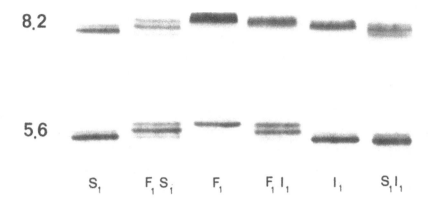

Fig. 1. Photographs of starch gels showing the six common phenotypes of placental alkaline phosphatase. The separation is performed at pH 8.2 and 5.6. The anode is at the top of the picture (reproduced by kind permission of Lars and Gunhild Beckman, University of Umeå, Sweden).

certain supporting media used for electrophoresis, such as starch gel. Such post-translational modifications of the enzyme could have a great impact on the classification systems used at present.

The molecular weight of the soluble form of the enzyme is close to 120,000. The enzyme is a dimer, with the subunit molecular weight of 60,000–65,000 (Holmgren and Stigbrand, 1976; Holmgren et al., 1977).

The enzyme, regardless of the phenotype expressed, is present in human serum in two forms that differ in size (Doellgast et al., 1977). One of the forms is a high molecular weight aggregate that is excluded on Sephadex or Sephrose gel filtration and does not enter polyacrylamide gels. The molecular weight of the fraction has been estimated to be > 600,000. Several investigations favor the idea that this component of the enzyme is membrane-associated and that the use of detergents such as Triton X-100 will solubilize the enzyme. The catalytic activity in these possible membrane fragments is of the same order of magnitude as that of the soluble enzyme (Doellgast et al., 1977). Preliminary results (Neuwald, personal communication) indicate that the subunit of the intact enzyme obtained from a cell line in vitro contains a fragment of approximately 2000 mw that is hydrophobic and binds detergent. Proteolytic degradation of the enzyme protein results in an apparent molecular weight reduction of the subunit from 63,000 to 61,000, and the binding of radiolabeled detergent is significantly reduced. Furthermore, the elution behavior on hydrophobic interaction chromatography is significantly modified. These results imply that the enzyme is bound by a hydrophobic part of the molecule to the cell membrane and that the release of the enzyme from the cell might owe both to membrane disintegration, resulting in a low molecular weight

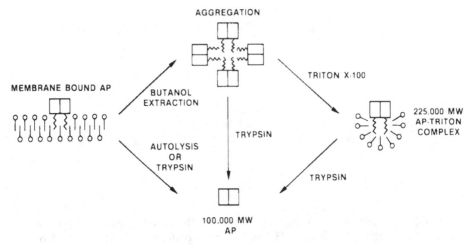

Fig. 2. Proposed mechanisms on the molecular events involved in solu-bilization of alkaline phosphatase from the JAR choriocarcinoma cell line (repro-duced by kind permission of Paul Neuwald, Frederick Cancer Research Center, Maryland, USA).

enzyme that has no exposed hydrophobic sites. The hypothesis is depicted in Fig. 2.

2.2. Assays

Serum normally contains low levels of alkaline phosphatases from several organs. To be able to distinguish between the different tissue types of phosphatases, it has been necessary to introduce assays capable of discrim-inating between the isoenzymes. This has been done in two ways: Catalytically (Posen et al., 1965; Fishman and Ghosh, 1967; Doellgast and Fishman, 1975) and immunochemically (Sussman et al., 1968; Usategui-Gomez, 1973; Fishman, 1974; Lehmann, 1975). Several cata-lytic or physicochemical properties distinguish the different alkaline phos-phatases, including pH-optimum, sensitivity to uncompetitive inhibitors (L-phenylalanine, L-tryptophan, L-homoarginine, L-leucine, levamisol, and imidazol), sensitivity to inactivation by heat or urea, and electro-phoretic migration in starch or agar gels (for a review, see Fishman, 1974). Great efforts have been made to establish sensitive techniques for the se-lective catalytic measurement of the placental type of enzyme in sera from tumor patients. In particular, heat inactivation and the use of uncompetitive inhibitors have been used to classify and describe the tumor-related phosphatases (Doellgast and Meis, 1979). Recently a very sensitive catalytic assay combining heat stability, phenylalanine inhibi-tion, and a long incubation time (15–20 h) has been described that is capa-ble of measuring two of the tumor-related variants of the placental form of the enzyme (Doellgast et al., 1981; Stigbrand and collaborators, unpublished observation).

Several of the catalytic assays described also reveal the presence of the placental isoenzyme in healthy individuals. Because of different cutoff limits for the upper level of normal, examination of tumor sera have resulted in very divergent conclusions about the presence and value of alkaline phosphatase in cancer. The first radioimmunoassays described for placental alkaline phosphatase were not sensitive enough to measure serum levels from more than a few tumor patients. The least detectable doses were those ranging from 5 to 20 ng/mL. The incidence of alkaline phosphatase in sera from several groups of cancer patients was consequently reported to be close to zero, as measured by these radioimmunoassays (Jacoby and Bagshawe, 1972; Chang et al., 1975; Holmgren et al., 1979).

Catalytic assays and radioimmunoassays, specifically measuring the placental type phosphatases, indicate that the mean level in healthy adults is 0.06 ± 0.08 µmol/min/L, corresponding to 0.3 ± 0.4 ng/mL (mean $\pm$ SD) with an upper limit for healthy persons amounting to 0.3 µmol/min/L (1.5 ng/mL) (Stigbrand and collaborators, unpublished observation). For comparison, the level during the last trimester of pregnancy amounts to 200–300 ng/mL. In sera from tumor patients, the level is generally below 25 ng/mL although concentrations up to 25 µg/mL have been reported.

The incidence of increased levels of placental alkaline phosphatase, measured both catalytically and radioimmunologically, is highest for tumors of trophoblastic origin, but also high for tumors from the reproductive tract in both males and females (Nathanson and Fishman, 1971; Stolbach el al., 1976; Holmgren et al., 1979; Wahren et al., 1979; Haije et al., 1979; Doellgast et al., 1981). Several other tumor groups tested show elevated levels in serum of 10–30% of the cases (Fishman and Stolbach, 1979; Wada et al., 1979). Recently a very sensitive sandwich enzyme-linked immunoassay has been developed with a detection limit of 0.5 ng/mL (Millan and Stigbrand, 1982). Future studies will reveal more clearly whether immunoassays with increased sensitivity, such as this one, will increase the diagnostic value of placental alkaline phosphatase in cancer.

2.3. Tumor-Related Alkaline Phosphatases

Placental alkaline phosphatase was the first enzyme described as an oncofetal or carcinoplacental antigen by Fishman et al. (1968a,b). It was found in the serum of a patient (Regan) with squamous cell carcinoma of the lung. The functional characteristics of the enzyme were indistinguishable from the placental enzyme by several catalytical and immunological criteria.

Other tumor-related forms have later been described; the Nagao variant (Nakayama et al., 1970), which is related to the rare placental D variant (Inglis et al., 1973). Another variant of the enzyme has also been described in a patient with hepatoma, the so called Kasahara variant, by Warnock and Reisman (1969). This was later partially purified and characterized by Higashino et al. (1972). The Kasahara variant has been shown to be related to the form found in Fl-amnion cells (Higashino et al., 1975).

In 1976 Fishman et al., described isoenzymes of placental alkaline phosphatase in placental tissue that seemed confined only to the first weeks of pregnancy (6–10 weeks). These enzymes have been called developmental phase-specific alkaline phosphatases, early-type placental alkaline phosphatases, or chorionic-type phosphatases. On electrophoresis, early placental alkaline phosphatases have been shown to consist of two heat-sensitive, L-homoarginine-inhibited bands, the slower of which possesses antigenic determinants shared with liver and bone phosphatases. The faster band seems to have unique antigenic determinants. These early placental isoenzymes are normally not expressed in the full-term placenta, and could be candidates for tumor markers. Indeed, some tumors have been shown to express enzymes with characteristics similar to these early types of phosphatases (Timperley et al., 1971; Warnes et al., 1972; Ehrmeyer et al., 1978). Expression of early-type placental alkaline phosphatase has been demonstrated by human carcinoma cell lines (Kottel and collaborators, unpublished observation). The main features of tumor-related alkaline phosphatases are summarized in Table 2.

The two most studied tumor-related forms of placental alkaline phosphatases are the Regan (Fishman et al., 1968a,b) and Nagao (Nakayama et al., 1970) variants. The Nagao isoenzyme has several documented properties of the Regan isoenzyme. However, it is sensitive to both L-phenyl-alanine and L-leucine, in contrast to Regan isoenzyme, which is inhibited only by L-phenylalanine. In addition, the electrophoretic mobilities and the sensitivities to inactivation by urea, EDTA, and some other mildly denaturing agents are slightly different. On the other hand, the immunological reactivity seems to be the same for the Regan and Nagao isoenzymes, at least when polyclonal antisera toward placental alkaline phosphatase are used. Seminoma tissues contain large amounts of placental alkaline phosphatase (Wahren et al., 1979), although the type has not been identified.

The extensive genetic polymorphism observed in placental tissues would also be expected to be present in tumor samples. However, this does not seem to be the case. Instead the very rare genetic variant of placental alkaline phosphatase with slow electrophoretic mobility, the so-called D-variant, was reported to be present in more than 50% of the tumor specimens. This D-variant was shown to be identical with the Nagao form of the

Table 2
Characteristics for Some Tumor-Related Alkaline Phosphatases

	Regan[a] (term placental type)	Nagao[b] (D variant)	Kasahara[c] (Regan variant)	Early placental phosphatases[d] (non-Regan isoenzyme)
Inactivated by heat, 5 min at 65°	No	No	Yes	Yes
Inhibition by L-phenylalanine, 5 mM	Yes	Yes	Yes	(No)
Inhibition by L-leucine, 0.5 mM	No	Yes	Yes	(No)
Determinants similar or identical to:				
Placental alkaline phosphatases	Yes	Yes	(Yes)	No
Liver alkaline phosphatases	No	No	No	Yes
Intestinal alkaline phosphatases	No	No	(Yes)	No

[a]Fishman et al., 1968a, b.
[b]Nakayama et al., 1970; Inglis et al., 1973.
[c]Warnock and Reisman, 1969; Higashino et al., 1972; Higashino et al., 1974, Higashino et al., 1975.
[d]Fishman, L., et al., 1976.

enzyme (Inglis et al., 1973). This identity has, however, been questioned (Beckman and Beckman, 1975).

The appearance of alkaline phosphatases in several malignant cell lines in vitro has been well documented. Many of these cell lines do synthesize placental alkaline phosphatase, in particular the Regan type (Singer and Fishman, 1974; Singer and Fishman, 1976; Singh et al., 1978; Hamilton et al., 1979; Chou, 1979). One osteosarcoma line was shown to produce bone-specific phosphatase, and the BeWo and Jar cell lines have been shown to synthesize both placental (Regan-type) and liver alkaline phosphatase (Speeg et al., 1977). HeLa cells and subclones of these also have been shown to produce both placental and other alkaline phosphatases (Singer and Fishman, 1974).

Some cell lines known to express the term placental alkaline phosphatase (Regan-type) in vitro switch their production to the early-type phosphatase (chorionic type) when grown as solid tumors in adult hamster cheek pouches (Singer et al., 1979). Other cell lines that produce the chorionic type in vitro have been shown to retain their isoenzyme profile when grown as solid tumors in nude mice (Kottel and collaborators, unpublished).

The re-expression of different embryonic phosphatases, as assayed by catalytic activity and electrophoretic mobility, has thus been documented both in cell lines in vitro and in human tumors in vivo. However, the chemical relationship between several of the tumor-related variants of alkaline phosphatase is still unknown. The future use of immunoassays and, in particular, the use of monoclonal antibodies may simplify the presently rather complex pattern of tumor-related alkaline phosphatases.

3. Histaminase (Diamine Oxidase)

Placenta has the highest level of histaminase among all human tissues tested. Furthermore, it has been known for a long time that histaminase is found in serum during pregnancy (Ahlmark, 1944). The level in pregnancy sera is several hundred to several thousand-fold higher than that of nonpregnancy sera (Southren et al., 1965).

The biological function of this enzyme is not entirely clear, although the fact that the enzyme degrades a wide range of biogenic amines in vitro suggests that it is involved in the metabolism of such amines. A possible physiological role in the degradation of excess amounts of histamine synthesized by the fetus, has also been proposed (Zeller, 1963).

Histaminase is an example of a placental protein that is not produced by the syncytiotrophoblast. Instead, the decidual cells present both on the endometrial and placental side of the blood barrier are responsible for histaminase production. Immunofluorescence studies (Lin et al., 1978) show that the enzyme is present in the cytoplasm of the decidual cell and in tissue spaces between the cells. The chorionic villi were completely lacking in fluorescent staining.

The affinity of histaminase for cadaverine has recently been utilized in the purification of the enzyme in a one-step affinity chromatography procedure (Lin et al., 1981). The enzyme has a subunit molecular weight of approximately 90,000 and is present in serum as a dimer with a molecular weight of 180,000–190,000 (Lin and Kirley, 1976).

Many methods for quantitation of the enzyme utilizing the enzymatic activity of histaminase have been decribed (Zeller, 1963; Buffoni, 1966; Kapeller-Adler, 1979; Bardsley et al., 1972; Neufeld and Chayen, 1971). Most of these methods, however, are neither highly specific nor sensitive.

The introduction of radioactive substrates provided more sensitive determinations of enzyme activity. Three radioassays have been decribed using ^{14}C-putrescine (Okuyama and Kobayashi, 1961), ^{3}H-histamine (Beaven and Jacobsen, 1971) and ^{14}C-histamine (Roscoe and Kupfer, 1972), respectively. The enzyme has its highest activity towards putrescine and the most sensitive radioassay has a detection limit of 0.01 unit, which corresponds to approximately 2 ng/mL (Lin and Angellis, 1981).

Several studies have shown elevated histaminase levels in human tumors (Benda and Miravet, 1960; Borglin and Willert, 1962; Baylin et al., 1972). Both biochemical and histochemical evidence indicate that elevated levels of the enzyme both in serum and effusion fluids of cancer patients are the results of production by the tumor (Atkins et al., 1973 ; Lin et al., 1979; Mendelsohn et al., 1978). The histaminase obtained from tumors or effusion fluids has furthermore been shown to be immunologically identical to that of the placenta (Lin et al., 1979). Using catalytic assays, Lin et al. (1979) demonstrated elevated histaminase levels in 72 out of 162 (44%) effusions (pleural, peritoneal, or pericardial) from patients with cancer. When compared to other tumor-associated markers simultaneously assayed in these fluids, tumors from the colon and stomach were often accompanied by elevated levels of CEA, whereas tumors of the ovary were associated with production of the β-subunit of human chorionic gonadotrophin. Table 3 summarizes the findings on the occurrence of these markers according to Lin et al. (1979). It is hoped that highly sensitive radioimmunoassays, such as the one recently described by Lin and Angellis (1981), will increase the usefulness of histaminase as a biochemical marker for cancer.

4. Human Chorionic Gonadotropin

Human chorionic gonadotropin (HCG) was first described as a serum factor secreted by the placenta and inducing functional changes in the ovaries (hyperemia, formation of corpus luteum, and induction of estrus) of virgin guinea pigs (Aschner, 1913; Aschheim and Zondek, 1927). Human

Table 3

Frequency of Elevated Levels[a] of Histaminase, CEA,
β-HCG, and Regan Isoenzyme in Effusion Fluids (Pleural, Peritoneal,
or Pericardial) from Cancer Patients[b]

	Histaminase	CEA	β-HCG	Regan
Breast	14/43 (33)[c]	20/34 (47)	6/41 (15)	4/43 (9)
Lung	13/45 (29)	19/45 (42)	17/45 (40)	6/45 (13)
Ovary	20/23 (87)	11/23 (48)	16/23 (70)	12/23 (52)
Colon	8/11 (73)	10/11 (91)	4/11 (36)	6/11 (55)
Stomach	7/8 (88)	6/8 (75)	5/8 (63)	2/8 (25)
Endometrium	4/8 (50)	2/9 (25)	3/8 (38)	4/8 (50)
Lymphoma	0/6 (0)	0/6 (0)	0/6 (0)	0/6 (0)
Others	6/18 (33)	2/18 (11)	5/18 (28)	4/18 (22)
Non Ca fluids	0/12 (0)	—	—	—
Normal sera	0/19 (0)	—	—	—

[a]Elevated levels for histaminase > 40 ng putrescine per hour per ml CEA > 25 ng/mL, β-HCG > 5 mUI/mL, Regan isoenzyme > 0.4 placental units/mL.

[b]According to Lin et al., 1979.

[c]Percentage of patients above the normal level.

chorionic gonadotrophin is a glycoprotein with a molecular weight of approximately 45,000 that shares chemical and immunological properties with several other human glycoprotein hormones—LH, TSH, and FSH—all of which are secreted by the anterior pituitary. Each of these hormones is composed of two different subunits, the so called α- and β-chains, which are held together noncovalently by hydrophobic interactions (Aloj et al., 1973). The alpha subunit of HCG, with a molecular weight of 15,000–20,000, has been sequenced and found indistinguishable from the α-chains of FSH, LH, and TSH.

The beta subunit, with a molecular weight of 24,000–30,000 contains portions that are unique to HCG (Carlsen et al., 1973; Bellisario et al., 1973; Morgan et al., 1973, 1975), e.g., the 30 amino acids at the carboxy terminal end. Thus, antisera used in radioimmunoassays have to be specific for the beta subunit or even the C-terminal part of the β-chain in order to give a specific assay (Vaitukaitis et al., 1972).

Placenta normally contains both HCG and excess free immunoreactive alpha chains (Vaitukaitis, 1974; Franchimont and Reuter, 1972). The amounts of free beta subunit and mRNA for this subunit have been found to be very low in normal placental extracts (Chatterjee et al., 1976). Similar observations have been made for other hormones in pituitary extracts (Kourides et al., 1975; Prentice and Ryan, 1975), i.e., that the α-chain is produced in excess of the β-chain.

4.1. Assays

Several qualitative and quantitative bioassays have been developed to measure HCG (Ross, 1973). Despite several obvious disadvantages, i.e, low sensitivity and interference by endogenous HPL, most of the early information regarding HCG as a tumor marker was elaborated by use of bioassays on concentrates of 24-h urine samples (Hertz et al., 1961; Ross et al., 1965).

Many different immunological assays using hemagglutination, latex particle agglutination, and agglutination inhibition have been developed for early diagnosis of pregnancy (Cargille, 1971). The sensitivity of these tests, however, was not sufficient for diagnostic purposes in cancer. Early radioimmunoassays (Bagshawe, 1973; Midgley et al., 1967; Maffezzoli et al., 1972; Kaplan et al., 1972), as well as the radioreceptor assays (Catt et al., 1971; Landesman and Saxena, 1976), were not absolutely specific for HCG and, consequently, the production of HCG by tumors was sparsely investigated (Weintraub and Rosen, 1971; Braunstein et al., 1973a). However, the development of radioimmunoassays specific for the β-subunit (Vaitukaitis et al., 1972; Chen et al., 1976) represented a major breakthrough in the area of tumor diagnosis as well as pregnancy detection. Assays specific for HCG are now available with a least detectable dose of 1 ng/mL, corresponding to 5 mIU/mL.

4.2. HCG as a Tumor Marker

The significance of HCG measurement both for diagnostic and prognostic purposes in gestational trophoblastic disease is well-documented (Lewis, 1976; Goldstein, 1976; Bagshawe, 1976). High initial levels of HCG or persisting levels after chemotherapy have been shown to yield valuable information both with regard to prognosis and resistance to chemotherapy (Ross et al., 1965; Hammond et al., 1973; Goldstein, 1974; Vaitukaitis and Ebersole, 1976; Lewis, 1976).

The germ cell tumors of the testis have been shown to secrete a number of both placental and fetal proteins. By use of β-HCG radioimmunoassays, the frequency of elevated levels in serum has been estimated to 15% for seminomas, 50% for embryonal carcinomas, 42% for teratocarcinomas, and 100% for choriocarcinomas (Braunstein et al., 1973a; Cochran, 1975; Perlin et al., 1976; Lange et al., 1976). Serial determinations of HCG have proven valuable for monitoring therapy of these tumors, and serum levels of HCG often parallel changes in the tumor burden (Patton et al., 1960; Perlin et al., 1976). Persisting high levels following surgery, radiation, or chemotherapy of testicular tumor is an indicator of residual disease.

Several nontrophoblastic as well as trophoblastic tumors have been shown to secrete HCG. The relative proportions of the β-chain, the α-chain and the intact hormone varies, which indicates independent synthesis of the subunits (Weintraub and Rosen, 1973; Rosen et al., 1975; Rosen and Weintraub, 1974).

Low but elevated levels of HCG in serum from patients with nontrophoblastic tumors have also been demonstrated, although the levels usually are below 10 ng/mL. Table 4 (as reproduced from Braunstein, 1979) summarizes the incidence of immunoreactive HCG in patients with different neoplasms. The highest incidence has been observed for ovarian (41%) and breast (30%) neoplasms. The overall incidence of ectopic HCG production in sera from tumor patients has been estimated to 16%. Immunohistochemical studies, however, have indicated that a higher incidence might be anticipated by use of more sensitive assays. McManus et al., 1976) thus demonstrated immunoreactive HCG in or at the surface of 89% of tumors or monolayers in tissue cultures. It should be emphasized, though, that a low percentage (1.8%) of normal persons have immunoreactive HCG in their serum (Braunstein, 1979), and HCG-like proteins have been demonstrated both in normal human testis (Braunstein et al., 1975), pituitary and concentrates of castrate male urine (Chen et al.,

Table 4

Incidence of Immunoreactive HCG in Sera of Patients with Neoplasma[a]

	Number of patients	Number positive by HCG	Percent
Ovarian	103	42	40.8
Breast	386	115	29.8
Melanoma	210	40	19.1
Gastrointestinal	654	109	16.7
Esophagus	12	0	0
Stomach	75	17	22.7
Pancreatic	45	15	33.3
Small intestine	23	3	13.0
Biliary tract	9	1	11.1
Liver	217	36	16.6
Large intestine/rectum	129	21	16.3
Sarcoma	51	7	13.7
Lung	311	41	13.5
Renal	69	7	10.1
Hematopoietic	661	34	5.1
Leukemia	262	12	4.6
Lymphoma	283	11	3.9
Multiple myeloma	116	11	9.5
Totals:	2445	395	16.2

[a]According to Braunstein 1979.

1976). HCG-like proteins have also been demonstrated in human lung, liver, spleen, intestine, and other organs (Yoshimoto et al., 1977; 1978 ; Braunstein et al., 1979).

Recently, a low molecular fragment (6000) of HCG has been demonstrated in urine from both pregnant females and tumor patients (Masure et al., 1981).

5. Pregnancy-Specific Glycoprotein (SP1)

Much interest has been focused recently on the placental protein SP1 in cancer (synonyms: Schwangerschafts Proteine 1, trophoblast specific β_1-glycoprotein, pregnancy specific β-globulin, PSβG). The protein was first described by Tatarinov and Masyukevich (1970) and was isolated and characterized by Bohn (1972a). With the availability of specific antisera to SP1, the quantitative expression of SP1 in pregnancy as well as in malignancy has been under intense investigation. Excellent reviews on SP1, covering its structure, possible function, and expression in pregnancy as well as in malignancy, have appeared recently (Bohn, 1978a; Tatarinov, 1978; Tatarinov, 1979).

SP1 is a glycoprotein of molecular weight approximately 100,000 containing about 30% carbohydrate (Bohn, 1972a). Its amino acid and carbohydrate composition is that of a typical acidic glycoprotein, and its isoelectric point is relatively low (Bohn et al., 1976). It is synthesized by the placenta during pregnancy and can be found in the maternal (but not fetal) circulation in amounts increasing with advancing pregnancy to reach approximately 300 µg/mL at term. After delivery, it rapidly disappears from the circulation.

5.1. Assays

Depending on the purpose, a variety of immunochemical assays are being used in the study of SP1. Table 5 summarizes some of the most commonly used assays and their approximate detection limits. Even the least sensitive immunoprecipitation assays are sensitive enough to monitor the high levels of SP1 found during the second and third trimesters of pregnancy. However, for apparent reasons, only the most sensitive assays, radioimmunoassay or enzyme immunoassay, are adequate for early diagnosis of pregnancy or for monitoring malignant disease.

5.2. Normal Tissue Origin of SP1

Several reports have shown that SP1 can be localized to the epithelium of the placental villi by immunofluorescence or immunoperoxidase techniques (Sedlacek et al., 1976; Lin and Halpert, 1976; Horne et al., 1976a;

Table 5
Immunochemical Assays for SP1

Type of assay	Detection limit, μg/L	Application	Reference
Immunoprecipitation or radial immunodiffusion	10	Pregnancy	Bohn (1974) Schultz-Larsen et al. (1979)
Rocket immunoelectrophoresis	10	Pregnancy	Teisner et al. (1978)
Nephelometry	10	Pregnancy	Wood et al. (1978)
Radioimmunoassay	0.001–0.010	Malignancy	Grudzinskas et al. (1977)
		Early pregnancy	Tatarinov and Sokolov (1978) Kaminska et al. (1979)
Enzyme immunoassay	0.001–0.010	Malignancy, pregnancy	McDonald et al. (1979)

Tatarinov, 1978). Most SP1 is localized to the superficial syncytiotrophoblast, but some also seems to be present in the cytotrophoblast (Tatarinov, 1978) and, to a lesser extent, in the stroma (Sedlacek et al., 1976) of the placental villi. Furthermore, short term cultures of immature placenta incorporate radioactive amino acids into immunoreactive material (Horne et al., 1976). Tissues such as liver, lung, and muscle from pregnant women did not incorporate radioactivity in a similar way (Tatarinov, 1978).

5.3. Tumors Associated with Elevated Levels of SP1

SP1 was first found in sera from patients with trophoblastic tumors by Tatarinov et al. (1974). The finding has since been confirmed and extended by several groups using different techniques of detection (Seppälä et al., 1978, Bagshawe et al., 1978; Searle et al., 1978; Rutanen and Seppälä, 1980; O'Brien et al., 1980).

High levels of SP1 are always found in patients with actual gestational trophoblastic disease. After successful treatment, the levels rapidly decrease. A recurrence of residual disease is mostly accompanied by rising or persistent SP1 in serum. Thus, it seems that SP1 is an excellent marker for such tumors. Future studies will tell whether it will be used mainly as an adjunct to HCG.

For the purpose of trophoblastic tumors, HCG has long been regarded as a model marker, because changes in the serum levels of HCG are an excellent and highly sensitive indicator of tumor activity. There are instances where assays for HCG are not sufficient for monitoring trophoblastic tumors. Even assays specific for the HCG β-chain suffer from cross-reactivity with other hormones. As a consequence, there is always some ambiguity of results with low levels of HCG, especially if it is both low and persistent. In these cases, a positive or negative SP1 test would add very valuable information.

Although in gestational trophoblastic disease both SP1 and HCG are found in the circulation in relatively high concentrations and both rapidly disappear after successful treatment, evidence exists that they are not indicators of the same cellular activity.

Seppälä et al. (1978) first showed discordant behavior of SP1 and HCG in the course of disease in individual patients with choriocarcinoma . In one patient, e.g., there was a dramatic increase in SP1 several months before HCG became positive and the tumor, assumed to be present on the basis of the HCG secretion, was treated again. In subsequent studies it was found that the correlation between SP1 and HCG values in patients with trophoblastic tumors "was not close" (Bagshawe et al., 1978) and Searle et al. (1978) demonstrated persistant SP1 levels after HCG had become undetectable following chemotherapy in several patients.

Although there is not enough information yet to draw any conclusions on the basis of presence or absence of SP1 from the circulation of patients with gestational trophoblastic tumors, further studies should be encouraged.

Expression of SP1 has also been reported to occur in nontrophoblastic ovarian tumors. Crowter et al. (1979) measured SP1, HCG, and placental lactogen (HPL) in 37 patients with primary epithelial carcinoma of the ovary. SP1 was detected in five of the patients, compared with 8 and 2 detections of HPL and HCG, respectively. An interesting finding in this group of patients was the complete discordance between HCG and SP1 expression in that, of those patients positive for any one of these three markers, none expressed SP1 and HCG simultaneously. This particular study was accompanied by a large normal control group. In none of 100 nonpregnant females could SP1 be detected (<10 ng/mL). In similar studies on ovarian cancer, the incidence of tumors expressing SP1 has not been significantly different from that of a control population (Würz, 1979; Searle et al., 1978; Tatarinov and Sokolov, 1977).

Germ cell tumors of the testis have recently been shown by Rosen et al. (1979a) to be associated with elevated SP1 levels in a significant number of patients. Tumors classified as choriocarcinomas, embryonal carcinomas, and teratocarcinomas, but not seminomas, produced high levels of SP1. Searle et al. (1978) in their study on SP1 in neoplastic disease found that 7 out of 8 patients with teratomas that were associated with high HCG levels also expressed SP1. Similarly, in the collaborative study on SP1 and HCG by Bagshawe et al. (1978), a few gonadal tumors secreting high levels of HCG were found also to secrete SP1.

Tatarinov and Sokolov (1977) also reported on the ectopic production of SP1 by nontrophoblastic tumors. A large percentage of their tumor patients with different kinds of common tumors had SP1 in their serum , detected by competitive double antibody radioimmunoassay. The levels were, compared to those found in pregnant women or in patients with trophoblastic tumors low, but represented significant inhibition in the assay. These findings by Tatarinov and Sokolov are another example substantiating the attractive hypothesis of re-expression of fetal genes in cancer. The study also seemed to confirm the somewhat controversial finding by Horne et al. (1976b) of the demonstration of SP1 in cancerous tissue of the breast. Later reports from several groups (Würz, 1979; Searle et al., 1978; Bagshawe et al., 1978) further confirm results by Tatarinov and Sokolov that SP1 can indeed be detected in the serum of patients with, for example, cancer of the breast and the gastrointestinal tract. However, some of the studies have not found complete absence of SP1 in sera of control individuals, which makes application of the SP1 test in cancer less practical. Engvall and Yonemoto (1979) could not find significantly elevated SP1 either in cancer patients or in patients with other diseases. No conclusion can yet be drawn from the somewhat conflicting data presently available. It is hoped that an exchange of assay reagents and critical samples could result in agreement on this matter.

5.4. SP1 In Vitro

A big surprise occured when Rosen and collaborators (1979b) reported on the production of SP1, as detected by radioimmunoassay in human fibroblasts. All established fibroblastic cell lines that were tested produced SP1. The highest production rate of SP1 was found in a cell line derived from a fibrosarcoma. The material reactive in the SP1 radioimmunoassay was shown to have the same apparent molecular weight as authentic SP1 and to give inhibition curves parallel to those of standard SP1. The finding of fibroblast SP1 has since been confirmed and extended by one of us (Engvall, unpublished) to include a large number of cell lines, as well as further characteristics of the SP1 produced by some cell lines. Table 6 summarizes some of these data. Several malignant cell lines of trophoblastic origin, known to produce HCG eutopically, did not produce SP1. On the other hand, two cell lines that produce HCG ectopically also produced SP1. One of these was derived from an ovarian carcinoma (Azer et al., 1980) and the other one from a cervical carcinoma (DOT). Without exception, all 16 fibroblastic cell lines tested to date have produced SP1 in easily detectable amounts. These cell lines have all been derived from skin biopsies of healthy adults.

At present there are no explanations for the apparent discrepancies found between the expression of SP1 in vivo and in vitro. Why would the

Table 6
Concentrations of SP1 in Culture Medium
of Confluent Cultures

Cultured cell type	SP1, ng/mL
Trophoblastic tumor cells (G-8, BeWo, JEG)	< 1
Teratocarcinoma (PA-1, Paxton)	< 1
Colon carcinoma (HT-29, SW 480)	< 1
Bladder carcinoma (RT-4, T24, 5637)	< 1
Cervical carcinoma (3 HeLa sublines) (DoT)	< 1
	1–10
Ovarian cystadenocarcinoma	10–100
Fibroblasts (16 lines)	10–100

trophoblast be the sole source of SP1 in vivo where in vivo fibroblasts seem to be the predominant SP1 producer? Further studies on the production of SP1 by cells and tissues in vitro and the precise localization and site of synthesis in vivo may reveal interesting insights into the regulation of expression of tissue-specific proteins.

6. Placental Proteins (PP)

The first observations on pregnancy-associated proteins, of which some were of placental origin, were made after immunization of rabbits with pregnancy sera followed by absorption with male serum. This procedure resulted in antisera with specificity toward at least four different proteins described elsewhere in this volume (Horne and Brenner, 1980).

Bohn (for review, see Bohn 1979) was the first to investigate systematically the possibility of using placental extracts as immunogens. The extraction procedures included both hydrophilic and organic solvents. The antisera obtained were directed toward soluble and insoluble antigens in the placental tissue, some of which are normally not secreted into the maternal blood stream. Bohn also was the first to partially purify and characterize several of these proteins, named placental proteins (PP1–PP7) (Bohn, 1972b; Bohn, 1979). The properties and characteristics of these soluble placental tissue proteins are summarized in Table 7. Several of these proteins turned out not to be absolutely specific for the placental tissue. PP2, for example, was identified as ferritin. At least one of them, PP5, could not be identified in any other fetal or adult tissue and has subsequently been most studied. PP5 is a glycoprotein, synthesized by the syncytiotrophoblast, with the molecular weight of 36,000 (Bohn and Winckler, 1977). The total amount in a mature placenta has been esti-

Table 7
Characteristics of Soluble Placental Tissue Proteins[a]

Placental protein	Name or function	Physicochemical properties, mw	Carbohydrate content,[b]%	Amounts found in extracts of term placentae,[b] mg/placenta
PP1		160,000	2.7	3
PP2	Ferritin	~500,000	—	18
PP3		~100,000	nd	nd
PP4		~ 30,000	nd	nd
PP5	Protease inhibitor	36,600	19.8	1.5
PP6		1,000,000	6.6	100
PP7		40,000	5.4	60

[a]According to Bohn (1979).
[b]nd = not determined.

mated to 1.5 mg, and compared to the other "placenta-specific" proteins, the content in placenta is low. A sensitive radioimmunoassay with a least detectable dose of 10 ng/mL has been developed for PP5 (Obiekwe et al ., 1979) and the levels during pregnancy reach a maximum concentration of 45 ng/mL in the 36th week. In normal sera, values below the detection limit (1.2 ng/mL) in a radioimmunoassay have been reported by Seppälä et al. (1979).

Radioimmunoassays have been used to demonstrate the occurrence of PP5 in sera from patients with trophoblastic tumors and testicular tumors (Obiekwe et al., 1979). Interestingly, Seppälä et al. (1979) demonstrated elevated levels only in two out of 19 samples with hydatidiform mole, and none of 77 serum specimens from patients with choriocarcinoma showed any detectable PP5 even when serum concentrations of HCG and SP1 were high. This may have an important implication in clinical practice with regard to differential diagnosis between normal pregnancy and invasive trophoblastic disease. Since PP5 can be demonstrated in the normal, but not in the malignant, trophoblast, it has been suggested that this protein may be involved in the regulation of trophoblastic invasiveness. In light of the proposed biological role for PP5 in exerting in vitro protease inhibitor activity (Bohn and Winckler, 1977), this observation is an attractive possibility. No results have so far been presented on the occurrence of this protein in other malignant diseases.

Bohn (1978b), in his systematic search for new antigens in placenta, also used a variety of detergents, high ionic strength buffers, and proteolytic enzymes to solubilize membrane-associated components from the placental tissue. Polyclonal antisera raised against such preparations resulted in antibodies with specificity against a number of known proteins, such as placental alkaline phosphatase, HPL, SP1, PP5, PP4, fibrinogen split products, and fibronectin. In addition, at least 11 new antigens—designated alphabetically A to L—were identified. Some of these may prove to be new oncoplacental proteins.

7. Final Remarks

The search for placental proteins suitable as tumor markers has progressed rapidly during recent years. Some of the markers have already proved of value in the monitoring of tumors, although assays with improved sensitivity and specificity will be needed to prove the value of others. Several new membrane-associated placental proteins that have encouraging properties as candidate tumor markers have been described during the last few years. It is likely that the use of monoclonal antibodies will lead to identification of an increasing number of placental antigens that will be of interest to tumor biologists and can serve as tumor markers.

Acknowledgments

We are greatly indebted to Dr. and Mrs. W. H. Fishman for providing the stimulating atmosphere at the La Jolla Cancer Research Foundation.

We want to thank the investigators who provided us with reprints and preprints of their work. The preparation of this review and some of the original work was supported by grants from the Swedish Medical Research Council (4217 and 5802), University of Umeå, and Lions Foundation, and grants CA 27464, CA 21967, and CA 22384 from the National Cancer Institute, DHHS.

We also want to thank Ms. Nancy Beddingfield and Mrs. Ulla-Britt Mattsson for helping with the manuscript and Drs. Wahren and Sell for their patience.

References

Ahlmark, A. (1944), *Acta Physiol. Scand.* 9 (28), 1.
Aloj, S. M., H. Edelhoch, K. C. Ingham, F. J. Morgan, R. E. Canfield, and G. T. Ross (1973), *Arch. Biochem. Biophys.* 159, 497.
Aschheim, S., and B. Zondek (1927), *Klin. Wochenschr.* 6, 1322.
Aschner, B. (1913), *Arch. Gynaecol.* 99, 534.

Atkins, F. L., M. A. Beaven, and H. R. Keiser (1973), *N. Engl. J. Med.* **289**, 545.

Azer, P. C., G. D. Braunstein, R. L. van de Velde, S. van de Velde, R. Kogan, and E. Engvall (1980), *J. Clin. Endocrin. Metab.* **50**, 234.

Bagshawe, K. D. (1973), in *Methods in Investigative and Diagnostic Endocrinology*, Part III, *Peptide Hormones* (Bearson, S. A., and R. S. Yalow, eds.) North-Holland, Amsterdam, p. 756.

Bagshawe, K. D. (1976), *Cancer* **38**, 1373.

Bagshawe, K. D., R. H. Lequin, Ph. Sizaret, Y. S. Tatarinov (1978), *Eur. J. Cancer* **14**, 1331.

Bardsley, W. G., M. J. C. Crabbe, J. S. Shindler, and J. S. Ashford (1972), *Biochem. J.* **127**, 875.

Baylin, S. B., M. A. Beaven, L. M. Buja, H. R. Keiser (1972), *Am. J. Med.* **53**, 723.

Beaconsfield, P., and J. Ginsburg (1979), in *Placenta—A Neglected Experimental Animal* (Beaconsfield, P., and C. Villee, eds.), Pergamon Press, p. 34.

Beaven, M. A., and S. Jacobsen, *J. Pharmacol. Exptl. Ther.* **176**, 52.

Beckman, G., and L. Beckman (1975), *Hereditas* **81**, 85.

Beckman, L., G. Björling, C. Cristodoulou (1966), *Acta Genet.* **16**, 59.

Bellisario, R., R. B. Carlsen, and O. P. Bahl (1973), *J. Biol. Chem.* **248**, 6796.

Benda, M. R., and L. F. Miravet (1960), *Bull. Mem. Soc. Med. Paris* **76**, 184.

Benham, F. J., M. S. Povey, and H. Harris (1977), *Clin. Chim. Acta* **86**, 201.

Bohn, H. (1971), *Arch. Gynaek.* **210**, 440.

Bohn, H. (1972a), *Blut* **24**, 292.

Bohn, H. (1972b), *Arch. Gynäk.* **212**, 165.

Bohn, H., R. Schmidtberger, and H. Zilg (1976), *Blut* **32**, 103.

Bohn, H. (1974), *Arch. Gynecol.* **217**, 219.

Bohn, H., and W. Winckler (1977), *Arch. Gynäk.* **223**, 179.

Bohn, H. (1978a), in *Chemistry of Tumor-Associated Antigens* (E. Ruoslahti and E. Engvall, eds.) *Scand. J. Immunol.*, **6**, suppl. 6.

Bohn, H. (1978b), in *Placental Proteins* (Klopper, A., and T. Chard, eds.), Springer-Verlag, Berlin, p. 119.

Bohn, H. (1979), in *Carcino-Embryonic Proteins*, Vol. 1 (Lehmann, F.-G ., ed.), Elsevier/North-Holland, p. 289.

Borglin, N. B., and B. Willert (1962), *Cancer* **15**, 271.

Boyer, S. H. (1961), *Science* **134**, 1002.

Braunstein, G. D., K. R. McIntire, and T. A. Waldmann (1973a), *Cancer* **31**, 1065.

Braunstein, G. D., J. L. Vaitukaitis, P. P. Carbone, and G. T. Ross (1973b), *Ann. Intern. Med.* **78**, 39.

Braunstein, G. D., J. Rasor, and M. E. Wade (1975), *N. Engl. J. Med.* **293**, 1339.

Braunstein, G. D. (1979), in *Immunodiagnosis of Cancer. Part I.* (Herberman, R. B., and K. R. McIntire, eds.), Dekker, New York.

Buffoni, F. (1966), *Pharmacol.* **18**, 1163.

Carlsen, R. B., O. P. Bahl, and N. Swaminathan (1973), *J. Biol. Chem.* **248**, 6810.

Cargille, C. M. (1971), in *Laboratory Diagnosis of Endocrine Diseases* (Sunderman, F. W., and F. W. Sunderman, Jr., eds.), Green, St. Louis, p. 152.

Catt, K. J., M. L. Dufau, and T. Tsuruhara (1971), *J. Clin. Endocrinol . Metab.* **32**, 860.

Chang, C.-H., S. Raam, D. Angellis, G. Doellgast, and W. H. Fishman (1975), *Cancer Res.* **35**, 1706.

Chatterjee, M., B. S. Baliga, and H. N. Munro (1976), *J. Biol. Chem.* **251**, 2945.

Chen, H. C., G. D. Hodgen, S. Matsura, L. J. Lin, E. Gross, L. E. Reichert, Jr., S. Birken, R. E. Canfield, and G. T. Ross (1976), *Proc. Natl. Acad. Sci. USA* **73**, 2885.

Chou, J. V. (1979), *In Vitro* **16**, 789.

Cochran, J. S., P. C. Walsh, J. C. Porter, T. C. Nicholson, J. D. Madden, and P. D. Peters (1975), *J. Urol.* **114**, 549.

Crowter, M. E., J. G. Grudzinskas, T. A. Poulton, and Y. B. Gordon (1979), *Obstetr. Gynecol.* **53**, 59.

Davies, I. J., and K. J. Ryan (1972), *Vitamins and Hormones* **30**, 223.

Doellgast, G. J., and W. H. Fishman (1975), *Isoenzymes. I*, Academic Press, New York, p. 293.

Doellgast, G. J., J. Spiegel, R. A. Guenther, and W. H. Fishman (1977), *Biochim. Biophys. Acta* **484**, 59.

Doellgast, G. J., and K. Benirschke (1979), *Nature* **280**, 601.

Doellgast, G. J., and P. J. Meis (1979), *Clin. Chem.* **25**, 1230.

Doellgast, G. J., C. C. Lemons, and H. D. Homesley (1981), (manuscript in preparation).

Ehrmeyer, S. L., B. L. Joiner, L. Kahan, F. C. Larson, and R. C. Metzenberg (1978), *Cancer Res.* **38**, 599.

Engvall, E., and R. H. Yonemoto (1979), *Int. J. Cancer* **23**, 759.

Fishman, W. H. (1974), *Am. J. Med.* **56**, 617.

Fishman, W. H., and N. K. Ghosh (1976), *Adv. Clin. Chem.* **10**, 255.

Fishman, W. H., L. L. Stolbach (1979), in *Immunodiagnosis of Cancer* Part 1 (Herberman, R. B., and K. R. McIntire, eds.) Dekker, New York p. 447.

Fishman, W. H., N. R. Inglis, S. Green, C. L. Anstiss, N. K. Ghosh, A. E. Reif, R. Rustigian,, M. J. Krant, and L. L. Stolbach (1968a), *Nature* **219**,697.

Fishman, W. H., N. R. Inglis, L. L. Stolbach, and M. J. Krant (1968b), *Cancer Res.* **28**, 150.

Fishman, W. H., N. R. Inglis, N. K. Ghosh (1968c), *Clin. Chim. Acta* **19**, 71.

Fishman, L., H. Miyayama, S. G. Driscoll, and W. H. Fishman (1976), *Cancer Res.* **36**, 2268.

Franchimont, P., and A. Reuter (1972), in *Protein and Polypeptide Hormones* (Margoulies, M., and F. Greenwood, eds.) Excerpta Medica, Amsterdam, p. 38.

Gardner, R. L. (1979), in *Placenta—A Neglected Experimental Animal* (Beaconsfield, P., and C. Villee, eds.) Pergamon Press, New York, p. 148.

Gibbons, J. M., M. Mitnick, and V. Chieffo (1975), *Am. J. Obstet. Gynecol.* **121**, 127.

Goldstein, D. J., C. E. Rogers, and H. Harris (1980), *Proc. Natl. Acad . Sci. USA* **77**, 2857.

Goldstein, D. J., and H. Harris (1979), *Nature* **280,** 602.

Goldstein, D. P. (1974) in *Controversy in Obstetric and Gynecology.* II. (Reid, D. R., and C. D. Christian, eds.) Saunders, Philadelphia, p. 219.

Goldstein, D. P. (1976), *Cancer* **38,** 453.

Gordon, Y. B., and T. Chard (1979), in *Placental Proteins* (Klopper, A., and T. Chard, eds.) Springer Verlag, Berlin p. 14.

Grudzinskas, J. G. Y. B. Gordon, D. Jeffrey, and T. Chard (1977), *Lancet* **1,** 333.

Haije, W. G., J. H. Meerwaldt, A. Talerman, T. J. Kuipers, L. Baggerman, A. H. Teeuw, W. B. van der Pompe, and J. van Driel (1979), *Int. J. Cancer* **24,** 288.

Hamilton, T. A., A. W. Tin, and H. H. Sussman (1979), *Exptl. Cell Res.* **122,** 31.

Hammond, C. B., L. G. Borchert, L. Tyrey, W. T. Creasman, and R. T. Parker (1973), *Am. J. Obstet. Gynecol.* **115,** 451.

Hershman, J. M., and W. R. Starnes (1971), *J. Clin. Endocrinol. Metab.* **32,** 52.

Hertz, R., J. L. Lewis, Jr., and M. B. Lipsett (1961), *Am. J. Obstet. Gyncol.* **82,** 831.

Higashino. K., M. Hashinotsume, K. Y. Yang, Y. Takahashi, and Y. Yamamura (1972), *Clin. Chim. Acta* **40,** 67.

Higashino, K., S. Kudo, and Y. Yamamura (1974), *Cancer Res.* **34,** 33 47.

Higashino, K., S. Kudo, R. Ohtani, Y. Yamamura, T. Honda and J. Sakurai (1975), *Ann. NY Acad. Sci.* **259,** 337.

Holmgren, P. Å., T. Stigbrand, and G. Beckman (1977), *Biochem. Genet.* **15,** 521.

Holmgren, P. Å., T. Stigbrand, M.-G. Damber, and B. von Schoultz (1979), *Scand. J. Immunol.* **54,** 5, 631.

Horne, C. H. W., C. M. Towler, R. G. P. Pugh-Humphreys, A. W. Thomson, and H. Bohn (1976a), *Experientia* **32,** 1197.

Horne, C. H. W., I. N. Reid, and G. D. Milne (1976b), *Lancet* **1,** 279/.

Horne, C. H. W., and R. D. Brenner (1980), in *Cancer Markers* (Sell, S., ed) Humana Press, Clifton, New Jersey, p. 225.

Inglis, N. R., S. Kirley, L. I. Stolbach, and W. H. Fishman (1973), *Cancer Res.* **33,** 1657.

Jacoby, B., and K. D. Bagshawe (1972), *Cancer Res.* **32,** 2413.

Josimovich, J. B. (1977), in *Endocrinology of Pregnancy,* 2nd ed (Fuchs , F., and A. Klopper eds.), Harper and Row, p. 191.

Kaminska, J., I. Calvert and S. W. Rosen (1979), *Clin. Chem.* **25,** 5 77.

Kaplan, G. N., R. D. Maffezzoli, and A. Chrambach (1972), *J. Clin. Endocrinol. Metab.* **43,** 370.

Kapeller-Adler, R. (1970), in *Amino Oxidases and Methods for Their Study,* Wiley-Interscience, New York.

Kourides, I. A., B. D. Weintraub, E. C. Ridgway and F. Maloof (1975). *J. Clin. Endocrinol. Metab.* **40,** 872.

Landesman, R., and B. B. Saxena (1976), *Fertil. Steril.* **27,** 367.

Lange, P. H., K. R. McIntire, T. A. Waldmann, T. R. Hakala and E. E. Fraley (1976), *New Engl. Med.* **295,** 257.

Lehmann, F.-G. (1975), *Clin. Chim. Acta* **65,** 257.

Lewis, J. L., Jr. (1976), *Cancer* **38,** 620.

Lin, C.-W., and S. D. Kirley (1976), in *Protides of the Biological Fluids* (H. Peters, ed.), Pergamon Press, New York p. 103.

Lin. C.-W., C. M. Chapman, R. A. Delellis, and S. D. Kirley (1978), *J. Histochem. Cytochem.* **26,** 1021.

Lin, C.-W., N. R. Inglis, A. H. Rule, R. N. Turksoy, C. M. Chapman, S. D. Kirley, and L. L. Stolbach (1979), *Cancer Res.* **39,** *4894.*

Lin, C.-W., S. D. Kirley, and M. S. Pierre, manuscript in preparation.

Lin, C.-W., and D. Angellis (1981), manuscript in preparation.

Lin, T.-M., and S. P. Halbert (1976), *Science* **193,** 1249.

Lin, T.-M., S. P. Halbert, W. N. Spellacy, and S. Gall (1976), *Am. J. Obstet. Gynaecol.* **124,** 382.

Maffezzoli, R. D., G. N. Kaplan, and A. Chrambach (1972), *J. Clin. Endocrinol. Metab.* **34,** 361.

Masure, H. R., W. L. Jaffe, M. A. Sickel, S. Birken, R. E. Canfield, and J. L. Vaitukaitis (1981), (Submitted to Endocrinology).

McComb, R. B., G. N. Bowers, and S. Posen (1979), *Alkaline Phosphatase ,* Plenum, New York.

McDonald, D. J., A. Belfield, C. J. Steele, D. S. Mack, and M. M. Shah (1979), *Clin. Chim. Acta* **94,** 41.

McKenna, M. J., T. A. Hamilton, and H. H. Sussman (1979), *Biochem. J.* **181,** 67.

McManus, L. M., M. A. Naughton, and A. Martinez-Hernandez (1976), *Cancer Res.* **36,** 3476.

Mendelsohn, G., J. C. Eggleston, W. R. Weisburger, D. S. Gann, and S. Baylin (1978), *Am. J. Pathol.* **92,** 35.

Midgley, A. R., Jr., I. F. Fong, and R. B. Jaffe (1967), *Nature* **213,** 733.

Millan, J. M., and T. Stigbrand (1982), *Clin. Chem.* (in press).

Morgan, F. J., S. Birken, and R. E. Canfield (1973), *Mol. Cell. Biochem.* **2,** 97.

Morgan, F. J., S. Birken, and R. E. Canfield (1975), *J. Biol. Chem.* **250,** 5247.

Nakayama, T., M. Yoshida, and M. Kitamura (1970), *Clin. Chim. Acta* **30,** 546.

Nathanson, L., and W. H. Fishman (1971), *Cancer* **27,** 1388.

Neufeld, E., and R. Chayen (1961), *Anal. Biochem.* **96,** 242.

Obiekwe, B., D. J. Pendlebury, Y. B. Gordon, J. G. Grudzinskas, T. Chard, and H. Bohn (1979), *Clin. Chim Acta* **95,** 509.

O'Brien, T. J., E. Engvall, J. B. Schlaert, and C. P. Morrow (1981), *Am. J. Obstet. Gyn.,* in press.

Okuyama, T., and Y. Kobayashi (1961), *Arch. Biochem. Biophys.* **95,** 242.

Opsahl, J. C., and C. N. H. Long (1951), *Yale J. Biol. Med.* **24,** 199.

Perlin, E., J. E. Engeler, Jr., M. Edson, D. Karp, K. R. McIntire, and T. A. Waldmann (1976), *Cancer* **37,** 215.

Petropoulos, E. A. (1973), *Acta Endocrin.* **73,** suppl. 176

Posen, S., F. C. Neale, and J. A. Club (1965), *Ann. Intern. Med.* **62,** 1234.

Prentice, L. G., and R. J. Ryan (1975), *J. Clin. Endocrinol. Metab.* **40,** 303.

Robson, E. B., and H. Harris (1965), *Nature* **207,** 1257.

Robson, E. B., and H. Harris (1967), *Ann. Hum Genet.* **30,** *219.*

Roscoe, H. G., and D. Kupfer (1972), *Anal. Biochem.* **47,** 418.

Rosen, S. W., and B. D. Weintraub (1974), *N. Engl. J. Med.* **290,** 1441.

Rosen, S. W., B. D. Weintraub, J. L. Vaitukaitis, H. H. Sussman, J. M. Hershman, and F. M. Muggia (1975), *Ann. Intern. Med.* **82,** 71.

Rosen, S. W., J. Kaminska, I. S. Calvert, and S. A. Aaronson (1979a), *Am. J. Obstet. Gynecol.* **134,** 734.

Rosen, S. W., N. Javadpour, I. Calvert, and J. Kaminska (1979b), *J. Natl. Cancer Inst.* **62,** 1439.

Ross, G. T., D. P. Goldstein, R. Hertz, M. B. Lipsett, and W. D. Odell (1965), *Am. J. Obstet. Gynecol.* **93,** 223.

Ross, G. T. (1973), in *Methods in Investigative and Diagnostic Endocrinology. Part III. Peptide Hormones* (Bearson, S. A., and R. S. Yalow, eds.), North-Holland, Amsterdam, p. 749.

Rutanen, E.-M., and M. Seppälä (1980), *J. Clin. Endocrin. Metab.* **50,** 57.

Schultz-Larsen, P., J. Lyngbye, J. G. Westergaard, and B. Teisner (1979), *Clin. Chim. Acta* **99,** 59.

Schultz-Larsen, P., J. Lyngbye, J. G. Westergaard, and B. Teisner (1979), *Clin. Chim. Acta* **99,** 59.

Searle, F., B. A. Leake, K. D. Bagshawe, and J. Dent (1978), *Lancet* **1,** 579.

Sedlacek, H. H., R. Rehkopf, and H. Bohn (1976), *Behring Inst. Mitt.* **59,** 81.

Seppälä, M., E.-M. Rutanen, M. Heikinheimo, H. Jalanko, and E. Engvall (1978), *Int. J. Cancer* **21,** 265.

Seppälä, M., T., Wahlström, and H. Bohn (1979), *Int. J. Cancer* **24,** 6.

Singer, R. M., and W. H. Fishman (1974), *J. Cell. Biol.* **60,** 777.

Singer, R. M., and W. H. Fishman (1976), in *Oncodevelopmental Gene Expression* (Fishman, W. H., and S. Sell eds.). Academic Press, New York p.177.

Singer, R. M., E. M. Leahy, and D. B. Harrrington (1979), in *Carcino-Embryonic Proteins.*, vol. II (F.-G. Lehmann, ed.), Elsevier North-Holland, p. 651.

Singh, I., K. Y. Isang, and W. S. Blakemore, (1978), *Cancer Res.* **38,**193.

Southren, A. L., Y. Kobayashi, P. Brenner, and A. B. Weingold (1965), *Appl. Physiol.* **20,** 1048.

Speeg, K. V., J. C. Azizkhan, and K. Stromberg (1977), *Exptl. Cell. Res.* **105,** 199.

Stolbach, L. L., N. Inglis, C. Lin, R. N. Turksoy, W. Fishman, D. Marchant, and A. Rule (1976), in *Oncodevelopmental Gene Expression* (Fishman, W. H., and S. Sell eds.), Academic Press, New York, p. 433.

Sussman, H. H., P. A. Small, Jr., and E. Cotlove (1968), *J. Biol. Chem.* **243,** 160.

Tatarinov, Y. S., and V. N. Masyukevich (1970), *Bull. Eksp. Biol. Med. USSR* **69,** 66.

Tatarinov, Y. S., N. V. Meshnankina, D. M. Nikulina, L. A. Novikova, B. O. Tolokonov, and D. M. Falaleeva (1974), *Int. J. Cancer* **14,** 548.

Tatarinov, Y. S., and A. V. Sokolov, (1977), *Int. J. Cancer* **19,** 161.

Tatarinov, Y. S., (1978), *Gynecol. Obstet. Invest.* **9,** 65.

Tatarinov, Y. S., (1979), in *Placental Proteins,* (Klopper, A., and T. Chard, eds.), Springer Verlag, Berlin, pp. 161-171.

Teisner, B., J. G. Westergaard, J. Folkersen, S. Husby, and S. E. Svehag (1978), *Am. J. Obst. Gynec.* **131**, 262.

Timperley, W. R., P. Turner, and S. Davies (1971), *J. Pathol.* **103**, 257.

Towler, C. M., C. H. W. Horne, V. Jandial, D. M. Campbell, and I. MacGillivray (1976), *Br. J. Obstet. Gynaecol.* **83**, 775.

Tuppy, H., and H. Nesvadba (1957), *Monatshilfe Chemie* **88**, 977.

Usategui-Gomez, M., F. M. Yeager, and A. Fernandez de Castro (1973), *Clin. Chim. Acta* **46**, 353.

Vaitukaitis, J. L., G. D. Braunstein, and G. T. Ross (1972), *Am. J. Obstet. Gynaecol.* **113**, 751.

Vaitukaitis, J. L. (1974), *J. Clin. Endocrinol. Metab.* **38**, 755.

Vaitukaitis, J. L., and E. R. Ebersole (1976), *J. Clin. Endocrinol. Metab.* **42**, 1048.

Vaitukaitis, J. L. (1977), in *Endocrinology of Pregnancy,* 2nd ed., (Fuchs, F., and A. Klopper, eds.), Harper and Row, New York, p. 63.

Wada, H. G., J. E. Shindelman, A. E. Orimeyer, and H. H. Sussman (1979), *Int. J. Cancer* **93**, 781.

Wahren, B., P. Å. Holmgren, and T. Stigbrand (1979), *Int. J. Cancer* **24**, 749.

Warnes, T. W., W. R. Timperley, P. Hine and G. Kay (1972), *Gut* **13**, 513.

Warnock, M. L., and R. Reisman (1969), *Clin. Chim. Acta* **24**, 5.

Weintraub, B. D., and S. W. Rosen (1971), *J. Clin. Endocrinol. Metab.* **32**, 94.

Weintraub, B. D., and S. W. Rosen (1973), *J. Clin. Invest.* **52**, 3135.

Westergaard, J. G., Ph. Sizaret, P. Hindersson, J. Folkersen, and B. Teisner (1981), *Acta Path. Microbiol. Scand.* (in press).

Wood, P. J., D. Cockett, and P. Mason (1978), *Clin. Chim. Acta* **90**, 87.

Würz, H. (1979), *Arch. Gynecol.* **227**, 1.

Yoshimoto, Y., A. R. Wolfsen, and W. D. Odell (1977), *Science* **197**, 575.

Yoshimoto, Y., A. R. Wolfsen, and W. D. Odell (1978), *Clin. Res.* **26**, 162A.

Zeller, E. A. (1963), in *The Enzymes,* vol. 8 (Boyer, P. D., H. Lardy, and K. Myrbäck, eds.), Academic Press, New York, p. 313.

13

Bladder and Renal Tumor Markers

Britta Wahren[1] and Peter Perlmann[2]

Radiumhemmet, Karolinska Hospital[1]
and [2]Department of Immunology, University of Stockholm,
Stockholm, Sweden

1. Introduction

The prognosis for bladder and renal cancer is often uncertain, although staging and histological or cytological grading do provide indications. It is therefore important to identify the patients who are going to develop invasive disease.

Malignant cells have several characteristics that serve to distinguish them from their normal counterparts. In this presentation, some recently established criteria are described, as well as tissue markers detectable by immunologic techniques. Serum and urinary markers that are potentially useful for monitoring patients with urothelial and renal tumors will be described. Such potential markers are tumor-associated enzymes, hormones, metabolites, and substances without other known functions. The present knowledge of immune reactivity to bladder or renal cancer cells in patients with these diseases is discussed.

2. Bladder Cancer

2.1. Morphological Markers
of Bladder Carcinoma Cells

Besides bladder carcinomas, for which several markers have been described (Irving, 1977; Lessing, 1978; Wahren, 1979) urothelial cell tumors include the more rare cancers of the renal pelvis, ureter, and urethra.

The diagnosis and monitoring of bladder cancer are based at present mostly on morphological criteria. Urothelial carcinoma cells display many changes when compared to the normal urothelium. Histopathological changes from normal are determined and graded according to conventional criteria (Sobin, 1978). Histopathologically, highly differentiated tumors have a near-normal growth pattern, a near-normal DNA pattern, cells and nuclei of slightly atypical size, little or no infiltration of surrounding tissue, and often a good prognosis when treated by surgery alone. Poorly differentiated or anaplastic tumors, on the contrary, have a considerable cell-size variation, DNA polymorphism, and often an infiltrative mode of growth.

Urothelial cells obtained by bladder washing can be graded in a similar way (Koss, 1968; Esposti and Zajicek, 1972; Koss et al., 1975). Since cystoscopy is usually performed frequently during followup of bladder cancer patients, repeated cytological analysis is a useful means of monitoring the patient and such cells are then easily available for other types of studies.

It is probable that some tumor cells obtained by bladder irrigation have a reduced adherence to surrounding tissue. Hence, the cytological sample may be more representative than histopathology of the population of cells with the greatest tendency to recur or metastasize. Cytology accordingly adds a new dimension to the diagnosis.

Microspectrophotometry and automated cytology of single cells are now being used for rapid identification of multiple parameters. This may be done on unstained native cell populations, after application of dyes with specific reactions, or with labeled immune sera. Computerization of data from tumor cell populations aid the description of growth patterns and of antigenic properties, and possibly also describe the aggressiveness of the tumor toward the host. DNA analysis shows the degree of ploidy of the tumor cells (Traganos et al., 1977) and has been used quite widely with bladder tumor cells or cells from bladder washings. The total DNA in large numbers of single cells has been analyzed, and showed aneuploidy to be an indication of malignancy (Tribukait and Esposti, 1978). Bladder cancers of grade 0–1 had 7% aneuploid cells, whereas grade 3 had 80%; noninvasive tumors were generally near-diploid.

Chromosomal defects also correlate with progression of the cancer (Lamb, 1967; Sandberg, 1977). Marker chromosomes are often found in bladder tumor cells and in many cases ring chromosomes are present. These findings are consistent with the aneuploidy that may be determined from total DNA measurements. Cytogenetic analyses show the existence of abnormal chromosomes in 60% of the patients. The prognosis of these patients is poor (Sandberg, 1977; Falor and Ward, 1978). Patients with no detectable abnormalities had a much better prognosis.

Electron microscopy has revealed alterations of surface membranes, cellular junctions, and microvilli in papillary tumors (Koss, 1977). Promising criteria for the evaluation of precancerous changes are chromatin texture, staining density of the nucleus, and optical density of the whole cell. Ultrastructural changes have been observed in chemical bladder carcinogenesis of rats. Pleomorphic villi may be related to invasiveness and it is conceivable that such investigation will lead to the diagnosis of precancerous lesions in humans (Jacobs et al., 1977).

Proliferation of a tumor is the function of relatively few progenitor cells. Cells from bladder tumors usually do not grow well in vitro, and cell analysis has therefore been limited. They can now be grown in soft agar, the so-called clonogenic assay (Buich et al., 1979). The progenitor cells of the tumor grow out to colonies that can be analyzed. The plating efficiency is not very high (<1%). However, the resulting colonies seem to represent the karyotype of the tumor quite well, while no normal cells grew in the assay.

2.2. Potential Tumor Markers in Bladder Cancer Tissue, Urine, and Serum

Several tumor markers have been described that occur in bladder carcinoma tissue or in the serum or urine of patients with this disease. They have been evaluated with a view to aiding the clinical staging and histological grading procedures for assessing the prognosis and for monitoring the individual patient.

2.2.1. Tumor Cell and Tissue Properties

2.2.1.1. Urothelial Organ Antigen. Intracellular urothelial-specific antigen(s) have been described (Nathrath et al., 1979) and antisera to these antigens have been prepared in rabbits. After absorption with a number of normal tissues, these antisera seemed to be specific for cells of urothelial origin. When bladder carcinoma cells were studied, they too appeared to possess the urothelial organ antigen, but to a lesser degree than normal urothelium. The chemical composition has not yet been analyzed, but the demonstration of such antigens may enable one to establish the origin of tumor cells and perhaps study their differentiation pattern.

2.2.1.2. Ek-2. A new series of surface antigenic determinants, Ek-1 to Ek-11, has been described recently (Espmark, 1978). The antigens do not belong to any of the known normal HLA transplantation antigens. One of the antigens, Ek-2, is common to several bladder carcinoma cell lines. It has now been shown on all of nine bladder carcinoma lines studied and on less than 10% of other tumor lines. It is not known whether the patients from whom the cell lines derive had this antigen in other somatic cells. The antigen is defined by selected sera from multiparous women. Only one serum out of 3000 tested contained antibodies to Ek-2. Sera of bladder cancer patients do not contain this antibody.

2.2.1.3. Carcinoembryonic Antigen. Carcinoembryonic antigen (CEA) occurs predominantly in adenocarcinomas of colon and rectum and in fetal gut tissue. It has been demonstrated to occur also in urothelial carcinoma tissue, but to a lesser extent (Wahren et al., 1977; Zimmerman and Hammarström, 1978; Zimmerman, 1979). The CEA from urothelial carcinoma seems to be identical to that of colon carcinomas.

Quantitative determination of the cellular CEA content is a new way to characterize the cancer cell population (Wahren et al., 1977). Urothelial tumor cells obtained by bladder washings were analyzed by immunofluorescence for the content of cellular CEA. Among the better differentiated cell populations, 61% had CEA positive cells in their smears. In poorly differentiated or anaplastic cell populations, CEA-containing cells were seen in only 24%. Using the immunoperoxidase technique, biopsies from bladder carcinomas were shown to contain CEA (Goldenberg and Wahren, 1978). Since no CEA is found in the normal urothelium, the raised urinary CEA content in bladder carcinoma probably derives from the bladder cancer cells (see below).

2.2.1.4. Blood Group Antigens. Urothelial cells possess the isoantigens A, B, and H, which are identical to the blood group antigens. One method for detecting those antigens is the red cell adherence assay, where the tissue is subjected to isoantibody. The binding of antibody is then demonstrated by adherence of red cells of the different blood groups. In 124 cases of bladder carcinomas, Davidsohn et al. (1973) found a correlation between histologic grade and adherence results. In dedifferentiated urothelial cells, the blood group isoantigens were usually lost.

A prognostic value has recently been ascribed to the blood group typing of the cancer cells (DeCenzo et al., 1974; Weinstein, 1976; Bergman and Javadpour, 1977; Lange et al., 1978; Alroy et al., 1978; Richie et al., 1980). Of 21 patients without detectable isoantigens on their tumor cells, 16 had invasive disease, while of 16 with isoantigens, only 2 developed invasive disease (Lange et al., 1978). All patients with early onset of invasive disease were isoantigen negative at the initial biopsy. In carcinoma *in situ,* a deletion of isoantigens could be demonstrated in most cases (Weinstein, 1976). Also with urothelial cancer cells obtained by bladder washing, blood group isoantigens could be determined, and deletion associated with poor differentiation of the cells (Sadoughi et al., 1980). The blood group antigens seem to be lost early during the tumor's natural history.

After radiotherapy, several invasive carcinoma tissues were found to be isoantigen positive (Alroy et al., 1978) suggesting that the treatment might have induced a differentiation of the cells.

2.2.2. Markers in Serum and/or Urine

2.2.2.1. Enzymes. Enzyme determinations in serum or urine are useful when isoenzymes specific for a certain organ exist. Organ-related isoenzymes have been described with many tumors, but not in bladder carcinoma. In the case of metastatic urothelial tumors, bone or liver alkaline phosphatase (ALP) may be raised in serum with skeletal metastasis and liver metastasis. Other types of serum enzyme determinations, such as γ-glutamyltransferase and lactic dehydrogenase (LDH), are also often sensitive means of detecting spread to the liver.

There are a number of enzymes that are raised in the urine of patients with bladder cancer as compared to healthy persons (Lessing, 1978). Such enzymes are urinary LDH and ALP (Schmidt, 1966). Lysozyme, cleaving glucosidic linkages in mucopolysaccahrides, is normally high in kidney and some body secretions apart from urine. Kovanyi and Letnansky (1971) showed it to be elevated in 28 out of 29 patients with bladder carcinomas, but not in 21 of 28 healthy persons or patients with benign tumors. However, patients with severe bacterial infections have raised lysozyme levels owing to the presence of leukocytes, which limits the usefulness of lysozyme demonstration. β-Glucuronidase has been shown to be elevated in a high percentage of urines from patients with bladder cancer (Abdel-Tawab et al., 1966a; Senda, 1971). Raised creatinine phosphokinase (Block et al., 1974) has also been demonstrated with malignant disease. None of the above enzymes are specific for tumor disease and their practical value has not yet been studied thoroughly.

2.2.2.2. Fetal Antigens. Several authors (Hall et al., 1972; Hall et al., 1973; Guinan et al., 1975; Wahren et al., 1975; Fraser et al., 1975) have found that urinary CEA is present in elevated amounts in the urine of patients with urothelial carcinoma. The level of urinary CEA increases with increasing size of the bladder tumor. CEA levels in the urine have thus shown a relationship to clinical stage, although not comparable to that obtained with gastrointestinal tumors (Gold et al., 1973). A correlation between rising urinary CEA and local recurrence has also been reported (Zimmerman et al., 1980). In patients who respond to treatment, urinary CEA values normalize. For screening healthy persons, no obvious benefits were seen in measuring urinary CEA (Turner et al., 1976).

A statistical evaluation of 294 patients with bladder cancer in various stages has shown that urinary CEA levels were significantly lower with small stage T1–T2 tumors than the larger T3–T4 tumors (Zimmerman et al., 1980). The urinary CEA levels decreased with successful radiotherapy. A high pretreatment CEA value was indicative of early recurrence, but this information was limited to the more advanced tumors.

In chronic urinary infections, substances occur that have CEA immunoreactivity. Provided that the urine is extracted with perchloric acid (to avoid inhibitory substances) and that heavy bacterial infections can be excluded, sequential urinary CEA was found to be a reliable method for monitoring patients with bladder carcinoma (Zimmerman et al., 1980).

Serum CEA levels are increased in around 50% of patients with bladder cancer in stages T3 and T4, but not to very high levels. A further increase is seen with metastasizing bladder tumors (Wahren et al., 1975; Ørjasaeter et al., 1978).

The clinical value of CEA determinations in urine and serum of patients with bladder cancer is controversial in early diagnosis, but has a place in followup during and after primary treatment. It adds information to the clinical T-classification and predicts early recurrence.

2.2.2.3. Metabolites.   There is evidence of a role for some metabolites in carcinogenesis of the bladder (Yoshida et al., 1970). Metabolites of the amino acid trytophan have been suspected of causing urinary bladder cancer in man. The small amounts of tryptophan that are present in normal human urine are elevated in patients with bladder cancer; furthermore, loading tests increase the metabolites in patients whose level is already high (Benassi et al., 1963). Yoshida et al. (1970) have followed patients with low stage bladder cancer for 5 years after resection. Recurrences occurred in all patients whose initial values were high, but in only half of those in whom they were not raised. The elevated level of metabolites in urine has been attributed to abnormalities in tryptophan metabolism, but other authors (Teulings et al., 1978) have found that an elevation may also reflect impaired renal function, such as is caused by an obstructed ureter. Tryptophan metabolite determinations may still be of value for tracing recurrences, but the etiological significance of tryptophan and its metabolites is thus debatable.

Nicotine, among other substances, is thought to be related to the development of bladder cancer. Analysis of the major metabolites of nicotine in the urine has shown that the ratio of cotinine to nicotine-1-*N*-oxide is significantly higher in patients with bladder cancer than in a control group (Gorrod et al., 1974). The variations between individuals were large, and the relation to grade or stage of the disease was not analyzed. The cause for the increased ratio of these metabolites in bladder cancer patients is as yet unknown, but may be a result of a changed metabolism in the tumor-affected bladder.

Tissue polypeptide antigen (TPA) is present in several human tissues. TPA serum and urinary levels are raised in patients with many types of malignancies, but usually not in healthy persons (Björklund, 1980). In patients with bladder cancer, the urinary TPA may be raised in around 40% of the patients, but the levels vary considerably among individuals.

Polyamines and nucleosides are byproducts of increased cellular metabolism. Urinary levels are raised in a number of malignancies. Polyamines have high levels in the urine and serum of cancer patients, and these levels may reflect the efficacy of treatment (Cohen, 1977).

2.2.2.4. Microbial Agents. Bilharzia is thought to be an etiological agent of squamous cell carcinomas of the bladder, which are frequent in Africa and the Middle East. The disease is more than 75% associated with previous infestation with *Schistosoma haematobium*, usually commencing one to several years before clinical detection of a tumor. The infection may give rise to an abnormal tryptophan metabolism (Abdel-Tawab et al., 1966b). Increased urinary β-glucuronidase is also found in the patient with bilharzia and bladder cancer (Abdel-Tawab et al., 1966a). Abnormal urinary contents of tryptophan metabolites and the enzyme may thus be induced by bilharzia, and perhaps precede the development of bladder cancer. No investigations have yet dealt with the possibility that bilharzial antigens may remain in bladder cells after transformation.

Virus infections of the urinary tract are known to be common in patients with immunological impairment, which is not uncommon in bladder cancer (Olsson et al., 1972). Virus particles similar to oncornavirus have been described in the cytoplasm of transitional cell carcinomas of the human renal pelvis, ureter, and bladder (Fraley et al., 1974). Other workers have not isolated such virus.

Cytomegalovirus is another virus of interest in the study of bladder cancer. It is ubiquitous in the human population and is often found in the urine. Some herpesviruses, including cytomegalovirus, can transform cells in tissue culture (Geder et al., 1976). The common feature of herpesviruses and oncornaviruses is their capacity for latency within host cells. It is known that chemical or physical carcinogens can induce the expression of RNA viruses of endogenous or exogenous origin, and this expression may result in cell transformation. Since chemical carcinogens have a definite role in the etiology of bladder cancers, one might speculate that chemicals and ubiquitous viruses or parasites cooperate to initiate and promote bladder tumors.

2.3. Disease-Associated Immune Response in Bladder Cancer

It is well-established that tumors in experimental animal systems frequently are immunogenic and may give rise to tumor-directed immune responses. The specificity of the tumor markers is defined by the humoral or cell-mediated immune response of the host. Hence, such tumors may be diagnosed and their development monitored by analyzing the tumor-specific or tumor-associated immune response of the tumor-bearing animal.

Despite extensive studies during the past decade, the extent of immunogenicity for the host of spontaneously arising malignancies in the human remains a controversial issue (Baldwin and Embleton, 1977). Antibodies reacting with bladder tumor cells in tissue culture have been described (Elliott et al., 1974; Hakala et al., 1974b), but the specificity of these reactions is unresolved. Some preliminary evidence for a possible cellular immunity to bladder carcinoma-associated antigens has been obtained by skin testing (Hollinshead et al., 1978) or by applying the leukocyte adherence inhibition assay (Guinan et al., 1978). More experiments are needed to establish the tumor-associated specificity of these reactions. The many problems involved in assessing and evaluating tumor-directed immune responses in humans are well-illustrated by in vitro studies of cell-mediated cytotoxicity in transitional cell carcinoma of the urinary bladder, one of the neoplastic diseases that has been studied most extensively in this respect. In the following, relevant findings made in this system will be discussed in some detail.

2.3.1. Determination of Cell-Mediated Reactions by Microcytotoxicity

In their initial studies, Bubenik et al. (1970a,b) used a microcytotoxicity assay to investigate the effect of blood leukocytes from patients with bladder cancer on the survival of tumor cells kept in short-term culture in vitro. Leukocytes from patients were found to be cytotoxic to target cells derived from either autologous or allogeneic bladder carcinomas. Leukocytes from normal donors or from patients with unrelated tumors appeared to be less cytotoxic to these target cells. Furthermore, control targets derived from unrelated tumors or normal fibroblasts were not lysed to a comparable degree. The results suggested the existence of a tumor-type specific immune response. These findings were corroborated and extended by O'Toole et al. (1972a,b), who used purified blood lymphocytes as cytotoxic effector cells. They established tumor cell strains from bladder carcinomas or other origins as the principal source of target cells. These authors also noted that the tumor-directed lymphocyte cytotoxicity was most pronounced in untreated patients with localized tumors. In patients with larger tumors, the reactivity was less frequent. Treatment with local radiotherapy greatly depressed existing cytotoxicity. This depression lasted as long as therapy was given, but a temporary cytotoxicity reappeared shortly thereafter. The exception occurred in some patients for whom residual tumors or distant metastases were detected within a few months after irradiation had been discontinued. When studied several years after radiotherapy, the existence of cytotoxic lymphocytes in a patient usually reflected presence of a tumor. In patients treated with surgery, successful removal of the tumor appeared to abolish lymphocyte cytotoxicity.

In the years following these initial studies, the usefulness of lymphocyte cytotoxicity for monitoring cancer patients has been debated extensively (Baldwin, 1975; Herberman and Oldham, 1975). Apart from technical considerations, the controversies arose mainly from the finding that
lymphocytes from both patients and healthy donors frequently lyse a large
variety of tumor cells without any obvious relationship to disease
(Herberman and Holden, 1978; Pross and Baines, 1977). These controversies also concerned bladder carcinomas (Bean et al., 1975). Thus, although several investigators confirmed that blood lymphocytes from patients with bladder cancer as a group did exhibit an elevated cytotoxicity to
bladder tumor cells compared with that of the lymphocytes from various
control groups (Bean et al., 1974; Bloom et al., 1974; Bloom and Seeger,
1976; Hakala et al., 1974a; Vilien and Wolf, 1978), they also reported that
lymphocytes from many control donors were cytotoxic to such cells. Similarly, lymphocytes from patients with bladder carcinoma were often found
to be cytotoxic to unrelated target cells. Moreover, in the studies of Bloom
et al., (1974), the tumor-associated specificity of the reactions became
questionable when it was found that lymphocytes from some patients with
nonmalignant diseases of the genitourinary tract were as cytotoxic to
urothelial tumor cells as those from patients with bladder cancer. Other
groups, using similar methods, were unable to detect any tumor-related
cytotoxicity in patients with bladder cancer (Bean et al., 1975; Bolhuis,
1977; Catalona et al., 1977; Moore and Robinson, 1977). These negative
results appear to have various explanations, such as increased susceptibility to lysis of some tumor cells (Moore and Robinson, 1977), reduced
cytotoxic activity of the patient's lymphocytes, or, conversely, a generally
elevated cytotoxicity of control lymphocytes.

In view of the many variables affecting the microcytotoxicity assay
(Bean et al., 1976), such discordant results are not surprising. It is clear
that demonstration of disease-related cellular cytotoxicity in cancer patients requires careful selection and matching of lymphocyte donors, titration of the effector cells, and the use of target cells that are equally susceptible to cell-mediated lysis (Bean et al., 1976). By cautiously scrutinizing
target cell selection and effector cell titration, Vilien et al. (1980a,b) were
recently able to confirm and extend several of the earlier observations by
O'Toole et al. (1972a,b) of a disease-related lymphocyte cytotoxicity in
bladder cancer. Among other findings, these authors reported that lymphocytes from patients with non-invasive tumors of grades 2 and 3 exhibit a
more pronounced cytotoxicity than those from patients with invasive tumors of the same grades. Followup studies of individual patients treated
with radiotherapy or surgery indicated a positive correlation between the
presence of tumor and lymphocyte cytotoxicity. Prospective followup
studies also revealed a significantly lower survival rate for patients with
low-grade specific cytotoxicity than for those whose lymphocytes displayed a high-grade specific cytotoxicity.

2.3.2. Determination of Cell-Mediated
Reactions by Isotope Release

All results referred to in the foregoing were obtained with the microcytotoxicity assay, which registers survival of target cells after prolonged in
vitro incubation (usually 36–48 h) of lymphocytes and tumor cells. Some
of the difficulties inherent in this assay are avoided by measuring release of
isotopic markers, usually ^{51}Cr, from labelled tumor cells exposed to
lymphocytes in vitro (Perlmann and Cerottini, 1979). This assay measures
target cell lysis more directly than the microcytotoxicity, requires shorter
incubation periods, and therefore permits more accurate assessment of
both intensity and specificity of lymphocyte induced tumor cell destruction. Troye et al. (1977a, 1980a) used this assay with lymphocytes from
several matched control groups and a panel of target cells of different origins. They fully supported earlier evidence of a disease-related lymphocyte cytotoxicity in bladder cancer patients. Thus, lymphocytes from the
patients, but not from the controls, displayed a significantly elevated mean
cytotoxicity to bladder tumor cells compared to targets from normal
urothelium or from unrelated tumors. Moreover, the cytotoxicity to bladder tumor cells of the patients' lymphocytes was, on average, significantly
higher than that of the control donors, including a matched group of patients with carcinoma of the prostate. The disease-related specificity of this
cytotoxicity was most pronounced for patients not treated for their disease
prior to testing. Analysis of complete cytotoxicity profiles indicated that
lymphocyte cytotoxicity in both patients with bladder cancer and controls
reflected multifactorial immune responses to a variety of antigens, shared
to different degrees by different target cells. In patients with bladder cancer there occurs, in addition, a superimposed cytotoxicity that is related to
their disease and probably reflects reactions against one or several tumor-
associated antigens. It remains to be established whether these antigens are
unique for bladder tumors or represent tissue specific molecules that are
well expressed on the surface of the tumor cells, but not on normal adult
urothelium.

2.3.3. Mechanisms of Cell-Mediated
Cytotoxicity in Bladder Carcinoma

Recent findings indicate that natural cell-mediated cytotoxicity in vitro often does not reflect immune recognition of target cell antigens (Kiessling
and Haller, 1978; Herberman and Holden, 1978). Natural cell-mediated
cytotoxicity in vitro is a heterogeneous phenomenon (Perlmann and
Cerottini, 1979). Analysis of the mechanisms involved in bladder cancer
has shown that a very significant fraction of the activity reflects an antibody dependent cellular cytotoxicity (ADCC) (Troye et al., 1977b,
1980b). In other words, in the majority of the cases, lymphocyte cytotoxicity of both patients with bladder cancer and controls is primarily (but not

exclusively) the expression of antigen recognition by either natural or disease-related antibodies, produced by the lymphocyte donors. Antibodies inducing ADCC by normal donors' lymphocytes to bladder tumor cells in tissue culture have also been found in the sera of some patients (Hakala et al., 1975; Troye et al., 1980c). However, the tumor-associated specificity of these serum antibodies remains to be established.

In the studies discussed above, the target cells used were mostly from established cell lines obtained from patients other than the lymphocyte donors. Available evidence indicates that cytotoxicity in these instances was not due to HLA-antigens. Also when tumor targets and lymphocytes were tested in autologous combinations, an elevated cytotoxicity was seen in a few cases (Troye et al., 1980b). These reactions were not correlated to those found when the lymphocytes from the same donors were tested with allogeneic bladder tumor targets. Moreover, the autologous reactions were not antibody-dependent and were displayed by a different type of lymphocyte. It remains to be established whether these autologous reactions reflected recognition of some tumor-specific antigens or an HLA-restricted activity of cytotoxic T lymphocytes.

In conclusion, although it has been shown that a bladder tumor-related lymphocyte cytotoxicity does exist and varies with the course of the disease and with treatment, the variable and sometimes high background of disease-unrelated reactions in many cases severely hampers the clinical use of these assays for monitoring individual patients. The demonstration that disease-related cytotoxicity in most patients appears to reflect humoral immune responses is of considerable practical importance, since it greatly facilitates further immunochemical elucidation of the molecular bases of these reactions (Schneider et al., 1980a,b). Characterization of the antigens involved will make it possible to develop more specific assays for monitoring individual patients with carcinoma of the bladder.

2.3.4. Nontumor-Specific Immunoglobulins in Bladder Carcinoma Patients

An increased incidence of organ antibodies has been described in patients with bladder cancer (Kurki et al., 1977), similar to the findings in other forms of tumors and in proper autoimmune disease. Patients with bladder carcinoma had antireticulin antibodies in 30%, smooth muscle antibody in 36%, and other types of autoantibodies in 8–24%. The size of the primary tumor did not seem to influence the antibody level; neither did removal of the tumor by operation. Since the same pattern of antitissue antibodies also occurs in patients with chronic renal inflammation, it was considered that inflammatory changes in the tumor might be the cause of antibody development. The presence of autoantibodies in patients with bladder cancer has to be taken into consideration also when assaying for tumor specific antibodies.

Patients with malignant tumors often have elevated urinary proteins of several kinds, although serum concentrations are normal. The urine seems to contain higher concentrations of immunoglobulins than in other urological diseases. In a study of bladder cancer patients, Johansson et al. (1971) reported elevated urinary IgM. The elevation was seen in 80% of patients with more malignant tumors compared with only 20% with less malignant tumors (Johansson et al., 1971; Johansson and Kistner, 1974). A local IgM synthesis may take place in patients with active bladder cancer. Urinary IgG elevations have also been described with bladder cancer (O'Brien et al., 1979). The specificity of these immunoglobulins is not known and Ig levels vary greatly between patients. No interpretation of this phenomenon can therefore be attempted at present.

3. Renal Cancer

A primary diagnosis of renal tumor is usually made with intravenous pyelography. The preoperative thin needle biopsy and an evaluation of the malignancy grading may help in selecting therapy. Exfoliated tumor cells in the urine are found only with tumors of the renal pelvis. Criteria similar to those for bladder carcinoma, such as variations in size of cells and nuclei, are evaluated. Cytology thus provides a non-invasive technique for preoperative analysis of renal cancer (von Schreeb et al., 1967).

3.1. Potential Tumor Markers in Renal Cancer

3.1.1. Hormones

Relatively few serum or urinary markers have been explored for renal cancer. Renal tumors may have ectopic hormone production. Ectopic adrenocorticotrophic hormone (ACTH) secretion, although most common with lung tumors, has also been noted in renal carcinomas (Liddle et al., 1969). It is important to differentiate the ectopic Cushing's syndrome that may occur with these tumors from that induced by primary adrenocortical tumors. Parathyroid hormone production by renal cell tumors may explain the finding of hypercalcemia even in the absence of bone metastases (Goldberg et al., 1964; Goodall, 1969). Other rare displaced hormones of kidney tumors are enteroglucagon, which gives malabsorption, and prolactin, giving galactorrhoea. Rarer syndromes have been described by Ratcliffe et al. (1976).

3.1.2. Erythropoietin

Erythropoietin is normally found in the kidney, and renal tumors may cause an abnormally high secretion (Thorling, 1972). Erythropoietin stimulates the maturation of red blood cells and a polycythemia may develop. Resection of the tumor leads to reduction or disappearance of the polycythemia. Only about 3% of renal tumors produce an excess of erythropoietin, while an elevated sedimentation rate is found in many more cases. The reason for this has been sought in serum protein abnormalities of diverse kinds, such as raised haptoglobin or globulins.

3.1.3. Mucopolysaccharide

The morphology of nephroblastoma is reminiscent of the developing embryonic kidney. An interesting substance from Wilms' renal tumor of childhood is a mucopolysaccharide that is also present in the blood and urine. It does not occur in the normal adult or fetal kidney, but is immunologically similar to calf fetuin (Wise et al., 1975). The clinical usefulness of this antigen has not yet been explored.

3.2. Immune Responses in Patients with Renal Cancer

Little evidence of renal tumor antigens has been presented (Stjernswärd et al., 1970; Bubenik et al., 1971; Diehl et al., 1971). Using the mixed lymphocyte-target interaction test, lymphocyte reactivity to renal carcinoma cells was described. The tumor cells significantly stimulated the patient's own lymphocytes in some cases, while normal renal tissue did not induce the same reaction. These results seen to be confirmed by studies demonstrating leukocyte inhibition by renal tumor extracts (Kjaer and Christensen, 1977; Schwarze et al., 1979). Cell-mediated reactivity to autologous tumor cells has also been described with Wilms' tumor (Hellström et al., 1968; Kumar et al., 1972). Antibodies with membrane reactivity or cooperating in cell-mediated killing have been described in a few children with this tumor (Kumar et al., 1977).

Immune complexes are deposited in the kidney in autoimmune and other diseases (Wilson, 1976). Presumably it is not only antibodies reacting with a conceivable renal tumor cell antigen that can be deposited there, but also circulating immune complexes derived from other antigen–antibody reactions (Robins and Baldwin, 1977). Antigen–antibody complexes can be found in a linear pattern along the glomerular basement membrane, indicating an immune reaction to this membrane as found in glomerulonephritis. Another pattern is irregular clumps in glomeruli and the mesangium, indicating trapping of circulating complexes. Antigenic substances that have been found in such deposits in connection with tumors are: CEA in neoplastic disease, EBV in Burkitt's lymphoma, oncornavirus-related antigen in leukemia.

Antitissue antibodies have been demonstrated in patients with renal disease (Kurki et al., 1977). Both antinuclear antibodies, and antibodies to smooth muscle, mitochondria and other antigens were detected in such patients. High frequencies of antibodies and a similar distribution of the various types were noted in patients with renal carcinomas and in those with chronic renal inflammation. Perhaps their appearance owes therefore to inflammatory reactions rather than the malignancy. Such antibodies generally do not change in titer after surgical treatment.

References

Abdel-Tawab, G. A., S. M. El-Zoghby, Y. M. Abdel-Samie, A. Zaki, and A. Sadd (1966a), *Int. J. Cancer* **1**, 383.

Abdel-Tawab, G. A., F. S. Kelada, and N. L. Kelada (1966b), *Int. J. Cancer* **1**, 377.

Alroy, J., K. Teramura, A, Miller, B. Pauli, J. Gottesman, M. Flanagan, I. Davidsohn, and R. Weinstein (1978), *Cancer* **41**, 1739.

Baldwin, R. W. (1975), *J. Natl. Cancer Inst.* **55**, 745.

Baldwin, R. W., and M. J. Embleton (1977), *Int. Rev. Exptl. Pathol.* **17**, 49.

Bean, M., and B. Bloom, R. Herberman, L. Old, H. Oettgen, G. Klein, and W. Terry (1975), *Cancer Res.* **35**, 2902.

Bean, M., B. R. Bloom, J. C. Cerottini, J. R. David, R. B. Herberman, H. S. Lawrence, I. C. M. MacLennan, P. Perlmann, and O. Stutman (1976), in B. R. Bloom and J. R. David eds., *In Vitro Methods in Cell-Mediated and Tumor Immunity*, Academic Press, New York, p. 27.

Bean, M., H. Pees, J. E., Fogh, H. Brabstald, and H. F. Oettgen (1974), *Int. J. Cancer* **14**, 186.

Benassi, C. A., B. Perissinoto, and G. Allegre (1963), *Clin. Chim. Acta* **8**, 822.

Bergman, S., and N. Javadpour (1977), *J. Urol.* **119**, 49.

Björklund, B. (1980), *Tumor Diagnostik* **1**, 9.

Block, N. L., J. Jaksy, and A. Tessler (1974), *Urology* **4**, 174.

Bloom, E. T., R. C. Ossario, and S. A. Brosman (1974), *Int. J. Cancer* **14**, 326.

Bloom, E. T., and R. C. Seeger (1976), *Cancer Res.* **36**, 1361.

Bolhuis, R. L. H. (1977), *Cancer Immunol. Immunother.* **2**, 245.

Bubenik, J., J. Jakoubková, P. Krákova, M. Baresová, P. Helbich, B. Viklichy, and V. Malasková (1971), *Int. J. Cancer* **8**, 503.

Bubenik, J., P. Perlmann, K. Helmstein, and G. Moberger (1970a), *Int. J. Cancer* **5**, 39.

Bubenik, J., P. Perlmann, K. Helmstein, and G. Moberger (1970b), *Int. J. Cancer* **5**, 310.

Buich, R. N., T. H. Stanisic, S. E. Fry, S. E. Salmon, J. M. Trent, and P. Krasovich (1979), *Cancer Res.* **39**, 5051.

Catalona, J. W., R. K. Oldham, R. B. Herberman, J. Y. Djeu, and G. B. Cannon (1977), *J. Urol.* **118**, 254.

Cohen, S. (1977), *Cancer Res.* **37**, 939.

Constanza, M., V. Pinn, R. Schwartz, and L. Nathanson (1973), *New Engl. J. Med.* **289**, 520.

Davidsohn, I., R. Stejskal, and P. Lill (1973), *Lab. Invest.* **28**, 382.

DeCenzo, J. M., P. Howard, and C. E. Irish (1974), *J. Urol.* **114**, 874.

Diehl, V., B. Jereb, J. Stjernswärd, C. O'Toole, and L. Åhström (1971), *Int. J. Cancer* **7**, 277.

Elliott, A. Y., P. C. Cleveland, J. Cervenka, A. E. Castro, N. Stein, T. R. Hakala, and E. E. Fraley (1974), *J. Natl. Cancer Inst.* **53**, 1341.

Espmark, Å. (1978), *Tissue Antigens* **11**, 287.

Esposti, P. L., and J. Zajicek (1972), *Acta Cytol.* **16**, 529.

Falor, W. H., and R. M. Ward (1978), *J. Urol.* **119**, 44.

Fraley, E. E., A. Y. Elliott, A. E. Castro, P. Cleveland, T. Hakala, and N. Stein (1974), *J. Urol.* **111**, 378.

Fraser, R. A., M. J. Ravry, J. W. Segura, and V. L. W. Go (1975), *J. Urol.* **114**, 226.

Geder, L., R. Lausch, F. J. O'Neill, and F. Rapp (1976), *Science* **192**, 1134.

Gold, P., T. Wilson, R. Romero, J. Shuster, and S. O. Freedman (1973), *Dis. Colon Rect.* **16**, 358.

Goldberg, M. F., A. H. Tashjian, Jr., S. E. Order, and G. J. Dammin (1964), *Am. J. Med.* **36**, 805.

Goldenberg, D., and B. Wahren (1978), *Urol. Res.* **6**, 211.

Goodall, C. M. (1969), *Int. J. Cancer* **4**, 1.

Gorrod, J. W., P. Jenner, G. R. Keysell, and B. R. Mikhael (1974), *J. Natl. Cancer Inst.* **52**, 1421.

Guinan, P., A. Dubin, I. Bush, H. Alsheik, and R. J. Ablin (1975), *Oncology* **32**, 158.

Guinan, P., C. Mickiel, M. Flanagan, R. Bhatti, D. Pessis, and R. Ablin (1978), *J. Urol.* **119**, 747.

Hakala, T. R., A. E. Castro, A. Y. Elliott, and E. E. Fraley (1974a), *J. Urol.* **111**, 382.

Hakala, T. R., P. H. Lange, A. Castro, A. Elliott, and E. E. Fraley (1974b), *Cancer* **34**, 1929.

Hakala, T. R., P. H. Lange, A. E. Castro, A. Y. Elliott, and E. E. Fraley (1975), *J. Urol.* **113**, 663.

Hall, R., D. Laurence, D. Darcy, U. Stevens, R. James, S. Roberts, and A. M. Neville (1972), *Brit. Med. J.* **3**, 609.

Hall, R., D. Laurence, A. M. Neville, and D. M. Wallace (1973), *Brit. J. Urol.* **45**, 88.

Hellström, I., K. Hellström, G. E. Pierce, and J. P. S. Yang (1968), *Nature* **220**, 1352.

Herberman, R. B., and H. F. Holden (1978), *Adv. Cancer Res.* **27**, 305.

Herberman, R. B., and R. K. Oldham (1975), *J. Natl. Cancer Inst.* **55**, 749.

Hollinshead, A., H. Miller, K. Tanner, O. Lee, and J. Klausia (1978), *Cancer Immunol. Immunother.* **5**, 93.

Irving, C. C. (1977), *Cancer Res.* **37**, 2872.

Jacobs, J. B., S. M. Cohen, M. Arai, and G. H. Friedell (1977), *Acta Cytol.* **21**, 3.

Johansson, B., and S. Kistner (1974), *Scand. J. Urol. Nephrol.* **9**, 52.

Johansson, B., S. Kistner, and R. Norberg (1971), *Scand. J. Urol.* **5**, 229.

Kiessling, R., and O. Haller (1978), *Contemp. Top. Immunobiol.* **8**, 171.

Kjaer, M., and N. Christensen (1977), *Cancer Immunol. Immunother.* **2**, 41.

Koss, L. G. (1968), *Diagnostic Cytology and Its Histopathologic Basis*, Lippincott, Philadelphia.

Koss, L. G. (1977), *Cancer Res.* **37**, 2824.

Koss, L. G., P. H. Bartels, M. Bibbo, S. Z. Freed, J. Taylor, and G. L. Wied (1975), *Acta Cytol.* **19**, 378.

Kovanyi, G., and K. Letnansky (1971), *Eur. J. Cancer* **7**, 25.

Kumar, S., G. Taylor, J. K. Steward, M. A. Waghe, and A. Pearson (1972), *Int. J. Cancer* **10**, 36.

Kumar, S., M. Waghe, and G. Taylor (1977), *Int. J. Cancer* **19**, 351.

Kurki, P., E. Linder, A. Miettinen, O. Althan, A. Heikkinen, and A. Pasternak (1977), *Int. J. Cancer* **19**, 33.

Lamb, D. (1967), *Brit. Med. J.* **1**, 273.

Lange, P. H., C. Limas, and E. E. Fraley (1978), *J. Urol.* **119**, 52.

Lessing, J. A. (1978), *J. Urol.* **120**, 1.

Liddle, G. W., W. E. Nicholson, D. P. Island, D. N. Orth, K. Abe, and S. C. Lowder (1969), *Recent Progr. Horm. Res.* **25**, 283.

Moore, M., and N. Robinson (1977), *Cancer Immunol. Immunother.* **2**, 233.

Nathrath, W., F. Detheridge, and L. Franks (1979), *J. Natl. Cancer Inst.* **63**, 1322.

O'Brien, P., J. Gozzo, W. Cronin, and A. Monaco (1979), *Invest. Urol.* **171**, 28.

Ørjasaeter, H., S. Fosså, S. Schjølseth, and K. Fjaestad (1978), *Cancer* **42**, 287.

O'Toole, C., P. Perlmann, B. Unsgaard, G. Moberger, and F. Edsmyr (1972a), *Int. J. Cancer* **10**, 77.

O'Toole, C., P. Perlmann, B. Unsgaard, L. E. Almgård, B. Johansson, G. Moberger, and F. Edsmyr (1972b), *Int. J. Cancer* **10**, 92.

Perlmann, P., and J. C. Cerottini (1979), in *The Antigens,* M. Sela, ed., vol. V, Academic Press, New York, p. 173.

Pross, H. F., and M. G. Baines (1977), *Cancer Immunol. Immunother.* **3**, 75.

Ratcliffe, J. G., J. Podmore, and B. McIlroy (1976), in *Cancer Related Antigens,* P. Franchimont, ed., North Holland, Amsterdam, p. 131.

Richie, J., R. Blute, and J. Waisman (1980), *J. Urol.* **123**, 22.

Robins, R. A., and R. W. Baldwin (1977), *Cancer Immunol. Immunother.* **2**, 205.

Sadoughi, N., A. Rubenstone, J. Mlsna, and I. Davidsohn (1980), *J. Urol.* **123**, 19.

Sandberg, A. A. (1977), *Cancer Res.* **37**, 2950.

Schmidt, J. D. (1966), *J. Urol.* **96**, 950.

Schneider, M. U., S. Paulie, M. Troye, and P. Perlmann (1980a), *Int. J. Cancer* **26**, 193.

Schneider, M. U., M. Troye, S. Paulie, and P. Perlmann (1980b), *Int. J. Cancer* **26**, 185.

Schwarze, G., R. Dietz, and A. Pappas (1979), *Eur. J. Cancer* **15**, 205.

Senda, H. (1971), *Nagoya J. Med. Sci.* **33**, 203.

Sobin, L. H. (1978), *Urol. Res.* **6**, 193.

Stjernswärd, J., L.-E. Almgård, S. Franzén, T. von Schreeb, and L. B. Wadström (1970), *Clin. Exptl. Immunol.* **6**, 963.

Teulings, F. A. G., H. A. Peters, W. C. J. Hop, W. Fokkens, W. G. Haije, H. Portengen, and B. van der Werf-Messing (1978), *Int. J. Cancer* **21**, 140.

Thorling, E. B. (1972), *Scand. J. Haematol. Suppl.* **17**, 1.

Traganos, F., Z. Darzynkiewicz, T. Sharpless, and M. R. Melamed (1977), *Int. J. Cancer* **20**, 30.

Tribukait, B., and P. L. Esposti (1978), *Urol. Res.* **6**, 201.

Troye, M., P. Perlmann, Å. Larsson, H. Blomgren, and B. Johansson (1977a), *Int. J. Cancer* **20**, 188.

Troye, M., P. Perlmann, G. R. Pape, H. L. Spiegelberg, I. Näslund, and A. Gidlöf (1977b), *J. Immunol.* **119**, 1061.

Troye, M., Y. Hansson, S. Paulie, P. Perlmann, H. Blomgren, and B. Johansson (1980a), *Int. J. Cancer* **25**, 45.

Troye, M., G. R. Pape, Å. Larsson, S. Paulie, M. Karlsson, P. Perlmann, H. Blomgren, and B. Johansson (1980b), *Cancer Immunol. Immunother.* **8**, 13.

Troye, M., M. Vilien, G. R. Pape, and P. Perlmann (1980c), *Cancer* **25**, 33.

Turner, A. G., H. Palmer, M. E. A. Powell, and A. M. Neville (1976), *Lancet* **2**, 308.

Vilien, M., and H. Wolf (1978), *J. Urol.* **119**, 338.

Vilien, M., H. Wolf, and F. Rasmussen (1980a), *Cancer Immunol. Immunother.* **8**, 189.

Vilien, M., H. Wolf, and F. Rasmussen (1981b), *Cancer Immunol. Immunother.*, in press.

von Schreeb, T., S. Franzén, and A. Ljungqvist (1967), *Scand. J. Urol. Nephrol.* **1**, 265.

Wahren, B. (1979), *Urol. Res.* **7**, 57.

Wahren, B., F. Edsmyr, and R. Zimmerman (1975), *Cancer* **36**, 1490.

Wahren, B., P. Esposti, and R. Zimmerman (1977), *Cancer* **40**, 1511.

Weinstein, R. S. (1976), *Cancer Res.* **36**, 2518.

Wilson, C. B. (1976), in *Textbook of Immunopathology*, P. A. Miescher and H. J. Müller-Eberhard, eds., vol. 1, Grune Stratton, New York, p. 529.

Wise, K. S., S. E. Allerton, G. Trump, D. Powars, and J. W. Beierle (1975), *Int. J. Cancer* **16**, 199.

Yoshida, O., R. R. Brown, and G. T. Bryan (1970), *Cancer* **25**, 773.

Zimmerman, R. (1979), Carcinoembryonic Antigen in Urothelial Carcinoma, Thesis, Stockholm.

Zimmerman, R., and S. Hammarström (1978), *Urol. Res.* **6**, 215.

Zimmerman, R., B. Wahren, and F. Edsmyr (1980), *Cancer*, **46**, 1802.

14

Endocrine Markers of Cancer

The Biological and Clinical Implications of Polypeptide Hormones

Geoffrey Mendelsohn[1] and Stephen B. Baylin[2]

Oncology Center and the Departments of Pathology[1] and Medicine,[2] The Johns Hopkins University School of Medicine and Hospital, Baltimore, Maryland

1. Introduction

Specific "endocrine" markers (polypeptide hormones and biogenic amines) have for several decades now played a vital role in the clinical evaluation and management of patients with a wide range of endocrine tumors. Some of these hormones, such as ACTH, gastrin, insulin, vasoactive intestinal peptide (VIP), and serotonin are responsible for the production of specific and often dramatic clinical syndromes. Others, such as calcitonin, a highly sensitive marker for the spectrum of thyroid C-cell proliferative disorders, are not associated with any known clinical syndromes. Ectopic (inappropriate) endocrine syndromes in patients with non-endocrine tumors have likewise been recognized for several decades. The earliest appreciation of inappropriate endocrine activity by tumors dates back to the 1920s (Klemperer, 1923; Brown, 1928), and over the ensuing years, numerous examples of inappropriate endocrine syndromes have been noted in patients with non-endocrine tumors (Meador et al., 1962; Lipsett et al., 1964; Liddle et al., 1969; Anderson, 1973; Ratcliff and Rees, 1974; Blackman et al., 1978; Trump and Baylin, 1979). In 1948, it was first appreciated that humoral factors might be involved in these endocrine syndromes (Albright and Reifenstein, 1948). During the past two decades, the development of sensitive bioassay, immunoassay, and receptor assay techniques has confirmed that excess quantities of circulating hormones were responsible for endocrine syndromes in patients with both endocrine and non-endocrine tumors (Meador et al., 1962; Amatruda et al., 1963; Liddle et al., 1969; Orth et al., 1973).

With the advent of these highly sensitive and specific assay techniques, it has also become apparent that many endocrine and non-endocrine tumors produce a variety of peptide hormones and amines either in quantities that are insufficient to produce clinical effects or in biologically inactive forms (Steiner et al., 1967; Steiner and Oyer, 1967; Berson and Yalow, 1968; Gorden et al., 1971; Yalow and Berson, 1971; Habener et al., 1972; Gewirtz and Yalow, 1973; Gewirtz and Yalow, 1974). By employing recently developed, highly sensitive immunohistochemical methods for the study of such tumors, it has become possible to localize many of these endocrine markers within tumor cells. Such assay and localization studies have played a major role in recognizing the enormous spectrum of endocrine activity in endocrine and non-endocrine tumors. These observations also suggest the potential that studies of tumor endocrine activity may have in understanding important aspects of tumor biology and in understanding many of the mechanisms involved in the synthesis, storage, and secretion of hormones in normal and neoplastic tissues.

During the course of this chapter, we will discuss the association of polypeptide hormones and biogenic amines with a variety of cancers. We will consider some of the known patterns of ectopic (inappropriate) hormone production by non-endocrine tumors and will consider theories and concepts that have been developed to explain such inappropriate endocrine activity. We will discuss briefly some of the mechanisms involved in synthesis, storage, and secretion of hormones in normal and neoplastic endocrine and non-endocrine tissues; and, finally, we will specifically address the clinical and biological implications of the presence of these endocrine markers in specific neoplastic diseases of endocrine and non-endocrine tissue.

2. Patterns of Inappropriate (Ectopic) Hormone Production by Tumors

It is apparent in addressing the clinical and biological relationships among tumors and the wide range of endocrine markers that tumors produce, that certain patterns of inappropriate endocrine activity exist. Bronchogenic squamous carcinoma, for example, is most often related to ectopic para-thyroid hormone-like activity, but does not cause hormonally mediated hypercalcemia. Bronchogenic small cell carcinoma, on the other hand, is the tumor most frequently associated with ectopic ACTH activity and yet rarely produces Cushing's syndrome (Blackman et al., 1978; Trump and Baylin, 1979). In a similar vein, carcinoid tumors arising in the lung, me-diastinum, and gastrointestinal tract may produce small polypeptide hor-mones, such as ACTH, in addition to their characteristic biogenic amines (Meador et al., 1962; O'Neal et al., 1968; Rees et al., 1974).

Similar patterns exist, also, for the "oncoplacental" hormones such as placental lactogen and human chorionic gonadotropin (HCG). Al-though several types of cancer are known to produce HCG, for example, it is apparent that high amounts of this hormone are most frequently associa-ted with gonadal tumors that have a major embryonal and/or trophoblastic cellular component (Braunstein et al., 1973; Rosen et al., 1975; Baylin and Mendelsohn, 1980).

It is pertinent, then, to consider briefly some of the concepts that have been proposed to explain these patterns of inappropriate hormonal activity in tumors. In this section, we will consider the current status of these con-cepts in the light of recent findings and advances.

2.1. Ectopic Small Polypeptide Hormone Production— The APUD (Amine Precursor Uptake and Decarboxylation)–Neural Crest Theory

It was largely through the work of Pearse and his colleagues during the past 15 years (Pearse, 1966a; Pearse, 1966b; Pearse, 1969; Pearse and Carvalheira, 1967; Pearse and Polak, 1971; Pearse et al., 1973), that the APUD cell–neural crest theory gained such prominence as a means of ex-plaining many of the patterns of small polypeptide hormone production by tumors. Pearse (1966a; 1966b; 1969) first noted that peptide hormone-producing cells in a number of different tissues shared certain biochemi-cal, cytochemical, and ultrastructural properties; he recognized the com-mon ability of such cells to take up amine precursors and to synthesize and/or store biogenic amines and coined the term "APUD" to highlight this phenomenon (1966a; 1966b). Utilizing the technique of formalde-hyde-induced fluorescence (Falck, 1962) and newly developed immuno-cytochemical methods, Pearse and others (Pearse, 1969; Pearse and Carvalheira, 1967; Pearse and Polak, 1971; Pearse et al., 1973) were able to map APUD cells and to show that in the mouse and dog, for example, some of the APUD cells were of neural crest origin. The APUD–neural crest theory was readily embraced because, in proposing the existence of widely dispersed neuroendocrine system related to a single tissue of origin (the neural crest), it presented a most convenient unifying concept for ex-plaining the propensity of a wide range of apparently unrelated endocrine and non-endocrine tumors to produce ectopic hormones. The frequent production of ectopic peptide hormones by small (oat) cell carcinoma of the lung, for example, might be explained by proposing that small cell carcinoma was a malignant tumor derived from the bronchial APUD cell, the K cell, which in turn was considered by some to be of possible neural crest origin (Bensch et al., 1968; Weichert, 1970; Bonikos and Bensch, 1977).

Because of the appeal of the APUD–neural crest theory, the terms APUD and neural crest became synonymous for many workers (Weichert, 1970; Ratcliff and Rees, 1974; Baylin, 1975); however, elegant experimental studies during the past 10 years have cast doubt on some aspects of the theory and have led to the appreciation that possession of APUD characteristics by cells does not necessarily imply origin from the neural crest or from any other neural tissue.

A detailed discussion of these experimental studies is beyond the scope of this chapter, but a brief review of the current status of the APUD theory is pertinent. APUD cells for which there is good supporting evidence for neural crest derivation are listed in Table 1. In the case of thyroid and ultimobranchial body C cells, a variety of cytochemical and immunocytochemical studies (Pearse, 1969; Pearse and Carvalheira, 1967; Pearse and Polak, 1971), together with the very elegant avian allograft chimera studies initiated by LeDouarin and LeLievre (1971) and subsequently used by other workers (Polak et al., 1974), have provided a substantial body of evidence supporting neural crest origin. Similar avian allograft studies and various histochemical studies have furnished good evidence, too, for the origin of sympathetic ganglion cells, carotid body chief (type I) cells, and adrenal medullary cells from the neural crest (Fontaine and LeDouarin, 1971; LeDouarin et al., 1972; Pearse et al., 1973; Teillet and LeDouarin, 1974).

It is less well known, however, that similar histochemical and transplant chimera studies, most notably those of Andrew (1974; 1975; 1976), LeDouarin and Teillet (1973), Pictet et al. (1976), and Fontaine and

Table 1

APUD Cells with Good Supporting Evidence for Neural Crest Derivation

Thyroid C cells
Ultimobranchial body C cells
Carotid-body chief cells (type I cells)
Adrenal medullary cells
   Adrenalin-secreting
   Noradrenalin-secreting
Small intensely fluorescent (SIF) cells of the sympathetic ganglia
Melanoblasts

LeDouarin (1977) have yielded a solid body of evidence demonstrating that many APUD cells, such as those of the gut and pancreas, are not, in fact, of neural crest origin. These workers suggest that the APUD endocrine cells of gut and pancreas probably differentiate from the endoderm of the developing gut wall. The studies of Cheng and Leblond (1974) support this concept and indicate that the endocrine cells may derive from a single type of progenitor basal crypt cell.

Pearse and Takor (1979) have recently addressed the APUD–neural crest theory in relation to the above findings. They have speculated that the endocrine cells that develop in endodermal tissues are "neuroendocrine-programmed" at an extremely early stage of embryogenesis, probably during their origin from the embryonic epiblast. The nature of such programming, however, remains speculative.

Not withstanding the embryological derivation of cells with APUD properties, the APUD theory still provides a valuable unifying concept for the study of hormone activity in tumors. Certainly, the majority of tumors associated with well-defined clinical syndromes resulting from excess production and secretion of small polypeptide hormones and/or biogenic amines (such as Cushing's, inappropriate ADH, watery diarrhea, and carcinoid) possess typical APUD properties, including characteristic neurosecretory granules. It has recently become apparent, however, that "non-APUD" tumors can contain significant amounts of peptides such as ACTH (Abe et al., 1977; Yalow, 1979). Most notably, ACTH and related peptides have been demonstrated in lung carcinomas of all histologic types (Gewirtz and Yalow, 1974; Yalow, 1979). Many of these peptides in non-APUD tumors, however, are present in large molecular weight forms that may represent metabolically inactive precursors (Ayvazian et al., 1975; Odell et al., 1979). In some tumors, a single precursor molecule gives rise to multiple active hormones, such as the precursor molecule for ACTH and beta-lipotropin (Bertagna et al., 1978a). Although it has been postulated, by some, that a single large protein may serve as the precursor for virtually all (ectopically produced) peptide hormones (Bertagna et al., 1978a; Deftos et al., 1978; Lips et al., 1978), subsequent studies have not substantiated this hypothesis (Bertagna et al., 1978a; Mendelsohn et al., 1979a; Nakanishi et al., 1979).

Recent studies of the pituitary gland are particularly important with regard to the biological aspects of the synthesis and secretion of several polypeptide hormones, such as ACTH, the melanocyte-stimulating hormones, the lipotropins, the endorphins and enkephalins, and calcitonin; and with regard to the production of multiple polypeptide hormones by many endocrine and non-endocrine tumors. During the past few years, much has been learned concerning the mechanisms involved in pituitary polypeptide hormone synthesis and secretion. Although the precise role of these mechanisms remains unclear as far as the ectopic production of pituitary hormones is concerned, awareness of these processes is critical for considering the entire spectrum of peptide hormone synthesis and/or secretion by human neoplasms.

It has been shown, during the past few years, that certain of the pituitary polypeptide hormones share a common molecular origin. There is compelling recent evidence to indicate that the lipotrophic hormones (LPH), α-LPH and β-LPH, the melanocyte-stimulating hormones (MSH), α-MSH and β-MSH, ACTH, and the peptides with opiate-like activity, the endorphins and enkephalins, are derived from a single 31,000-dalton (31K) glycoprotein precursor molecule (Guillemin et al., 1977; Mains et al., 1977; Nakanishi et al., 1977; Roberts and Herbert, 1977; Eipper and Mains, 1980). Immunocytochemical studies have shown that in rat and human pituitary, these peptides are present within the same cells (Phifer et al., 1974; Bloom et al., 1977), and experimental studies in the rat have shown that ACTH and β-endorphin, for example, are secreted concomitantly (Guillemin et al., 1977). More recently, there have been several studies that have shown a calcitonin-like peptide within the rat and human pituitary (Deftos et al., 1978; Mendelsohn et al., 1979a; Cooper et al., 1980; Lee et al., 1980). Although, on the basis of initial investigations (Deftos et al., 1978) it was suggested that the entire calcitonin molecule might be part of the 31K precursor molecule, it would appear that the immunoreactive calcitonin-like material present in the pituitary differs from that in normal and neoplastic thyroid C cells (Mendelsohn et al., 1979a; Cooper et al., 1980; Lee et al., 1980). Also, no intact calcitonin was found in sequence studies of the bovine 31K precursor to ACTH/β-LPH (Nakanishi et al., 1979). Notwithstanding the uncertainty surrounding calcitonin and the pituitary gland, there is ample evidence that many of the pituitary hormones, including those frequently produced ectopically, are cleaved from a single precursor molecule. An appreciation of this important biological principle is crucial in considering the presence of multiple peptide hormones in both endocrine and non-endocrine tumors. For example, the simultaneous presence within certain lung carcinomas of ACTH, β-endorphin, and β-LPH is now readily explained by these recent studies of hormone synthesis in the pituitary.

It is interesting to suggest, on the basis of available information, that all tumors have the potential to produce small polypeptide hormones. However, for a given tumor to be associated with clinically evident endocrine syndromes, such as Cushing's syndrome and the carcinoid syndrome, specific complex "machinery" must be manifest in the tissues. These specific biochemical properties include the presence of dense-core secretory granules and the capacity for amine synthesis, both of which have become the sine qua non for the identification of APUD cells.

What seems crucial, then, is an appreciation that the possession of APUD characteristics does not necessarily imply origin from the neural crest. Rather, the development of APUD characteristics may be one of several pathways of differentiation available to immature, uncommitted epithelial cells of multiple embryologic derivations. We will, during the course of our discussion of endocrine markers in certain non-endocrine tumors, such as bronchogenic carcinoma and prostatic carcinoma, examine the experimental evidence that suggests this possibility. We will also carefully consider the clinical and biological implications of these findings.

2.2. Ectopic "Oncoplacental" Hormone Production

The so-called placental or "oncoplacental" tumor markers include hormones such as human placental lactogen (HPL) and human chorionic gonadotropin (HCG). As with the small polypeptide hormones discussed above, the ectopic production of oncoplacental hormones is not entirely random, and certain patterns exist for the production of these hormones by tumors. Although production of oncoplacental hormones has been noted in almost every type of cancer, it is clear that the highest amounts and most frequent occurrence are associated with gonadal germ cell tumors with a major embryonal and/or trophoblastic cellular component (Braunstein et al., 1973; Rosen et al., 1975; Baylin and Mendelsohn, 1980). In contrast, elevated circulating amounts of HCG in patients with non-epithelial tumors, such as sarcomas and hematological or lymphoid malignancies, are extremely uncommon. Data obtained from the studies of Braunstein et al. (1973) and Rosen et al. (1975) indicate that elevated levels of the beta-subunit of HCG are found in 56% of patients with ovarian or testicular germ cell tumors having prominent embryonal components, in 15% of patients with non-germ cell carcinomas, such as bronchogenic carcinoma, mammary carcinoma, and gastrointestinal carcinoma, in only 6% of patients with sarcomas, and in only 2% of patients with hematological cancers. Similarly, levels of HPL are increased in tumors, either gonadal or extragonadal, which have trophoblastic differentiation; circulating HPL is increased in fewer than 5% of patients with nontrophoblastic tumors (Rosen et al., 1975). Thus, a level of differentiation that is present most often in germ cell or epithelial tumors and that involves trophoblastic components is associated with the presence of HCG and HPL.

3. Proposed Mechanisms of Inappropriate Hormone Production by Non-Endocrine Tumors

The precise mechanisms determining the appearance of various hormones, such as small polypeptides and oncoplacental proteins, in different types of tumors are not known. In this section, we will consider briefly various genetic and nongenetic mechanisms that have been proposed to explain ectopic production of hormones by non-endocrine tumors.

In most hormonally active endocrine tumors, endocrine activity is the result of retention of the ability to secrete a product normally produced by the parent cell. The peptide hormone secretion patterns in insulinoma, glucagonoma, and medullary thyroid carcinoma are typical examples of this type of endocrine activity.

The mechanisms underlying the inappropriate (ectopic) production of hormones by non-endocrine tumors are not, as yet, well understood. There has been much speculation in recent years in this regard, and several concepts have been proposed to explain the phenomenon. At present, there is little firm supporting experimental evidence for any of the theories advanced to explain ectopic hormone production. However, the recent advances in the field of molecular genetics give great promise that such information will be forthcoming. For example, the expanding capabilities for the isolation of the DNA responsible for peptide hormone expression and for the study of mRNA synthesis and processing (Crick, 1979; Nathans, 1979; Setlow and Hollander, 1979), should facilitate further study of the mechanisms involved in the expression of ectopic endocrine activity.

Below, we will briefly consider some of the major theories that have been proposed for ectopic hormone production.

3.1. "Sponge" Theory

According to the sponge theory, some circulating hormones may be selectively taken up and concentrated within tumors (Unger et al., 1964). Release of bound hormone by dying tumor cells would, according to this theory, account for increased circulating hormone concentrations. Although there is abundant evidence that some tumor cells possess receptors for certain peptides (Schorr et al., 1971) and steroids (McGuire, 1978) and may specifically bind these hormones, this does not offer an adequate explanation for most examples of tumor-associated endocrine activity. During the past several years, a convincing body of evidence has accumulated indicating active production and secretion of hormones by certain tumors. The most convincing evidence validating synthesis of hormones by tumor cells themselves includes in vitro evidence of hormone production (George et al., 1972; Rabson et al., 1973; Bertagna et al., 1978a) and immunocytochemical localization of hormone within tumor cells in culture (Acevedo et al., 1978).

3.2. Genetic Mechanisms

Several genetic mechanisms have been implicated in the complex process of ectopic hormone production; these include random genetic mutation, gene derepression, and dedifferentiation.

If the appearance of hormones in tumors was related to random *genetic mutation* occurring during the complex process of "neoplastic transformation," then one would predict random expression of endocrine activity by tumors and the presence of unusual protein forms. As discussed above, however, there are certain nonrandom patterns of inappropriate activity. Furthermore, there is much evidence to indicate that the synthesized hormones within tumors represent normal initial gene products. The presence within tumors of precursor molecules (Gordon et al., 1971; Gewirtz and Yalow, 1974; Bertagna et al., 1978a; Odell et al., 1979; Yalow, 1979), fragments of peptide hormones (Orth et al., 1973) and subunits of certain hormones such as the glycoprotein hormones (Rosen et al., 1975) does indicate a considerable degree of post-transcriptional and post-translational disorder. These peptide products of tumor cells, however, appear to be structurally and biochemically identical to the precursor forms or metabolic fragments in normal cells, thus pointing towards structural integrity of the initial gene product.

There is no experimental evidence to support major mutational events during the process of neoplastic transformation. Studies have failed to demonstrate generalized emergence of abnormal DNA sequences in tumor cells; in a recent survey of evidence for mutational events in tumors, Uriel (1975) concluded that extensive recent studies had failed to identify new antigens, enzymes, or molecules that logically would be expressed by the progeny of mutated cells.

According to the widely discussed and popular concept of *gene derepression* (Gellhorn, 1969), portions of DNA that are "inactive" and not available for transcription in the parent cell become "activated"— i.e., certain genetic control mechanisms are lost during the process of neoplastic transformation. Such a theory would predict an overall increase in gene transcription during tumor evolution. There is, however, some recent evidence to indicate that, in point of fact, there may be no significant change, or even a loss, in DNA transcription during the evolution of some tumors in culture (Shields, 1977; Shearer and Dodge, 1977).

Odell and others (1977) have postulated that in normal adult non-endocrine tissues, transcriptional activity for many proteins, most notably the small polypeptide hormones, may never be completely repressed. The finding of small amounts of peptides, such as ACTH and HCG, in normal tissues supports such a postulate (Yoshimoto et al., 1977). The exact identity of the molecules accounting for displacement in the immunoassays used for such studies need attention. Furthermore, mRNA for peptide hormones in normal non-endocrine epithelial cells must be identified. Amplification of peptide hormone production in carcinomas and in states of increased epithelial proliferation, such as hepatic regeneration and inflammatory bowel disease may, according to Odell et al., (1977), indicate that cell proliferation might per se result in "less effective" gene repression. This postulation also requires direct confirmation. In short, no direct experimental evidence for derepression of peptide hormone genes in neoplastic cells has yet been provided.

The *"dedifferentiation"* theory (Uriel, 1975; Shields, 1977) that has gained considerable popularity during the past several years implies that during the process of neoplastic transformation, the cancer tissue reverts to a more primitive state of gene expression. This concept suggests a regression along the embryological pathway by which the parent tissue differentiated. As for derepression, the mechanism of dedifferentiation would be consistent with many of the patterns of ectopic hormone production we have discussed. These theories would, for example, support the APUD–endocrine cell hypothesis, which postulates that APUD tissues in many areas of the body are embryologically related to a primitive neuroendocrine organ, the neural crest; these cells, at many differentiation stages then contain the genetic machinery for the production of multiple polypeptide hormones and biogenic amines. Thus, it would be postulated that in a given type of endocrine cell there is a selective repression of many of these properties as the normal cell differentiates towards its mature state. Neoplastic transformation would lead to a reversal along the particular pathway of neuroendocrine differentiation, with concomitant loss of the genetic repression that had occurred during embryogenesis. Such APUD tumors would then be capable of producing multiple peptide hormones or biogenic amines. However, although the dedifferentiation theory offers a plausible explanation for many examples of ectopic endocrine activity in tumors, there is a considerable body of evidence against retrograde differentiation. Within the hematopoietic system, for example, in which the pathways of cell differentiation are being well-characterized, there is no firm evidence in either normal or neoplastic states that backward movement can occur (Cline and Gold, 1979; Quesenberry and Levitt, 1979a,b,c). Although the same may not necessarily hold true for epithelial tissues, caution must be exercised when considering the possible role of these genetic mechanisms in relation to ectopic endocrine activity.

Recently, it has been suggested that ectopic endocrine activity in non-endocrine tumors may be related to abnormal differentiation or *"dysdifferentiation"* (Abelev, 1974); that the expression of endocrine activity in the non-endocrine tumors is related to altered "forward movement" rather than "backward movement." Recent studies of certain tumor models and tumor systems have lent some support for this latter hypothesis. In the forthcoming sections in which we will discuss endocrine markers, polypeptide hormones, and biogenic amines in certain specific tumors, our prejudice for this concept will emerge. Thus, we will, in addition to addressing the clinical implications of the endocrine expression of various tumors, consider the relationships to the above biological concepts and hypotheses.

4. Markers in Endocrine Tumors

4.1. Calcitonin in Medullary Thyroid Carcinoma and Other Human Cancers

Medullary thyroid carcinoma (MTC) presents a classic situation in which an endocrine biomarker can be employed to diagnose and precisely monitor patients with a cancer. Several features of this tumor allow for this situation. First, the precise cell of origin of the tumor has been identified and the endocrine biochemistry of that same cell has been elucidated. Thus, it is now well established that the C cell of the thyroid gland has, as its major endocrine function, the secretion of the small polypeptide hormone, calcitonin (Foster et al., 1964; Hirsch and Munson, 1969; Hoyt et al., 1973). In turn, medullary thyroid carcinoma is a tumor of this same cell and maintains a high capacity for synthesis and secretion of the parent endocrine product. Thus, the presence of an abnormal circulating level of calcitonin is almost universal in patients with clinically evident MTC (Tashjian et al., 1970; Wells et al., 1978b). Second, some 10–20% of patients with MTC develop the tumor in a unique familial setting in which the neoplasms are inherited via a Mendelian dominant trait. These multiple neoplasia syndromes have been well-defined (Schimke and Hartman, 1965; Schimke et al., 1968; Steiner et al., 1968; Khairi et al., 1975) and have allowed individuals at direct risk for development of the tumors to be identified. Studies of circulating calcitonin levels in these patients provide the situation in which a clinically occult neoplasm can be identified through abnormal circulating levels of its specific endocrine product (Tashjian et al., 1970; Melvin et al., 1971; Jackson et al., 1973). In doing so, a spectrum of C-cell proliferation has been defined in which C-cell hyperplasia is the benign precursor of MTC (Wolfe et al., 1973; Mendelsohn et al., 1978) and the use of provocative testing for calcitonin secretion to identify even very young children with preneoplastic stages of familial MTC has now been well-defined (Wells et al., 1978b; Baylin et al., 1979a). Thus, in the present setting, we will not dwell on these maneuvers in detail. It is important to stress, however, that the screening of any individuals at risk for developing familial MTC or in the post-operative setting for evaluation of disease status should not depend on measurement of basal calcitonin levels alone. Provoked secretion of circulating calcitonin with the newly described short calcium infusions (Parthemore et al., 1974), pentagastrin injections (Hennessy et al., 1974) or, in our opinion, a combination of the two (Wells et al., 1978a; Baylin et al., 1979a) should be utilized. Patients with very early forms of familial disease, i.e., C-cell hyperplasia and microscopic MTC, often have normal basal levels of calcitonin with abnormalities becoming apparent only during provoked secretion (Wells et al., 1978b). Similarly, those patients with known MTC in the pre-operative setting can best be assessed if their response to provocative testing is compared with results obtained following surgery. Longitudinal studies of such secretory responses seem more accurate than following basal levels alone in the majority of patients with MTC (Baylin et al., 1979a; Trump et al., 1979).

Since the value of calcitonin as a biomarker in MTC has now been well defined, it may be useful to consider briefly some new nuances of the relationship of this biomarker to the tumor which, at present, may be most important for considering the biology of the disease, but which may also come to have impact upon the clinical care of patients with this cancer. In its early stages, and during the total course of the disease in many patients, MTC appears to be a slow growing neoplasm that may maintain a relatively high level of differentiation. Thus, particularly in the setting of small lesions, the relationship between an increasing tumor size and an increasing basal and/or provoked level of calcitonin appears to be a rather precise one (Tashjian et al., 1970; Wells et al., 1978b). However, in a smaller number of patients, MTC can behave as a very virulent neoplasm, with the capacity for rapid widespread dissemination and resultant death of the patient (Woolner, 1971; Chong et al., 1975). In this regard, there is increasing evidence to suggest that the anaplastic characteristics of the virulent tumor are manifested by a marked change in cellular differentiation. The efficacy for calcitonin production appears to be diminished in tumors that achieve a large size and/or come to behave in an aggressive manner (Trump et al., 1979; Mendelsohn et al., 1980b). The evidence for this lies in a relatively decreased concentration of calcitonin in larger as opposed to smaller lesions, and an absolutely diminished total content of hormone in lesions from some patients with very virulent disease (Baylin et al., 1979b; Trump et al., 1979). At the histologic level, one also sees a progressive heterogeneity of cell staining for calcitonin in the tumor lesions; in contrast to the early, small lesions where most cells appear to contain significant quantities of hormone (Mendelsohn et al., 1978), there are regions of nonstaining cells and/or total lack of cellular staining in occasional metastatic lesions (Trump et al., 1979; Mendelsohn et al., 1980b). This facet of tumor biology can present a problem for the interpretation of circulating calcitonin levels in a minority of patients with MTC; in some patients with virulent disease, the levels of circulating calcitonin can be much lower than would be expected for the large tumor burden (Trump et al., 1979). Thus, in an occasional patient, a diminuition either in basal blood calcitonin levels or in response to provocative testing over a period of time may correlate with a worsening clinical status rather than being indicative of improvement.

Finally, it should be remembered that the secretion of polypeptide hormones other than calcitonin has now been well-described in patients with MTC (Donahower et al., 1968; Szijj et al., 1969; Melvin, 1974; Birkenhäger et al., 1976; Iwanaga et al., 1978). The most commonly described situation has been that of ectopic Cushing's syndrome with increased levels of circulating and tumor tissue ACTH (Donahower et al., 1968; Szijj et al., 1969; Melvin et al., 1971; Iwanaga et al., 1978). The exact frequency with which MTC tissue can synthesize and/or secrete polypeptide hormones other than calcitonin has not yet been documented. For example, it is not known, in the minority of patients who exhibit increasing virulence of disease, whether a diminution of the efficiency for calcitonin production may coincide with production of other polypeptide hormones by the tumor cells. Also, the question of whether one tumor cell type is responsible for the simultaneous secretion of calcitonin plus other polypeptide hormones is not yet entirely settled, and conflicting evidence exists in this regard (Abe et al., 1977; Kameya et al., 1977; Capella et al., 1978). A more precise quantitation of the relationships between tumor growth patterns and the presence or absence of hormones other than calcitonin in MTC should help clarify these questions; the results of such studies should also have much relevance for the biology of other types of human cancers.

Lastly, the presence of calcitonin in cancers other than MTC must be considered. It has now been well-documented that significant quantities of immunoreactive calcitonin can be detected in such tumors as carcinoids (DeLellis and Wolfe, 1976; Dayal et al., 1980), pheochromocytomas (Voelkel et al., 1973; Heath and Edis, 1979), lung cancers (Silva et al., 1974; Becker et al., 1978; Baylin et al., 1978) and neuroblastic tumors (Trump et al., 1977). Similarly, increased circulating levels of calcitonin have been described, particularly in patients with lung cancer (Coombes et al., 1974; Milhaud et al., 1974; Silva et al., 1976; Becker et al., 1978; Roos et al., 1980) and breast cancer (Coombes et al., 1974; Milhaud et al., 1974; Silva and Becker, 1976; Roof et al., 1979). Several important qualifications must be considered before speculating upon the clinical significance of these observations. First, the precise chemical identification of the immunoreactive material as calcitonin needs to be pursued in most of the examples cited above. It is now well-recognized that even specific radioimmunoassays can be subject to artefacts in certain situations. Thus, peptides other than the one directly being measured may share certain amino acid sequences or structural homologies that allow partial displacement in the standard curve. As mentioned previously, such a situation appears to account for the identification of a calcitonin-like peptide in human and rat pituitary glands (Deftos et al., 1978; Mendelsohn et al., 1979a; Cooper et al., 1980) and for the presence of β-endorphin-like immunoreactivity in human placenta (Julliard et al., 1980). Therefore, more studies are needed to characterize precisely the calcitonin immunoreactivity present in tumor tissues and in the circulation of patients with cancers other than MTC.

Whatever the source of the immunoreactivity for calcitonin in patients with certain tumors other than MTC, there does seem to be some potential for utilizing the levels to monitor patients with some non-MTC cancers. We discuss elsewhere this possibility with reference to lung cancer, and other investigators have been actively pursuing this question in breast carcinoma (Silva and Becker, 1976; Roof et al., 1979). The exact value of measuring calcitonin in patients with cancer in general should await the outcome of these and other research investigations. In general, the presence of immunoreactive calcitonin in the circulation should not be confusing in terms of making the diagnosis of MTC vs other neoplasms. First, the levels of calcitonin in patients with tumors other than MTC are usually quite low. Second, patients with non-MTC cancers generally fail to show significant increases in calcitonin during provocative testing (Roof et al., 1979). Finally, the most exquisite use of calcitonin as a biomarker, namely for the diagnosis of familial MTC, usually does not present a confusing clinical circumstance with regard to the presence of other cancers.

In summary, calcitonin is an elegant biomarker for monitoring patients with MTC, particularly in the setting of familial disease. There are situations in which tumor burden and blood calcitonin levels do not correlate even for this neoplasm; those situations appear to involve aggressive forms of MTC. Increased quantities of an immunoreactive calcitonin do appear to be involved with some neoplasms other than MTC; the precise nature of the immunoreactive material in each setting needs further investigation. The clinical significance of increased calcitonin immunoreactivity in patients with cancers other than MTC requires further investigation; such studies may verify that the monitoring of circulating calcitonin levels in patients with cancers other than MTC has clinical utility. Finally, MTC is capable of synthesizing and secreting other polypeptide hormones; the relationship of this activity to disease status and the clinical signficance of monitoring other peptide hormones in patients with MTC also remains to be defined.

4.2. Islet Cell Tumors of the Pancreas

The islet cells of the pancreas represent a fascinating cell system in which multiple tumors with different types of predominant hormonal output probably arise in a common cell lineage. The hormonal phenotype of a given islet cell neoplasm, as may be true for tumors arising in the bronchial epithelium, probably reflects the level of differentiation of the cell in which neoplastic transformation has occurred, or of the direction and degree of maturation that the neoplastic cell has pursued. An understanding of the derivation of the different types of cells that comprise the pancreatic islets and of their specific hormonal synthesis is, as for other tumors with endocrine function, essential for understanding the biology of these neoplasms and for fully appreciating their spectrum of clinical activity as well. In this section, therefore, we will briefly consider the current thinking about the origin of the pancreatic islets and the hormonal relationships between the different types of normal cells present. In this setting, we can then discuss the unique spectrum of tumors that can emanate from this endocrine system.

It is now well-appreciated that the pancreatic islet cells may be classified in the APUD series of endocrine cells, which have neurosecretory type granules and some capacity for biogenic amine synthesis and for secretion of specific small polypeptide hormones (Pearse, 1966a; 1966b; 1969). This complex of biochemical activity made the islet cells a prime candidate for embryologic origin in the neural crest, in the setting of the initial thinking about APUD cells (Pearse, 1969; Weichert, 1970; Baylin, 1975); over the past six years, however, the pancreatic islets have been one of the endocrine tissues for which evidence has been garnered against an origin in the neural crest. Several studies (LeDouarin and Teillet, 1973; Andrew, 1975; Andrew, 1976; Pictet et al., 1976; Fontaine and LeDouarin, 1977) have failed to provide any direct evidence for neural crest contribution to pancreatic islet embryogenesis. Furthermore, the data generated from these studies suggest that the islet cells are formed from the epithelium of the developing pancreatic ducts that are clearly of endodermal origin. If this is the case, the formation of the islets and their subsequent differentiation into multiple cell types might be viewed in the context of recent studies of the gastrointestinal mucosa (Cheng and Leblond, 1974). These investigations suggest that all intestinal mucosal cells, including the Kulchitzky cell, appear to be derived from the basal crypt cells. Thus, a single type of progenitor cell with the capability of multipotential differentiation may give rise to the pancreatic ducts and to cells with endocrine differentiation that constitute the islets. Such a concept would embody a fascinating scheme of differentiation in which the different types of islet cells emerge with quantitatively different expressions of polypeptide hormone content.

In the setting of the above thinking about the development of the pancreatic islets, the spectrum of tumors that would evolve from such cells might encompass the entire range of differentiation expression found among the normal islet cells. This concept would be similar to that which, in later sections, we discuss for the development of carcinoid tumors in the gastrointestinal tract and bronchial epithelium and for lung cancers in the bronchial epithelium. Indeed, the spectrum of islet cell lesions and the predominant hormone secretion from each type do reflect the endocrine biochemistry of normal islets of Langerhans. Islet cell tumors, for the most part, represent highly differentiated neoplasms and, despite some overlap among the types of hormones present in a given lesion, a predominant hormonal secretion and a predominant endocrine syndrome characterize these lesions. Even in a genetic setting, and within a single family inheriting a predeliction for islet cell tumors and other associated endocrine lesions, the full spectrum of islet cell differentiation can be seen (Hutcheon et al., 1979). Individual patients usually have an islet cell tumor with a single or predominant peptide hormone product, but the tumors may differ among individuals in the same family (Hutcheon et al., 1979). Thus, it is not uncommon to find families in which some members have a β-cell islet lesion and the resultant syndrome of hypoglycemia, while other members will have a non-β-cell lesion with Zollinger-Ellison disease (Vance et al., 1972; Hutcheon et al., 1979).

The clinical use of biomarkers for diagnosing and monitoring patients with islet cell tumors often depends on identifying the syndromes that result from excess secretion of a given hormone; the presence of certain symptom complexes directs the clinician towards obtaining quantitative verification of excess circulating levels of a specific hormone. With this philosophy, a high insulin level in a patient with an islet cell tumor only confirms the etiology of the low blood sugar present. Similarly, in a patient with peptic ulcer disease and a suspicion of the Zollinger-Ellison complex, a high circulating gastrin level or abnormal responses of gastrin to specific provocative tests, provides the confirming information (Lamers and van Tongeren, 1977).

Special mention should be made of the symptom of chronic diarrhea in patients with islet cell tumors. Three types of lesions, and perhaps some overlap in biochemical expression among such tumors, may account for this symptom complex in patients with islet cell neoplasms. Approximately 20% of patients with Zollinger-Ellison disease have diarrhea as a prime symptom in the absence of any peptic ulcers being demonstrated (Isenberg et al., 1973). The diarrhea apparently results from the excess gastric acid secretions emptying into the intestine, and the diagnosis can be confirmed by demonstrating abnormal blood gastrin levels, and/or cessation of the diarrhea with the institution of cimetidine therapy or chronic gastric suctioning. However, voluminous watery diarrhea is also a symptom in patients with islet cell tumors not secreting significant quantities of gastrin, but rather excess vasoactive intestinal peptide or other less well-identified peptide hormones that cause active small bowel secretion (Verner and Morrison, 1974; Said and Faloona, 1975; Jaffe et al., 1977; Hutcheon et al., 1979). These tumors must be diagnosed by ruling out abnormal blood gastrin levels, documenting increased circulating levels of vasoactive intestinal peptide, or as a diagnosis of exclusion when the Zollinger-Ellison syndrome is ruled out and no other cause for diarrhea can be identified. Finally, the multipotential nature of islet cell tumors has been well shown to include the capability for biogenic amine synthesis (Sayle et al., 1965; Patchefsky et al., 1972); in this setting, islet cell lesions represent an infrequent cause of the carcinoid syndrome (Dollinger et

al., 1967; Appleyard and Losowsky, 1970). Tumors of the pancreatic islets should be considered in the approach to patients who appear to have
the carcinoid syndrome; similarly, in patients with a high suspicion for islet cell tumor, the demonstration of abnormal levels of 5-hydroxyindole
acetic acid (5-HIAA) in the urine and/or elevated levels of blood serotonin
occasionally can be helpful in establishing the diagnosis.

Most islet cell tumors fall into one of the precise tumor syndrome categories such as insulinoma, Zollinger-Ellison disease, the watery diarrhea
syndrome, and the glucagonoma syndrome. However, many islet cell tumors appear to be nonfunctioning in terms of excess hormone secretion.
The recent recognition of the so-called somatostatinoma, or non-β islet
cell tumor that contains and secretes large quantities of somatostatin
(Ganda et al., 1977; Larsson et al., 1977; Galmiche et al., 1978) raises the
possibility that many islet cell tumors not fitting into the other major categories may represent such tumors. The diagnosis of a somatostatinoma is
extremely difficult and is usually a retrospective finding in a patient with
progressively difficult to control diabetes mellitus. The diabetes results
from apparent inhibition of insulin secretion by the excess quantities of
somatostatin (Alberti et al., 1973; Koerker et al., 1974). In patients with
suspected pancreatic neoplasms and the new onset of diabetes, the diagnosis of somatostatinoma must be considered.

It must be remembered that the endocrine potential of islet cell tumors
includes their ability to synthesize and secrete excess quantities of polypeptide hormones that are the predominant products of other endocrine tissues. The most common example of this appears to be the secretion of
ACTH and, in some patients, a resultant ectopic Cushing's syndrome
(Law et al., 1965; Sayle et al., 1965; Azzopardi and Williams, 1968).
Thus, identification of abnormal dynamics of cortisol secretion and/or abnormal blood levels of ACTH should be a consideration in all patients with
documented islet cell tumors. Similarly, it has been recently demonstrated
that the secretion of the α-subunit of human chorionic gonadotropin may
be a frequent occurrence in islet cell lesions (Kahn et al., 1977). This tumor activity appears to be more characteristic of islet cell carcinomas than
of benign islet cell lesions (Kahn et al., 1977).

Finally, the role of quantitating the hormonal content of surgically removed islet cell lesions, either by extraction of the hormones for radioimmunoassay or by appropriate immunohistochemical techniques, should
not be overlooked. Screening for the presence of all the peptides discussed
above should be considered for any islet cell lesion; this may be most expe-
ditiously done by using immunohistochemical techniques on frozen or
fixed tissue sections if appropriate antibodies are available. The knowledge of which hormones are present in any given tumor may greatly aid the
clinician; appropriate circulating hormones may then be selected to monitor completeness of tumor removal in some instances or the response to

other therapeutic modalities in patients with inoperable or residual islet cell tumors. Similarly, in patients at genetic risk for developing islet cell tumors, the spectrum of hormones that may be secreted can serve as circulating markers to identify those patients who may have early lesions.

In summary, the islet cells of the pancreas represent a fascinating aspect of cellular differentiation in which multiple endocrine cell types evolve in a single geographical unit. The parent hormones for each of the cell types that evolve may be secreted from neoplasms arising in this cell system. Although a single hormone usually appears to predominate, often in the presence of a defined clinical syndrome, overlap between the hormones occurs and any single neoplasm may contain significant quantities of several polypeptide hormones. Our understanding of the biology of the pancreatic islets has increased our knowledge about the hormonal content of tumors that arise in these endocrine cells and has simultaneously increased our ability to employ polypeptide hormone markers to diagnose and monitor patients with islet cell tumors.

4.3. Carcinoid Tumors

The carcinoid syndrome resulting from excess tumor production of serotonin, kinins, and probably polypeptide hormones is one of the most striking complex of symptoms attributable to hormonal activity in tumors. The finding of elevated levels of urinary 5-hydroxyindole acetic acid (5-HIAA), the major metabolite of serotonin, remains the key criterion for the diagnosis of carcinoid tumors, which may occur throughout the gastrointestinal tract, in the lung, pancreas, and mediastinum, and occasionally in the ovary or genitourinary tract (Dollinger et al., 1967; Patchefsky et al., 1972; Rosai and Higa, 1972; Godwin, 1975; Salyer et al., 1975; Robboy et al., 1977). Likewise, monitoring urinary 5-HIAA levels may play a valuable role in assessing completeness of tumor removal and course of disease.

It has recently been demonstrated that, in addition to serotonin and its metabolites, carcinoid tumors are also able to produce and secrete a variety of polypeptide hormones. Cushing's syndrome resulting from ACTH production has been recognized in association with carcinoid tumors for many years (Azzopardi and Williams, 1968). It has recently become apparent, however, that other polypeptide hormones, including β-MSH, calcitonin, somatostatin, substance P, and enteroglucagon, for example, may be produced by carcinoid tumors and some immunohistochemical studies have, in fact, localized these peptides within tumor cells (Pearse et al., 1974; Nakao et al., 1975; Sonksen et al., 1976; Abe et al., 1977; Wilander et al., 1977; Lechago, 1978; Skrabanek et al., 1978; Solcia et al., 1978; Wilander et al., 1979; Dayal et al., 1980). Currently, in practice, these peptide hormones are not being used as markers for carcinoid tumors; it is possible, however, that the ongoing assay and immunohistochemical studies of tumor tissue may identify for the oncologist a variety of peptides that are consistently produced by these tumors and that may serve as markers for following response to therapy and course of disease. These polypeptides might be particularly valuable as markers in the evolution of carcinoid tumors, which are "inert" from the standpoint of biogenic amine production. Functional interaction between the peptide hormones and amines is also a possibility. Recently, infusions of somatostatin have been shown to prevent the symptoms evoked by secretagogues such as pentagastrin (Frölich et al., 1978).

With regard to their ability to produce both biogenic amines and polypeptide hormones, carcinoid tumors obviously resemble pancreatic islet cell and other endocrine tumors. It is thus pertinent at this point to consider the embryologic derivation of the cells from which these tumors arise. The gastrointestinal and bronchial serotonin-producing K cells, the putative parent cells of carcinoid tumors, have characteristic APUD properties (Pearse, 1966a; 1966b; 1969) and have been considered by some (Bensch et al., 1968; Weichert, 1970; Bonikos and Bensch, 1977) to be of neural crest origin. As we have stressed in previous sections, however, there is good experimental evidence against origin of gastrointestinal K cells in the neural crest (LeDouarin and Teillet, 1973; Andrew, 1974; 1975; 1976; Cheng and Leblond, 1974; Pictet et al., 1976; Fontaine and LeDouarin, 1977; Pearse and Takor, 1977). These studies would, in fact, indicate that gastrointestinal K cells are of endodermal origin. There is also reason to believe that, in addition to the K cells, gastrointestinal polypeptide-producing endocrine cells (Lechago, 1978; Solcia et al., 1978) also differentiate within the developing endoderm. The precise origin of bronchial K cells in not yet known; since the tracheobronchial tree is an endodermal derivative, it is likely that bronchial K cells also differentiate within the endodermal epithelium. In the lung, recent studies have demonstrated immunoreactive calcitonin within normal bronchial K cells (Becker et al., 1980) and the presence of polypeptides in carcinoid tumors, both in the gastrointestinal tract and in the lung, may, therefore, not be truly ectopic or inappropriate. Rather, the production of these peptides should be considered in relation to the earlier discussion of pancreatic islet cell tumors and the discussion on mechanisms of hormone production by non-endocrine tumors. The production of biogenic amines and polypeptides by carcinoids, and occasionally the production of multiple hormones, may, as for pancreatic islet cell tumors, reflect different levels of differentiation within the tumors; such levels of ongoing differentiation within a tumor might then decide the spectrum of endocrine activity expressed.

In summary, serotonin production remains the diagnostic hallmark of carcinoid tumors. However, recent evidence indicates that polypeptide hormone elaboration is an integral part of the gene expression of these tumors; measurement of these polypeptides may come to play an important role in patient management.

5. Markers in Non-Endocrine Tumors

5.1. Carcinoma of the Lung

The relationship of endocrine activity to carcinoma of the lung has a rich history. Lung cancer is by far the leading cause of ectopic endocrine syndromes resulting from excess secretion of small polypeptide hormones. Thus, the syndrome of inappropriate antidiuretic hormone (ADH) secretion and that of Cushing's syndrome are both most commonly seen in patients with lung cancer (Baylin and Mendelsohn, 1980). Also, patients with hormonally induced gynecomastia have now been well-described in the setting of lung cancer (Faiman et al., 1967; Rosen et al., 1968). In addition to these clinically recognized syndromes, an increasing body of information has arisen concerning the direct measurement of polypeptide hormones in the circulation and tissues from patients with lung cancer. The high frequency with which multiple hormones can be detected has generated considerable interest with regard to the potential use of polypeptide hormones as biomarkers for diagnosing and monitoring the clinical progression of patients with carcinoma of the lung.

The association of specific polypeptide hormones with specific histologic types of lung cancer has generated intense biologic interest as well as clinical emphasis. The bronchial epithelium is somewhat unique among human tissues, which are highly associated with neoplastic transformation. From this single epithelium, at least four major histopathologic types of cancer are now well-recognized, and each has a major impact on man. The spectrum of endocrine activity that emerges from these tumor types is not only of clinical significance, but also has bearing on the relationships between the different histologic types of lung cancer. Indeed, the histogenesis and cellular origin of an important lung cancer, small (oat) cell carcinoma (SCC), has been closely linked to its endocrine activity and much debated in recent years. It is, therefore, worthwhile to review in some detail the history of the relationship of SCC to endocrine expression and to examine the current views concerning the relationship of this lung cancer to the other major histopathologic types. In this setting, the biologic implications of endocrine activity in lung tumors and the potential use of polypeptide hormones as biomarkers can then be addressed.

Small cell lung carcinoma (SCC) has long been known to exhibit growth patterns and biologic behavior that are somewhat different from the other major histologic types of lung cancer (Matthews, 1976; Hirsch et al., 1977; Hansen et al., 1978), as well as notable differences in response to therapy (Abeloff et al., 1976; Bunn et al., 1977; Weiss, 1978). SCC maintains a relatively high growth fraction relative to the other lung cancers and has the potential for extremely early metastatic dissemination (Hirsch et al., 1977); at the same time, SCC exhibits a higher sensitivity to radiation therapy and/or chemotherapy than the other tumors (Abeloff et al., 1976; Bunn et al., 1977; Weiss, 1978). Specifically, for the purpose of the present discussion, SCC has more propensity for secretion of biologically active small polypeptide hormones, such as ACTH and ADH, than the other lung cancer types. Thus, it is SCC among the major lung neoplasms that accounts for the high incidence of ectopic hormone syndromes in patients with lung cancer (Lipsett et al., 1964; Liddle et al., 1969; Anderson, 1973; Trump and Baylin, 1979; Baylin and Mendelsohn, 1980).

The propensity for endocrine activity in SCC, together with the presence of dense-core neurosecretory granules within tumor cells led Pearse (1969) and others (Bensch et al., 1968; Weichert, 1970; Baylin, 1975; Bonikos and Bensch, 1977) to include SCC as a neoplasm of "APUD" endocrine cells. The major facet of this theory, the joint ability of a cell to produce biologically active small polypeptide hormones and to have the capacity for biogenic amine production, was indeed identified in SCC tissues by a number of investigators (Azzopardi and Williams, 1968; Salyer and Eggleston, 1975; Baylin et al., 1978; Yesner, 1978; Baylin and Mendelsohn, 1980). A concomitant of the classification of SCC as an APUD tumor was the speculation that this tumor might arise from a neural crest cell in the bronchial mucosa (Bensch et al., 1968; Weichert, 1970; Bonikos and Bensch, 1977). This postulation stemmed from the original theory that most APUD endocrine cells probably had an embryologic origin in the neural crest (Pearse, 1969). Such a distinctive cellular origin for SCC would have placed this tumor in a separate category from the other types of human lung cancer that arise in the endodermally derived bronchial mucosa.

Over the past six years, a body of evidence has emerged that severely challenges the theory of a neural crest origin for SCC. First, as we have previously discussed, there is excellent evidence that not all APUD endocrine cells indeed arise in the neural crest. The strongest data in this regard involve the endocrine cells of the gastrointestinal tract (LeDouarin and Teillet, 1973; Andrew, 1974; 1975; 1976; Pictet et al., 1976; Fontaine and LeDouarin, 1977) and the postulation of Cheng and Leblond (1974) that a single type of progenitor cell gives rise to all of the major types of intestinal mucosal cells including the endocrine cells. Second, numerous investigators have reported that significant quantities of immunoreactive small polypeptide hormones such as ACTH, β-lipotropin, and calcitonin can be detected in all types of lung cancer, and thus are not restricted to SCC (Gewirtz and Yalow, 1974; Coombes et al., 1974; Silva et al., 1976; Odell et al., 1979; Schwartz et al., 1979; Silva et al., 1979). Third, increasing attention has been paid to the fact that mixed lung cancers exist, and features of the major histologic types of lung cancer, including SCC, have been shown to coexist in the same patient and even within the same tumor lesion (Brereton et al., 1978; Yesner, 1978; Abeloff et al., 1979). Each of these pieces of information, then, severely challenges a separate neural crest origin for SCC, and these points raise important questions about the precise relationship of endocrine biochemistry to the spectrum of human lung cancer. This relationship is important to the consideration of using endocrine markers to diagnose and monitor lung cancer patients.

Some recent work from our own group is relevant to the occurrence of endocrine activity in human lung cancer. Our first studies (Baylin et al., 1975; Baylin et al., 1978), which were restricted to SCC, further documented the heterogeneous nature of this tumor. This heterogeneity includes a variable presence of endocrine features such as concentrations of polypeptide hormones and even a key feature of the APUD concept, the enzyme L-dopa decarboxylase (the "D" in APUD). These features are different from patient to patient, from lesion to lesion in the same patient, and even from different regions of the same tumor mass (Baylin et al., 1978). Furthermore, we have found that the presence of each of the endocrine parameters investigated is shared to a degree, between each of the major histopathologic types of lung cancer (Baylin et al., 1980; Berger et al., 1980). For each marker investigated in tumor tissues, including the dopa-decarboxylase activity, much overlap in values occurred among the cancer types (Baylin et al., 1980; Berger et al., 1980). The frequent finding of a particular marker in a tumor and the chance for a high value occurring did favor SCC over the other tumor types. An endocrine index unit was constructed that represented a multiple value for four different markers in each tumor lesion; a high value for this index did separate SCC lesions from the other types except for unusual instances (Berger et al., 1980). These unusual cases were important, however, in that occasional adenocarcinomas were found to have an endocrine index unit as high as the highest values measured in SCC lesions (Berger et al., 1980).

We felt that the significance of our data lay in the further confirmation that endocrine activity is a shared property between the major types of human lung cancer. The data seem most consistent with the fact that each histologic subtype of lung cancer, including SCC, probably represents a neoplastic transformation occurring within a common cell lineage. In this cell lineage, the situation may be analogous to the gastrointestinal tract; a common basal cell progenitor in the bronchial mucosa has several directions of differentiation that it may normally take. These would include the major types of cells found in the bronchial mucosa, such as the ciliated columnar cell and the mucus-producing cell; it would also include the occasional bronchial epithelial cell with endocrine differentiation, the Kulchitzky (K) cell, and possibly the cells closely involved with the development of SCC (Baylin and Mendelsohn, 1980).

In the setting of normal bronchial mucosal differentiation discussed above, the endocrine expression of lung cancers might be closely involved with the levels of differentiation represented in the histologic tumor in question. If, within a common cell lineage, various levels of differentiation commitment involved some overlapping of cell types, then the tumors would be expected to share differentiation features to a variable degree. Such a sharing might account for the fact that endocrine-related properties would be found throughout the spectrum of lung cancer, but with a quantitative distribution favoring small cell lung carcinoma. The role of differentiation in the appearance of peptide hormones in lung cancer might also explain the high frequency with which ectopic hormone clinical syndromes occur in association with SCC. If SCC truly involves greater differentiation towards an endocrine cell, then it might be expected that the full packaging mechanisms for preparation of a biologically active small polypeptide hormone from its larger biologically inactive precursor molecule might be more intact. Indeed, as we have stated above, the existence of true ectopic hormone syndromes, such as Cushing's and inappropriate ADH secretion, are almost exclusively related to SCC among the lung cancers. We should, however, reiterate that squamous-cell carcinomas may infrequently produce a peptide with parathormone-like activity, causing significant hypercalcemia (Ratcliff and Rees, 1974; Trump and Baylin, 1979). The precise relationship of these particular tumors to the histological and biochemical spectrum of lung cancer requires further elucidation.

Having considered, in some detail, thoughts about the relationship of endocrine biochemistry to the different types of lung cancer, we must now turn to the clinical significance of endocrine biomarkers in these common forms of cancer. Numerous reports have now appeared that demonstrate a potential usefulness for measuring circulating endocrine products as a means to diagnose and/or monitor the course of lung cancer. Measurements of ACTH, ADH, calcitonin, and other hormones have all shown an appreciable incidence of increased quantities in the circulation (Amatruda et al., 1963; Liddle et al., 1969; Gewirtz and Yalow, 1974; Coombes et al., 1974; Milhaud et al., 1974; Silva et al., 1976; Silva et al., 1976; Silva et al., 1979; Roof et al., 1979; Roos et al., 1980). In some cases, there is a suggestion that the levels of each marker might parallel the course of the tumor, including responses to therapy (Silva et al., 1979). In general, the precise tracking of a tumor with any one individual marker has been disappointing (Baylin et al., 1978). For example, several different studies show that circulating levels of peptide hormones, such as ACTH, in patients with lung cancer, may not significantly differ between patients with limited disease and those with extensive disease and may not track with clinical course (Hansen and Hummer, 1979; Yalow, 1979). It is apparent, therefore, that much research is necessary to define the exact use of endocrine biomarkers in patients with lung cancer. These avenues of investigation might be divided into those involving direct measurements of the markers in the cancer tissues themselves and those aimed at investigating the utility of circulating levels of the hormones.

Studies of the tumor tissues might be directed at questioning whether profiles of endocrine-related biochemistry may, in any way, correlate with the type of histology present and, more importantly, the prognosis and/or treatment sensitivity of the particular tumor involved. For example, it has long been known that SCC transiently responds much better to irradiation and/or chemotherapy than the other types of lung cancer (Abeloff et al., 1976; Bunn et al., 1977; Weiss, 1978). However, it is being increasingly recognized that some patients with nonsmall cell bronchogenic carcinoma may also respond initially to such therapeutic modalities (Eagan, 1979; Perez et al., 1979). Could it be that a combination of endocrine related biomarkers, such as those we have discussed previously, might be a useful adjunct to histologic techniques in defining the sensitive tumors? For example, does an adenocarcinoma with a high quantity of endocrine biomarkers tend to behave more like SCC or more like the usual adenocarcinoma in terms of therapeutic response? At present, such a potential use for endocrine biomarkers in lung cancer remains the question and not a definitive answer. The current evidence certainly suggests that no single marker will correlate with a particular type of histology and, therefore, will not in any way predict prognosis or therapeutic response. A battery of such markers might define more precisely the differentiation status of any given lung tumor lesion and may be of much more value in this regard.

Tissue studies of endocrine biomarkers are also germane to consideration of using circulating levels of hormones as biomarkers in patients with lung cancer. No single hormone, such as ACTH, ADH, or calcitonin, seems likely at present to be positive in every patient with lung cancer or to necessarily follow the course of the disease. At best, more longitudinal studies with large numbers of patients must be performed with each of the circulating markers to reach definitive conclusions about the value of each marker for such purposes. Again, from the data obtained from tissue studies, it would seem likely that a battery of such markers would be (a) more likely to be positive in any given patient with lung cancer; (b) truly reflect the changes in tumor burden occurring with any treatment modality; and (c) be of prognostic significance in predicting the type of tumor present and its eventual course. Studies to address this question must be forthcoming and will have to involve large enough populations of patients to make accurate predictions in this regard.

Finally, the existence of endocrine syndromes in patients with lung cancer will always be important to the clinician. In patients with SCC, awareness of the potential for the abnormal electrolyte values that accompany excess secretion of ADH and/or ACTH, and their clinical ramifications must always be part of patient management. Evidence is also increasing, however, that the more subtle presentation of such syndromes may have prognostic value in patients with lung cancer. With proper provocative testing, delineation of abnormal water loading responses or abnormal diurnal variations in plasma cortisol values may predict a situation of poor clinical response in patients with all types of lung cancer. Studies on the use of endocrine biomarkers should, therefore, involve continued efforts to delineate precise syndromes that result from their presence, more sophisticated means to identify subclinical variations of these syndromes, and a quantitation of the prognostic significance of the presence of the subclinical variant.

In summary, the relationship of endocrine biochemistry to lung cancer is a complex and still poorly understood one. Evidence is accumulating that such endocrine parameters are important features of lung tumor differentiation and of the relationships between the major histopathologic types of lung cancer. The development of increasingly sensitive immunoassay and immunohistological techniques may provide valuable methods whereby the presence of various peptide hormones in normal, metaplastic, and neoplastic bronchial epithelium can be studied; and whereby the relationship of hormones to tumor evolution can be evaluated further.

5.2. Neural Tumors

Neural tumors, particularly those occurring in infancy and childhood, are not infrequently associated with ectopic endocrine activity. Diarrheal syndromes (Rosenstein and Engelman, 1963; Hamilton et al., 1968; Fausa et al., 1973; Swift et al., 1975; Mitchell et al., 1976), hypertension (Kogut and Kaplan, 1962), and Cushing's syndrome (Kogut and Donnell, 1961) have been encountered. In addition, hormones such as calcitonin and the biogenic amines may be produced by these tumors in the absence of clinically evident syndromes (Trump et al., 1977). The study of ectopic hormone production and of hormonally mediated syndromes in patients with a variety of neural and neuroblastic tumors has yielded some extremely interesting results, which have important implications for the relationship between the expression of ectopic endocrine activity and tumor differentiation.

Hormonally mediated diarrhea is the commonest endocrine syndrome encountered in patients with neural tumors, particularly during infancy and childhood (Rosenstein and Engelman, 1963; Hamilton et al.,

1968; Fausa et al., 1973; Swift et al., 1975; Mitchell et al., 1976; Trump et al., 1977; Mendelsohn et al., 1979b). For many years, there was considerable doubt concerning the precise hormonal agent responsible for the diarrhea in patients with neural tumors. These neural tumors have long been known to produce catecholamines and initially the biogenic amines were implicated (Rosenstein and Engelman, 1963). It seemed unlikely, even then, that the biogenic amines alone were responsible for the diarrhea since diarrhea is not a feature of patients with pheochromocytoma, despite the presence of very high levels of these products. Furthermore, many patients with neuroblastic tumors have diarrhea, but normal catecholamine levels (Peterson and Collins, 1967). Following reports of the watery diarrhea–hypokalemia–hypochlorhydria (WDHH or "pancreatic cholera") syndrome in patients with pancreatic islet cell tumors (Verner and Morrison, 1958) and the discovery that many cases could be attributed to the production of excess polypeptides, including vasoactive intestinal peptide (VIP), by the tumors (Gjone et al., 1970; Semb et al., 1970; Bloom et al., 1973; Said and Faloona, 1975), it was shown that some patients with neural tumors had typical WDHH syndrome. The diarrheal syndrome in these patients is characterized by unrelenting diarrhea, hypokalemia resulting from profound fecal potassium loss, hypochlorhydria or achlorhydria; less frequent features include hyperglycemia, hypercalcemia, and occasionally marked vasodilatation leading to flushing and hypotension (Verner and Morrison,1958; 1974). The diarrhea is caused by massive water and electrolyte secretion by gastrointestinal epithelial cells, resulting from stimulation of the adenyl cyclase system, a well known property of VIP (Schwartz et al., 1974). In many cases, serum and tumor tissue assays have revealed large quantities of VIP (Said and Faloona, 1975; Swift et al., 1975; Mitchell et al., 1976; Udall et al., 1976; Jansen-Goemans and Engelhardt, 1977; Trump et al., 1977); furthermore, in some cases, it has been possible to demonstrate VIP within tumor cells using immunohistochemical techniques (Mendelsohn et al., 1979b).

Recent immunohistochemical studies of neural tissue and, most recently, studies of tumors in cell culture have provided important information relative to the presence of polypeptide hormones in normal and neoplastic tissues. Several groups have localized VIP within neurons and nerve fibers of the central and peripheral nervous system using immunohistochemical techniques (Bryant et al., 1976; Larsson et al., 1976a; 1976b; Fuxe et al., 1977; Hökfelt et al., 1977; Mendelsohn et al., 1979b). In a recent study from our laboratory (Mendelsohn et al., 1979b), we were able to demonstrate VIP within normal sympathetic ganglion cells and nerve fibers, and within differentiating and mature neoplastic ganglion cells in a spectrum of neuroblastic tumors including ganglioneuroblastomas, ganglioneuromas, and an unusual composite ganglioneuroma–pheochromocytoma. We could not demonstrate VIP in (undifferentiated) neuroblasts, Schwann cells, or in pheochromocytes. The presence of VIP in ganglion cells of several ganglioneuromas, including some with typical WDHH syndrome, is certainly consistent with a role for the peptide in the production of the diarrheal syndrome. More significant from a biological standpoint, however, is the association of the peptide with ganglion cell differentiation. Recent evidence from other groups supports these findings. Tischler and Greene (1975; 1978) have reported on a rat pheochromocytoma cell line that, when exposed in culture to nerve growth factor, acquires morphological and cytochemical neuronal properties. In subsequent studies, Tischler and his co-workers (1980) have been able to show the appearance of increased VIP immunoreactivity occurring as part of this neuronal transformation of the pheo-chromocytoma tissue; their assay and immunohistochemical studies have shown abundant immunoreactive VIP in the transformed cells while little was present in the unaltered pheochromocytes.

The above studies must, however, be considered in the light of recent reports of polypeptide hormone production by pheochromocytomas. Although assayable immunoreactive VIP has been reported in pheo-chromocytoma tissue (Said and Faloona, 1975), cellular localization of the peptide has not been demonstrated. Findings with respect to other peptide hormones in pheochromocytoma are also important. Ectopic secretion of ACTH has been reported in this tumor (Forman et al., 1979; Sparks et al., 1979) and calcitonin, a peptide frequently reported to be present in a wide variety of tumors, including neural tumors (Trump et al., 1977; Mendel-sohn et al., 1979b), has also has been demonstrated in increased amounts (Voelkel et al., 1973; Rause et al., 1978; Heath and Edis, 1979). In some reports (Heath and Edis, 1979) there has indeed been good biochemical evidence for calcitonin production by pheochromocytoma, but in none of these reported cases have localization studies been undertaken. In an immunohistochemical study of calcitonin in several pheochromocytomas from patients with and without medullary thyroid carcinoma, we were unable to demonstrate immunoreactive calcitonin in pheochromocytes (Mendelsohn et al., 1980a). The only pheochromocytomas in which we could demonstrate immunoreactive calcitonin were those with deposits of metastatic medullary thyroid carcinoma; the calcitonin was present within the medullary carcinoma cells. The question of whether amine-producing pheochromocytes and adrenal medullary cells can synthesize and secrete peptides such as VIP, ACTH, and calcitonin is a most important one and deserves further investigation. Certainly, it would be extremely interesting to know whether in polypeptide-producing pheochromocytomas such as that recently reported by Heath and Edis (1979), the polypeptides can be localized using immunohistochemical methods. It is quite possible that the differences which have been encountered in the various neuroblastic and neural tumors are quantitative rather than purely qualitative; that peptide production is amplified in those neuroblastic tumors with ganglion cell differentiation while biogenic amine production is amplified in elements with pheochromocytomatous or paragangliomatous differentiation. A variety of polypeptides other than those mentioned above, such as gastrin and cholecystokinin, have been shown to normally be present in small quantities in neural tissue (Vanderhaegen et al., 1975; Dockray, 1976). The appearance of these peptides in increased amounts in neural tumors may thus likewise reflect an amplification of normal activity, occurring within the tumor, rather than an entirely abnormal or inappropriate phenomenon.

The study of peptide hormones in neurogenic tumors has thus provided important biological information concerning the relationships between directions and degrees of cellular differentiation and hormone elaboration. From these studies, hormonal syndromes in patients with neural tumors are being better understood; and, finally, it is hoped that peptide hormone markers, valuable in the clinical arena, might be forthcoming.

5.3. Prostatic Carcinoma

Despite the apparently remote differentiation relationships of the prostate to the pituitary gland, there are several well-documented cases of Cushing's syndrome occurring in patients with prostatic carcinoma (Newmark et al., 1973; Lovern et al., 1975; Wenk et al., 1977; Vuitch and Mendelsohn, 1980). Such cases are extremely uncommon and peptide hormone endocrine markers, unlike steroid hormones, have little clinical or practical impact in the management of patients with prostatic carcinoma. From a biological standpoint, however, the occurrence of ectopic endocrine activity in prostatic carcinomas has important implications with regard to underlying mechanisms of ectopic (inappropriate) hormone production. It is important, at the outset, to indicate that ectopic ACTH production has not been restricted to any single morphologic variant of prostatic carcinoma. Although the majority of prostatic carcinomas associated with ACTH production have been ''small cell'' carcinomas (Newmark et al., 1973; Wenk et al., 1977), others have been characteristic adenocarcinomas (Lovern et al., 1975).

Some workers have attempted to explain the ectopic production of ACTH in prostatic carcinomas by incriminating the APUD–neural crest theory (Wenk et al., 1977). As discussed earlier, hormone producing tumors would be derived from APUD cells normally present within the prostate; these, in turn, would be of neural crest origin (Pearse, 1966; 1969; Weichert, 1970). Azzopardi and Evans (1971) were the first to demonstrate APUD (argyrophilic and argentaffinic) cells within the normal prostate and in prostatic adenocarcinomas. In addition to noting the presence of such cells in approximately 10% of prostatic adenocarcinomas, they mention two cases of mixed adenocarcinoma–''carcinoid tumor'' occurring in the prostate. They explained the occurrence of argentaffinic cells on the basis of "divergent differentiation" within the prostatic carcinomas. Vuitch and Mendelsohn (1980), recently reported a case which strongly supports their contention and provides further evidence that APUD characteristics and the ability to produce polypeptide hormones do not necessarily imply origin from an endocrine progenitor cell. The case in question is that of a patient with prostatic carcinoma who developed Cushing's syndrome during the course of his illness. There was a clear progression from a moderately well-differentiated adenocarcinoma to a dimorphic tumor with moderately well-differentiated and anaplastic components. Immunoreactive ACTH could be demonstrated only within the anaplastic component of the tumor, suggesting a relationship of ectopic endocrine activity to a particular level of differentiation within the tumor.

Reports of ectopic peptide hormone production and Cushing's syndrome occurring in patients with carcinoma of the uterine cervix also exist (Shane and Naftolin, 1975; Jones et al., 1976; Matsuyama et al., 1979; Lojek et al., 1980). Again, such cases have been explained by incriminating APUD cells of neural crest origin. In this regard, it must be emphasized that there is no conclusive evidence in support of neural crest-derived cells within the female genitourinary tract.

It is highly likely, then, that mechanisms other than "endocrine cell origin" are operable in the expression of endocrine activity by tumors such as prostatic carcinoma and cervical carcinoma. Although the peptide-producing tumor cells and argyrophilic or argentaffinic cells normally present in these organs manifest true "endocrine" characteristics, this need not necessarily reflect specific embryologic origin. It seems likely, as discussed above, that the endocrine cells arise through differentiation processes ongoing in the normal or neoplastic epithelium in these tissues.

6. Summary

In this review, we have attempted to outline some of the important characteristics of peptide hormone production by endocrine and non-endocrine tumors; and in so doing, we have considered some clinical and biological implications of this endocrine activity in neoplasms. We have not attempted to cover all peptide hormone-producing tumors, nor have we discussed all the peptide hormones that tumors may produce; many of those we have not discussed are covered in other chapters. We have considered some of the theories that have been advanced to explain inappropriate (ectopic) endocrine activity in tumors and have related these theories to the various patterns of inappropriate hormone production. In discussing the association of peptide hormones with specific tumors, we have attempted to show that, in many tumors, the expression of specific endocrine activity may be related to ongoing differentiation processes within the tumors. These processes, in turn, may be closely related to cellular events in the normal tissues in which the tumors arise. The hormones and clinical syndromes discussed are of increasing importance in the clinical arena, and many of the tumors, such as medullary thyroid carcinoma and neurogenic tumors, provide important targets for the study of peptide hormone biosynthesis and secretion. Continued studies should yield pivotal information about the mechanisms involved in the expression of such endocrine activity in tumors, and these findings may also develop insight into the regulatory events that guide cellular differentiation and the control of gene expression. In turn, the information may enhance our understanding of the evolution of cell populations in tumors, and thus aid our efforts to refine existing therapeutic and diagnostic approaches and to define new ones.

References

Abe, K., I. Adachi, S. Miyakawa, M. Tanaka, K. Yamaguchi, N. Kameya, and Y. Shimosato (1977), *Cancer Res.* **37**, 490.

Abelev, G. I. (1974), *Transplant Rev.* **20**, 3.

Abeloff, M. D., D. S. Ettinger, S. B. Baylin, and T. Hazra (1976), *Cancer* **38**, 1394.

Abeloff, M. D., J. C. Eggleston, G. Mendelsohn, D. S. Ettinger, and S. B. Baylin (1979), *Am. J. Med.* **66**, 757.

Acevedo, H. F., M. Sliskin, and G. R. Pouchet (1978), in *Detection and Prevention of Cancer, Part 2* (Nieburgs, H. E., ed.), Dekker, New York, pp. 1, 937.

Alberti, K. G. M. M., N. J. Christensen, and S. E. Christensen (1973), *Lancet* **2**, 1229.

Albright, F., and E. C. Reifenstein, eds. (1948), in *The Parathyroid Glands and Metabolic Bone Disease—Selected Studies*, Williams and Wilkins, Baltimore.

Amatruda, T. T., Jr., P. J. Murlow, J. C. Gallagher, and W. H. Sawyer (1963), *N. Engl. J. Med.* **269**, 544.

Anderson, G. (1973), in *Recent Advances in Medicine*, (Baton, D. N., N. H. Compston, A. M. Dawson, eds.), Churchill Livingston, Edinburgh, p. 1.

Andrew, A. (1974), *J. Embryol. Exptl. Morphol.* **31**, 589.

Andrew, A. (1975), *Gen. Comp. Endocrinol.* **26**, 485.

Andrew, A. (1976), *J. Embryol. Exp. Morphol.* **35**, 577.

Appleyard, T. N., and M. S. Losowsky (1970), *Postgrad. Med. J.* **46**, 159.

Ayvazian, L. G., B. Schneider, G. Gewirtz, and R. S. Yalow (1975), *Ann. Rev. Resp. Dis.* **111**, 279.

Azzopardi, J. G., and E. D. Williams (1968), *Cancer* **22**, 274.

Azzopardi, J. G., and D. J. Evans (1971), *J. Pathol.* **104**, 247.

Baylin, S. B. (1975), *Hosp. Pract.* **10**, 117.

Baylin, S. B., M. D. Abeloff, K. C. Wieman, J. W. Tomford, and D. S. Ettinger (1975), *N. Engl. J. Med.* **293**, 1286.

Baylin, S. B., W. R. Weisburger, J. C. Eggleston, G. Mendelsohn, M. A. Beaven, M. D. Abeloff, and D. S. Ettinger (1978), *N. Engl. J. Med.* **299**, 105.

Baylin, S. B., G. Mendelsohn, and M. A. Levine (1979a), *Johns Hopkins Med. J.* **145**, 201.

Baylin, S. B., G. Mendelsohn, W. R. Weisburger, D. S. Gann, and J. C. Eggleston (1979b), *Cancer* **44**, 1315.

Baylin, S. B., and G. Mendelsohn (1980), *Endocrine Rev.* **1**, 45.

Baylin, S. B., M. D. Abeloff, G. Goodwin, D. N. Carney, and A. F. Gazdar (1980), *Cancer Res.* **40**, 1990.

Becker, K. L., R. H. Snider, O. L. Silva, and C. F. Moore (1978), *Acta Endocrinol.* **89**, 89.

Becker, K. L., K. G. Monoghan, and O. L. Silva (1980), *Arch. Pathol. Lab. Med.* **104**, 196.

Bensch, K. G., B. Corrin, R. Parienta, and H. Spencer (1968), *Cancer* **22**, 1163.

Berger, C. L., G. Mendelsohn, J. C. Eggleston, M. D. Abeloff, and S. B. Baylin (1980), *Proceedings of the 62nd Annual Meeting, The Endocrine Society* **273**, Abstr. 795.

Berson, S. A., and R. S. Yalow (1968), *J. Clin. Endocrinol. Metab.* **28**, 1037.

Bertagna, X. Y., W. E. Nicholson, G. D. Sorensen, O. D. Pettengill, G. D. Mount, and D. N. Orth (1978a), *Proc. Natl. Acad. Sci. USA* **75**, 5160.

Bertagna, X. Y., W. E. Nicholson, O. S. Pettergill, G. D. Sorenson, C. D. Mount, and D. N. Orth (1978b), *J. Clin. Endocrinol. Metab.* **47**, 1390.

Birkenhäger, J. C., G. V. Upton, H. J. Seldenrath, D. T. Krieger, and A. H. Tashjian, Jr. (1976), *Acta Endocrinol.* **83**, 280.

Blackman, M. R., S. W. Rosen, and B. D. Weintraub (1978), *Adv. Int. Med.* **23**, 85.

Bloom, F., E. Battenberg, J. Rossier, N. Ling, J. Lepparluoto, T. M. Vargo, and R. Guillemin (1977), *Life Sci.* **20**, 43.

Bloom, S. R., J. M. Polak, and A. G. E. Pearse (1973), *Lancet* **2**, 14.

Bonikos, D. S., and K. G. Bensch (1977), *Am. J. Med.* **63**, 765.

Braunstein, G. D., J. L. Vaitukaitis, P. P. Carbone, and G. T. Ross (1973), *Ann. Int. Med.* **78**, 39.

Brereton, H. D., M. M. Matthews, J. Costa, H. Kent, and R. E. Johnson (1978), *Ann. Int. Med.* **88**, 805.

Brown, W. H. (1928), *Lancet* **2**, 1022.

Bryant, M. D., J. M. Polak, I. Modlin, S. R. Bloom, R. H. Alburquerque, and A. G. E. Pearse (1976), *Lancet* **1**, 991.

Bunn, P. A., M. H. Cohen, and D. C. Ihde (1977), *Cancer Treat. Rept.* **61**, 333.

Capella, C., C. Bordi, G. Monga, R. Buffa, P. Fontana, S. Bonfani, G. Bussolati, and E. Solcia (1978), *Virch. Arch. A. Path. Anat.* **377**, 111.

Cheng, H., and C. P. Leblond (1974), *Am. J. Anat.* **141**, 537.

Chong, G. C., O. H. Beahrs, G. W. Sizemore, and L. B. Woolner (1975), *Cancer* **35**, 695.

Cline, M. J., and D. W. Golde (1979), *Blood* **53**, 157.

Coombes, R. C., P. B. Greenberg, C. Hillyard, and I. MacIntyre (1974), *Lancet* **1**, 1080.

Cooper, C. W., T. C. Peng, J. F. Obie, and S. C. Garner (1980), Endocrinol. **107**, 98.

Crick, F. (1979), *Science* **204**, 264.

Dayal, Y., D. S. O'Briain, H. J. Wolfe, and S. Reichlin (1980), *Lab. Invest.* **42**, 111 (Abstr.).

Deftos, L. J., D. Burton, B. D. Catherwood, H. G. Bone, J. G. Parthemore, R. Guillemin, W. B. Watkins, and R. Y. Moore (1978), *J. Clin. Endocrinol. Metab.* **47**, 457.

DeLellis, R. A., and H. J. Wolfe (1976), *Arch. Pathol. Lab. Med.* **100**, 340 (Letter).

Dockray, G. J. (1976), *Nature* **264**, 568.

Dollinger, M. R., L. H. Ratner, C. A. Shamoian, and B. D. Blackbourne (1967), *Arch. Int. Med.* **120**, 575.

Donahower, G. F., O. P. Schumacher, and J. B. Hazard (1968), *J. Clin. Endocrinol. Metab.* **28**, 1199.

Eagan, R. T. (1979), in *Lung Cancer: Progress in Therapeutic Research* (Muggia, F. M. and M. Rozencweig, eds.), Raven Press, New York, pp. 383–392.

Eipper, B. A., and R. E. Mains (1980), *Endocrine. Rev.* **1**, 1.

Faiman, C., J. A. Colwell, R. J. Ryan, J. M. Hershman, and T. W. Shields (1967), *N. Engl. J. Med.* **277**, 1395.

Falck, B. (1962), *Acta. Physiol. Scand.* **56**, (Suppl.) **197**, 1.

Fausa, O., B. Fretheim, K. Elgjo, L. S. Semb, and E. Gjone (1973), *Scand. J. Gastroenterol.* **8**, 713.

Fontaine, J., and N. M. LeDouarin (1971), *C. R. Acad. Sci. (Paris)* **273**, 1299.

Fontaine, J., and N. M. LeDouarin (1977), *J. Embryol. Exptl. Morphol.* **41**, 209.

Forman, B. H., E. Marban, R. D. Kayne, N. M. Passarelli, S. N. Bobrow, V. A. Livolsi, M. Merino, M. Minor, and L. R. Farber (1979), *Yale J. Biol. Med.* **52**, 181.

Foster, G. V., I. MacIntyre, and A. G. E. Pearse (1964), *Nature* **203**, 1029.

Fröhlich, J. C., Z. T. Bloomgarden, J. A. Oates, J. E. McGuigan, and D. Rabinowitz (1978), *New Engl. J. Med.* **299**, 1055.

Fuxe, K., T. Hökfelt, S. I. Said, and V. Mutt (1977), *Neurosci. Lett.* **5**, 241.

Galmiche, J. P., R. Colin, P. M. DuBois, J. A. Chayvialle, F. Descos, C. Paulin, and Y. Geffroy (1978), *New Engl. J. Med.* **299**, 1252.

Ganda, O. P., G. C. Weir, J. S. Soeldner, M. A. Legg, W. L. Chick, Y. C. Patel, A. M. Ebeid, K. H. Gabbay, and S. Reichlin (1977), *New Engl. J. Med.* **296**, 1977.

Gellhorn, A. (1969), *Adv. Int. Med.* **15**, 299.

George, J. M., C. C. Capen, and A. S. Phillips (1972), *J. Clin. Invest.* **51**, 141.

Gewirtz, G., and R. S. Yalow (1973), *Endocrinol.* **92** (Suppl), A-53.

Gewirtz, G., and R. S. Yalow (1974), *J. Clin. Invest.* **53**, 1022.

Gjone, E., B. Fretheim, A. Nördoy, C. D. Jacobsen, and K. Elgjo (1970), *Scand. J. Gastroenterol.* **5**, 401.

Godwin, J. D. (1975), *Cancer* **36**, 560.

Gorden, P., B. Sherman, and J. Roth (1971), *J. Clin. Invest.* **50**, 2113.

Guillemin, R., T. M. Vargo, J. Rossier, S. Minick, N. Ling, C. Rivier, W. Vale, and F. Bloom (1977), *Science* **197,** 1367.

Habener, J. R., B. Kemper, and J. T. Potts (1972), *Science* **178,** 630.

Hamilton, J. R., I. C. Radde, and G. Johnson (1968), *Am. J. Med.* **44,** 453.

Hansen, H. H., P. Dombernowsky, and F. R. Hirsch (1978), *Semin. Oncol.* **5,** 280.

Hansen, M., and L. Hummer (1979), in *Lung Cancer: Progress in Therapeutic Research* (Muggia, T. M., and M. Rozencweig, M., eds.), New York, Raven Press, p. 207.

Heath, H., and A. J. Edis (1979), *Ann. Int. Med.* **91,** 208.

Hennessy, J. F., S. A. Wells, Jr., D. A. Ontjes, and C. W. Cooper (1974), *J. Clin. Endocrinol. Metab.* **39,** 487.

Hirsch, P. F., and P. L. Munson (1969), *Physiol. Rev.* **49,** 548.

Hirsch, P. F., and H. H. Hansen, P. Dombernowsky, and B. Hainan (1977), *Cancer* **39,** 2563.

Hökfelt, T., L. G. Elfvin, M. Schultzberg, S. I. Said, V. Mutt, and M. Goldstein (1977), *Neuroscience* **2,** 885.

Hoyt, R. F., Jr., D. W. Hamilton, and A. H. Tashjian, Jr. (1973), *Anat. Rec.* **176,** 1.

Hutcheon, D. F., T. M. Bayless, J. L. Cameron, and S. B. Baylin (1979), *Ann. Int. Med.* **90,** 932.

Isenberg, J. I., J. H. Walsh, and M. I. Grossman (1973), *Gastroenterol.* **65,** 140.

Iwanaga, T., H. Koyama, S. Uchiyama, Y. Takahashi, S. Nakano, T. Itoh, T. Horai, A. Wada, and R. Tateishi (1978), *Cancer* **41,** 1106.

Jackson, C. E., A. H. Tashjian, Jr., and M. A. Block (1973), *Ann. Int. Med.* **78,** 845.

Jaffe, B. M., D. F. Kopen, K. DeSchryver-Kecskemeti, R. L. Gingerich, M. Greider (1977), *N. Engl. J. Med.* **297,** 817.

Jansen-Goemans, A., and J. Engelhardt (1977), *Pediatrics* **59,** 710.

Jones, H. W., III, S. Plymak, F. B. Gluck, P. A. Miles, and J. F. Greene, Jr. (1976), *Cancer* **38,** 1629.

Julliard, J. H., T. Shibasaki, N. Ling, and R. Guillemin (1980), *Science* **208,** 183.

Kahn, C. R., S. W. Rosen, B. D. Weintraub, S. S. Fajans, and P. Gorden (1977), *N. Engl. J. Med.* **297,** 565.

Kameya, T., Y. Shimosato, I. Adachi, K. Abe, N. Kasai, K. Kimura, and K. Baba (1977), *Am. J. Pathol.* **89,** 555.

Khairi, M. R. A., R. N. Dexter, N. J. Burzynski, and C. C. Johnston, Jr. (1975), *Medicine* (Baltimore) **54,** 89.

Klemperer, P. (1923), *Surg. Gynecol. Obstet.* **36,** 11.

Koerker, D. J., W. Ruch, and E. Chideckel (1974), *Science* **184,** 482.

Kogut, M. D., and G. N. Donnell (1961), *Pediatrics* **28,** 566.

Kogut, M. D., and S. A. Kaplan (1962), *J. Pediatr.* **60,** 694.

Lamers, C. B. H., and J. H. M. van Tongeren (1977), *Gut* **18,** 128.

Larsson, L.-I., J. Fahrenkrug, O. Muckadell de Schaffalittzky, F. Sundler, R. Håkansson, and J. F. Rehfeld (1976a), *Proc. Natl. Acad. Sci. USA* **73,** 3197.

Larsson, L.-I., L. Edvinsson, J. Fahrenkrug, R. Håkansson, C. H. Owman, O. Muckadell de Schaffalittzky, and F. Sundler (1976b), *Brain Res.* **113,** 400.

Larsson, L. I., J. J. Holst, C. Kühl, G. Lundquist, M. A. Hirsch, S. Ingemansson, S. Lindkaer-Jensen, and J. F. Rehfeld (1977), *Lancet* 1, 666.

Law, D. H., G. W. Liddle, H. W. Scott, Jr., and S. D. Tauber (1965), *N. Engl. J. Med.* 273, 292.

Lechargo, J. (1978), *Pathol. Ann.* 13, 2, 329.

LeDouarin, N. M., and C. LeLievre (1971), *C. R. Assn. Anat.* 152, 558.

LeDouarin, N. M., and M. A. Teillet (1973), *J. Embryol. Exptl. Morphol.* 30, 31.

LeDouarin, N. M., C. LeLievre, and J. Fontaine (1972), *C. R. Acad. Sci.* (*Paris*) 275D, 583.

Lee, A. K., H. J. Wolfe, R. F. Gagel, R. A. DeLellis, A. H. Tashjian, Jr., and L. S. Adelman (1980), *Lab. Invest.* 42, 131 (abstr.).

Liddle, G. W., W. E. Nicholson, D. P. Island, D. N. Orth, K. Abe, and S. C. Lowder (1969), *Rec. Progr. Hormone Res.* 25, 283.

Lips, C. J. M., J. Veer Sluys Vander, J. A. van der Donk, R. H. van Dam, and W. H. L. Hackeng (1978), *Lancet* 1, 16.

Lipsett, M. B., W. D. Odell, L. E. Rosenberg, and T. A. Waldman (1964), *Ann. Int. Med.* 61, 733.

Lojek, M. A., M. F. Fer, A. G. Kasselberg, A. D. Glick, L. S. Burnett, C. G. Julian, F. A. Greco, and R. K. Oldham (1980), *Am. J. Med.* 69, 140.

Lovern, W. J., B. L. Fariss, J. N. Wettlanfer, and S. Hane (1975), *Urology* 5, 817.

Mains, R. E., B. A. Eipper, and N. Ling (1977), *Proc. Natl. Acad. Sci.* 74, 3014.

Matsuyama, M., T. Inoue, Y. Ariyoshi, M. Doi, T. Suchi, T. Sato, K. Tashiro, and T. Chihara (1979), *Cancer* 44, 1813.

Matthews, M. J. (1976), in *Lung Cancer, Natural History, Prognosis and Therapy*, Ch. 2, Israel, L. (ed), London, Academic Press.

McGuire, W. L. (1978), *Semin. Oncol.* 5, 428.

Meador, C. K., G. W. Liddle, D. P. Island, W. E. Nicholson, C. P. Lucas, J. G. Nuckton, and J. A. Leutscher (1962), *J. Clin. Endocrinol. Metab.* 22, 693.

Melvin, K. E. W., H. H. Miller, and A. H. Tashjian, Jr. (1977), *New Engl. J. Med.* 285, 1115.

Melvin, K. E. W. (1974), *Ann. NY Acad. Sci.* 230, 378.

Mendelsohn, G., J. C. Eggleston, W. R. Weisburger, D. S. Gann, and S. B. Baylin (1978), *Am. J. Pathol.* 32, 35.

Mendelsohn, G., R. D'Agostino, J. C. Eggleston, and S. B. Baylin (1979a), *J. Clin. Invest.* 63, 1297.

Mendelsohn, G., J. C. Eggleston, J. L. Olson, S. I. Said, S. B. Baylin (1979b), *Lab. Invest.* 41, 144.

Mendelsohn, G., S. B. Baylin, and J. C. Eggleston (1980a), *Cancer* 45, 498.

Mendelsohn, G., S. H. Bigner, J. C. Eggleston, S. B. Baylin, and S. A. Wells, Jr. (1980b), *Am. J. Surg. Pathol.* 4, 333.

Milhaud, G., C. Calmette, J. Taboulet, A. Julienne, and M. S. Moukhtar (1974), *Lancet* 1, 462.

Mitchell, C. H., F. R. Sinatra, F. W. Crast, R. Griffin, and P. Sunshine (1976), *J. Pediatr.* 89, 593.

Nakanishi, S., A. Inoue, S. Taii, and S. Numa (1977), *FEBS Lett.* 84, 105.

Nakanishi, S., A. Inoue, T. Kita, M. Nakamura, A. C. Y. Chang, S. N. Cohen, and S. Numa (1979), *Nature* **278**, 423.

Nakao, Y., M. Tsuruzawa, H. Kanaoka, K. Tanioka, and M. Sudo (1975), *Clin. Endocrinol.* (Tokyo) **23**, 603.

Nathans, D. (1979), *Science* **203**, 903.

Newmark, S. R., R. G. Dluhy, and A. H. Bennett (1973), *Urology* **2**, 666.

Odell, W. D., A. Wolfsen, Y. Yoshimoto, R. Weitzman, D. Fisher, and F. Hirose (1977), *Trans. Assoc. Am. Phys.* **90**, 204.

Odell, W. D., A. R. Wolfsen, I. Bachelot, and F. M. Hirose (1979), *Am J. Med.* **66**, 631.

O'Neal, L. W., D. M. Kipnis, and S. A. Luse (1968), *Cancer* **21**, 1219.

Orth, D. N., W. E. Nicholson, W. M. Mitchell, D. P. Island, and G. W. Liddle (1973), *J. Clin. Invest.* **52**, 1756.

Parthemore, J. G., D. Bronzert, and G. Roberts (1974), *J. Clin. Endocrinol. Metab.* **39**, 108.

Patchefsky, A. S., R. Solit, L. D. Phillips, M. Cradlock, W. V. Harrer, H. E. Cohn, and O. D. Kowlessar (1972), *Ann. Int. Med.* **77**, 53.

Pearse, A. G. E. (1966a), *Nature* **211**, 598.

Pearse, A. G. E. (1966b), *Vet. Rec.* **79**, 587.

Pearse, A. G. E. (1969), *J. Histochem. Cytochem.* **17**, 303.

Pearse, A. G. E., and A. F. Carvalheira (1967), *Nature*, **214**, 929.

Pearse, A. G. E., and J. M. Polak (1967), *Histochem.* **27**, 96.

Pearse, A. G. E., J. M. Polak, F. W. D. Rost, J. Fontaine, C. LeLievre, and N. M. LeDouarin (1973), *Histochemistry*, **34**, 191.

Pearse, A. G. E., J. M. Polak, and C. M. Heath (1974), *Virch. Arch. Zellpathol.* **16**, 95.

Pearse, A. G. E., and T. T. Takor (1979), *Fed. Proc.* **38**, 2288.

Perez, C. A., K. Stanley, and W. Mietlowski (1979), in *Lung Cancer: Progress in Therapeutic Research* (Muggia, F. M., and M. Rozencweig, eds.), Raven Press, New York, pp.295–314.

Peterson, H. D., and O. D. Collins (1967), *Arch. Surg.* **95**, 934.

Phifer, R. F., D. N. Orth, and S. S. Spicer (1974), *J. Clin. Endocrinol. Metab.* **39**, 684.

Pictet, R. L., L. B. Rall, P. Phelps, and W. J. Rutter (1976), *Science* **191**, 191.

Polak, J. M., A. G. E. Pearse, C. LeLievre, J. Fontaine, and N. M. LeDouarin (1974), *Histochemistry* **40**, 209.

Quesenberry, P., and L. Levitt (1979a), *N. Engl. J. Med.* **301**, 755.

Quesenberry, P., and L. Levitt (1979b), *N. Engl. J. Med.* **301**, 819.

Quesenberry, P., and L. Levitt (1979c), *N. Engl. J. Med.* **301**, 868.

Rabson, A. S., S. W. Rosen, A. H. Tashjian, Jr., and B. D. Weintraub (1973), *J. Natl. Cancer Inst.* **50**, 669.

Ratcliff, J. G., and L. H. Rees (1974), *Brit. J. Hosp. Med.* **1**, 658.

Raue, F., J. M. Bayer, K. H. Rahn, C. Herfarth, H. Minne, and R. Ziegler (1978), *Klin. Wochenschr.* **56**, 697.

Rees, L. H., G. A. Bloomfield, G. M. Rees, B. Corrin, C. M. Franks, and J. G. Ratcliff (1974), *J. Clin. Endocrinol. Metab.* **38**, 1090.

Robboy, S. J., R. E. Scully, and H. J. Norris (1977), *Obstet. Gynecol.* **49**, 202.

Roberts, J. L., and E. Herbert (1977), *Proc. Natl. Acad. Sci. USA* **74**, 5300.

Roof, B. S., R. Weinstein, I. Vujic, and N. M. Burdash (1979), *Biomedicine* **30**, 82.

Roos, B. A., A. W. Lindall, S. B. Baylin, J. A. O'Neil, A. L. Frelinger, R. S. Birnbaum, and P. W. Lambert (1980), *J. Clin. Endocrinol. Metab.* **50**, 659.

Rosai, J., and E. Higa (1972), *Cancer* **29**, 1061.

Rosen, S. W., C. E. Becker, S. Schlaff, J. Easton, M. C. Gluck (1968), *N. Engl. J. Med.* **279**, 640.

Rosen, S. W., B. D. Weintraub, J. L. Vaitukaitis, H. H. Sussman, J. M. Hershman, and F. M. Muggia (1975), *Ann. Int. Med.* **82**, 71.

Rosenstein, B. J., and K. Engelman (1963), *J. Pediatr.* **63**, 217.

Said, S. I., and G. R. Faloona (1975), *N. Engl. J. Med.* **293**, 155.

Salyer, D. C., and J. C. Eggleston (1975), *Arch. Pathol.* **99**, 513.

Salyer, D. C., W. R. Salyer, and J. C. Eggleston (1975), *Cancer* **36**, 1522.

Sayle, B. A., P. A. Lang, W. O. Green, Jr., W. C. Bosworth, and R. Gregory (1965), *Ann. Int. Med.* **63**, 58.

Schimke, R. N., and W. H. Hartman (1965), *Ann. Int. Med.* **63**, 1027.

Schimke, R. N., W. H. Hartman, T. E. Prout, and D. L. Rimoin (1968), *New Engl. J. Med.* **279**, 1.

Schorr, I., P. Rathnam, B. B. Saxena, and R. L. Ney (1971), *J. Biol. Chem.* **246**, 5806.

Schwartz, C. J., D. V. Kimberg, H. E. Sheerin, M. Field, and S. I. Said (1974), *J. Clin. Invest.* **54**, 536.

Schwartz, K. E., A. R. Wolfsen, B. Forster, and W. D. Odell (1979), *J. Clin. Endocrinol. Metab.* **49**, 438.

Semb, L., E. Gjone, and W. S. Rosenthal (1970), *Scand. J. Gastroenterol.* **5**, 409.

Setlow, J. K., and A. Hollaender, eds. (1979), *Genetic Engineering,* Plenum Press, New York.

Shane, J. M., and F. Naftolin (1975), *Am. J. Obstet. Gynecol.* **121**, 133.

Shearer, R. W., and A. H. Dodge (1977), *Proc. Am. Assoc. Cancer Res.* **18**, 243 (abstr.).

Sheilds, R. (1977), *Nature* **269**, 752.

Silva, O. L., K. L. Becker, A. Primack, J. L. Doppman, and R. H. Snider (1974), *New Engl. J. Med.* **209**, 1122.

Silva, O. L., and K. L. Becker (1976), *Brit. Med. J.* **1**, 460.

Silva, O. L., K. L. Becker, A. Primack, J. L. Doppman, and R. H. Snider (1976), *Chest* **69**, 495.

Silva, O. L., L. E. Broder, J. L. Doppman, R. H. Snider, C. F. Moore, M. H. Cohen, and K. L. Becker (1979), *Cancer* **44**, 680.

Skrabanek, P., D. Cannon, J. Kirrane, and D. Powell (1978), *Ir. J. Med. Sci.* **147**, 47.

Solcia, E., C. Capella, R. Buffa, L. Usellini, P. Fontana, and B. Frigerio (1978), *Adv. Exptl. Med. Biol.* **106**, 11.

Sonksen, P. H., A. B. Ayres, M. Braimbridge, B. Corrin, D. R. Davies, G. M. Jeremiah, S. W. Daten, C. Lowy, and T. E. West (1976), *Clin. Endocrinol.* **5**, 503.

Sparks, R. F., P. B. Connolly, D. S. Gluckin, R. White, B. Sacks, and L. Landsberg (1979), *N. Engl. J. Med.* **301,** 416.

Steiner, D. F., D. Cunningham, L. Spigelman, and B. Aten (1967), *Science* **157,** 697.

Steiner, D. F., and P. E. Oyer (1967), *Proc. Natl. Acad. Sci.* USA **57,** 473.

Steiner, A. L., A. D. Goodman, and S. R. Powers (1968), *Medicine* (Baltimore) **47,** 371.

Swift, P. G. F., S. R. Bloom, and F. Harry (1975), *Arch. Dis. Child.* **50,** 896.

Szijj, I., Z. Csapo, F. A. Laszlo, and K. Kovacs (1969), *Cancer* **24,** 167.

Tashjian, A. H., Jr., B. G. Howland, K. E. W. Melvin, and C. S. Hill (1970), *N. Engl. J. Med.* **283,** 890.

Teillet, M. A., and N. M. LeDouarin (1974), *Arch. Anat. Micr. Morph. Exp.* **63,** 51.

Tischler, A. S., and L. A. Greene (1975), *Nature* **258,** 341.

Tischler, A. S., and L. A. Greene (1978), *Lab Invest.* **39,** 77.

Tischler, A. S., R. A. DeLellis, B. Biales, G. Nunnemacher, V. Carabba, and H. J. Wolfe (1980), *Lab. Invest.* **42,** 155.

Trump, D. L., N. Livingston, and S. B. Baylin (1977), *Cancer* **40,** 1526.

Trump, D. L., and S. Baylin (1979), in *Complications of Cancer: Diagnosis and Management* (Abeloff, M. D., ed.), The Johns Hopkins University Press, Baltimore, p. 211.

Trump, D. L., G. Mendelsohn, and S. B. Baylin (1979), *N. Engl. J. Med.* **301,** 253.

Udall, J. N., D. B. Singer, and C. T. L. Huang (1976), *J. Pediatr.* **88,** 819.

Unger, R. H., J. dev Lochner, and A. M. Eisentraut (1964), *J. Clin. Endocrinol. Metab.* **24,** 823.

Uriel, J. (1975), in *Cancer: A Comprehensive Treatise,* Vol. 3, *Biology of Tumors: Cellular Biology and Growth* (Becker, F. F., ed.), Plenum Press, New York, pp. 21–55.

Vance, J. E., R. W. Stoll, A. E. Kitbachi, K. D. Buchanan, D. Hollander, and R. H. Williams (1972), *Am. J. Med.* **52,** 211.

Vanderhaegen, J. J., J. C. Signeau, and W. Gepts (1975), *Nature* **257,** 604.

Verner, J. V., and A. B. Morrison (1958), *Am. J. Med.* **25,** 374.

Verner, J. V., and A. B. Morrison (1974), *Clin. Gastroenterol.* **3,** 595.

Voelkel, E. F., A. H. Tashjian, F. F. Davidoff, R. B. Cohen, C. P. Perlia, and R. J. Wurtman (1973), *J. Clin. Endocrinol. Metab.* **37,** 297.

Vuitch, M. F., and G. Mendelsohn (1981), *Cancer* **47,** 296.

Weichert, R. F. (1970), *Am. J. Med.* **49,** 232.

Weiss, R. B. (1978), *Ann. Int. Med.* **88,** 522.

Wells, S. A., Jr., S. B. Baylin, W. M. Linehan, R. E. Farell, E. B. Cox, and C. W. Cooper (1978a), *Ann. Surg.* **188,** 139.

Wells, S. A., Jr., S. B. Baylin, D. S. Gann (1978b), *Ann. Surg.* **188,** 377.

Wenk, R. E., B. S. Bhagavan, R. Levy, D. Miller, and W. R. Weisburger (1977), *Cancer* **40,** 773.

Wilander, E., G. Portela-Gomes, L. Grimelius, G. Lundquist, and V. Skoog (1977), *Virch. Arch. Cell. Pathol.* **25,** 117.

Wilander, E., L. Grimelius, G. Portela-Gomes, G. Lundquist, V. Skoog, and P. Westermark (1979), *Scand. J. Gastroenterol.* **14** (Suppl) **53,** 19.

Wolfe, H. J., K. E. W. Melvin, S. J. Cervi-Skinner, A. A. Alsaadi, J. F. Juliar, C. E. Jackson, and A. H. Tashjian, Jr. (1973), *N. Engl. J. Med.* **289,** 437.

Woolner, L. B. (1971), *Semin. Nucl. Med.* **1,** 481.

Yalow, R. S. (1979), in *Progress in Cancer Research and Therapy,* Vol. 11, *Lung Cancer: Progress in Therapeutic Research* (Muggia, F. M. and M. Rozencweig, eds.), Raven Press, New York, pp. 209–216.

Yalow, R. S., and S. A. Berson (1971), *Biochem. Biophys. Res. Commun.* **44,** 439.

Yesner, R. (1978), *Pathol. Ann.* **13,** 217.

Yoshimoto, Y., A. P. Wolfsen, and W. D. Odell (1977), *Science* **197,** 575.

15

Lung Cancer Markers

K. Robert McIntire

*Diagnosis Branch, Division of Cancer Biology and Diagnosis,
National Cancer Institute, Bethesda, Maryland*

1. Introduction

Circulating marker substances with specificity for any of the histologic types of lung cancer have not yet been identified despite considerable investigation. However, a large number of identifiable molecules has been reported to be abnormal in patients with lung cancer.

Lacking a universal or specific lung cancer marker, there may be possibilities for utilizing the nonspecific substances that are abnormal in this disease. This will require a type of analysis that has not yet been widely used. The first step is to find the right (optimal) marker for each patient with cancer. This might be done by analyzing the patient's serum, plasma, or urine by a battery of assays to discover which markers are significantly abnormal. During the initial phases of therapy those markers that were abnormal before therapy would be serially quantitated at frequent intervals to determine which appeared to correlate with the clinical evaluation of change in tumor size. The sampling of blood or urine should be collected at sufficiently frequent intervals to describe the correlation between changes in the tumor and changes in the markers. This will also provide an opportunity to learn more of the biology of the tumor being studied.

It is possible for tumor markers to have more than one clinical application and any single marker will probably not be useful for all situations (McIntire et al., 1979). The different applications can be described as follows: *(a)* screening or detection of lung cancer in asymptomatic individuals, usually in populations defined as high risk owing to factors such as age, family history, smoking, occupational exposure, etc.; *(b)* diagnosis of lung cancer in persons with symptoms or signs suggestive of lung cancer; *(c)* prognosis and staging that indicates the spread of disease even while it may still be microscopic or subclinical; *(d)* monitoring the course of lung cancer during treatment that includes aiding the selection of adjuvant therapy, determining the completeness of remission, and early detection of recurrent tumor activity after a period of clinical remission.

Other applications that might be considered valuable uses of lung cancer markers are: *(e)* localization of small metastatic tumor by injecting radiolabeled antibodies to tumor markers into the patient and allowing accumulation of the radioactivity to be visualized by nuclear medicine scanning techniques (Goldenberg et al., 1978); *(f)* classification of lung tumors by their biochemical and antigenic characteristics as well as by conventional morphology. This might be accomplished by immuno- or enzymo-histologic staining (Sternberger, 1979; Katoh et al., 1979) of the tumor cells directly as well as by quantitating markers in available body fluids.

The association of various serum components (markers) with bronchogenic carcinoma has been frequently described and yet none of these (with the exception of CEA) have as yet been employed as a marker for a careful clinical study of lung cancer.

The review of published work describing markers in lung cancer has been infrequently attempted (Primack, 1974; Chretien et al., 1979; Weiss et al., 1979), although reviews of lung tumor-associated antigens have appeared frequently in the past several years (Veltri et al., 1977; McIntire, 1979; Kelly and Levy, 1980; Gold and Goldenberg, 1980). The distinction between tumor marker and tumor-associated antigen may be a semantic one, but for the purpose of this article a marker will be a substance demonstrable in the blood or urine (as well as in the tumor) in abnormal amounts, while a tumor-associated antigen will be demonstrable primarily in the tumor. A tumor-associated antigen may subsequently become a tumor marker by development of a more sensitive assay that facilitates detection of the component in blood or urine.

The present review makes the optimistic assumption that any substance found in abnormal amounts in the blood or urine of patients with lung cancer might prove to be a useful marker with one or more applications (see above) in the management of this disease. For many of the markers, further work is necessary to confirm the relationship of marker and tumor and to describe the clinical correlation. This article is intended to be as inclusive as possible with the expectation that future studies will provide the necessary appropriate evaluation.

The markers will be described in five categories: oncofetal proteins, hormones, serum proteins, enzymes, and other substances.

2. Oncofetal Proteins

2.1. Carcinoembryonic Antigen (CEA)

The antigen described by Gold and Freedman, CEA, associated with adenocarcinoma of the large bowel (Gold and Freedman, 1965a, b) has also been demonstrated in association with carcinomas of other organ sites, including lung cancer (Thomson et al., 1969; LoGerfo et al., 1971; Reynoso et al., 1972; Vincent and Chu, 1973; Concannon et al., 1974) of all histologic types (Plow and Edgington, 1979). The frequency of elevated serum CEA appears to increase with increasing extent of disease (Vincent et al., 1975) and also appears greater in association with adenocarcinoma and large cell undifferentiated carcinoma than with squamous cell and small cell types (Plow and Edgington, 1979). The correlation of CEA elevation with size of tumor cannot be used in an absolute sense since there have been many exceptions found in clinical experience (Vincent et al., 1975).

Measurement of serum CEA as a screening technique for the early detection of lung cancer is not worthwhile for the same reasons that operate with respect to colorectal cancer: a high proportion of patients with small or ''early'' cancers have normal CEA (Vincent et al., 1975). There is the further problem that about 10-20% of patients with chronic obstructive pulmonary disease and other benign lung diseases have a rise in serum CEA (LoGerfo et al., 1971; Reynoso et al., 1972), as do about 10% of chronic smokers (Hansen et al., 1974; Cullen et al., 1976; Alexander et al., 1976) (which appears to be reversible with cessation of smoking).

Serum CEA may be useful in the evaluation of patients with lung cancer since it is usually higher in those with metastatic disease. Some studies have shown that patients with serum CEA above a certain level have shorter survival after resection of the tumor than those with CEA below that level (Concannon et al., 1978; Dent and McCulloch, 1979). Since the CEA value in serum is the result of not only the size of the tumor or number of cells, but also of the rates of synthesis and degradation, it would seem unwise to rely entirely on the CEA value as a prognostic indicator.

The clearest value of serum CEA in patients with lung cancer is for monitoring the effectiveness of therapy (Vincent and Chu, 1973; Vincent et al., 1975; Ford et al., 1979) in those patients for whom CEA is an appropriate marker; initially to evaluate the completeness of surgical resection, later to anticipate the presence of recurrent tumor before it is clinically apparent and to determine the efficacy of adjuvant therapy. The studies of Vincent, Chu, and colleagues (1979) have demonstrated that serial CEA determinations are not only helpful in judging the completeness of surgery, but can also lead to repeated surgery where a post-operative progressive CEA elevation may be the only sign of recurrent cancer.

Recently, the serial study of patients with small cell carcinoma during therapy has shown a remarkable correlation between changes in serum CEA and response to therapy and a value greater than 10 ng/mL was frequently found to be an indication of extrathoracic spread of the disease (Waalkes et al., 1980; Goslin et al., 1980).

2.2. Alphafetoprotein (AFP)

Despite the availability of sensitive radioimmunoassay methods capable of accurately measuring the normal serum AFP, there have been almost no reports of elevated values in association with primary lung cancer. In a series of 150 patients with lung cancer of all histologic types, 10 had elevated serum AFP (Waldmann and McIntire, 1974), but only one had the degree of elevation that strongly suggested synthesis by the tumor (125,000 ng/mL). The nine other elevations of AFP were quite modest and could conceivably have been related to liver dysfunction. Other studies have indicated that an occasional patient with lung cancer may have elevated serum AFP (Corlin and Tompkins, 1972). At this time, no studies have actually demonstrated synthesis of AFP by lung cancer cells.

It would appear that the oncofetal protein AFP may occasionally be a marker for lung cancer, but not with sufficient frequency to warrant routine serum AFP determinations on all patients with lung cancer.

2.3. Pancreatic Oncofetal Antigen (POA)

The POA, which was discovered by an antiserum developed against human fetal pancreas tissue (Banwo et al., 1974), is now known to be elevated in the sera of many patients with pancreatic cancer and also in patients with other cancers, including lung cancer (Gelder et al., 1979). Almost one-fourth of 53 patients with bronchogenic carcinoma had elevated serum POA with 15% having significant elevations, whereas only 1 of 12 patients with benign lung disease had an elevation of POA, and even in this case, the elevation was not a significant one. The levels of POA found in lung cancer sera were comparable to those found in pancreatic cancer. Several patients were followed serially and POA was found to decrease following successful therapy and to increase as tumor mass grew (Gelder et al., 1979).

POA is antigenically distinct from CEA and AFP (Gelder et al., 1979). Further work is now needed to determine the patterns of correlation with these two other oncofetal antigens. POA might prove helpful as a confirmation of CEA elevations or as a marker to monitor tumor changes in patients who do not have elevated CEA.

3. Hormones

3.1. Adrenocorticotropic Hormone (ACTH)

ACTH was first recognized in association with lung cancer by the clinical syndrome produced by adrenocortical hyperactivity (Brown, 1928). The ectopic production of hormones, such as ACTH, has for almost 50 years been described as an interesting anomaly in association with tumors that were thought to share a common origin from the neural crest, possibly owing to a derepression of genetic information during malignant transformation (Pearse and Polak, 1974). ACTH in certain patients could be quantitated by bioassay and was known to correlate with tumor activity sufficiently well that it could be used as an aid to monitoring therapy (Rees and Ratcliffe, 1974; Gilby et al., 1975).

Prior to 1974, the association between ACTH production and lung cancer had been primarily, but not exclusively, with the small cell anaplastic carcinoma (oat cell) type. Yalow and Berson (1971) had noted that patients with Cushing's syndrome resulting from ectopic ACTH production had significantly higher immunoreactive ACTH plasma levels than patients with pituitary Cushing's disease. This led to studies on the heterogeneity of ACTH which demonstrated that the molecular species produced by lung cancer was predominantly a larger (big ACTH), biologically inactive precursor (pro-hormone) of the functional hormone and was found in association with all the histologic types of primary lung cancer, but not with other carcinomas metastatic to the lungs (Gewirtz and Yalow, 1974). These studies have been confirmed by Odell and coworkers (Odell el al., 1977; Odell and Wolfsen, 1978) who found elevated plasma big ACTH in over 70% of patients with all types of lung cancer, and this differed significantly from the levels seen in normal subjects and benign lung disease patients. Several groups have demonstrated the correlation of diminishing plasma ACTH levels with decrease in tumor size following therapeutic measures (Gewirtz and Yalow, 1974; Odell and Wolfsen, 1978; Gropp et al., 1979).

Despite the very high percentage of lung tumors that appear to have elevated amounts of ACTH in tumor tissue (Wolfsen and Odell, 1979), there are still one-third or more of patients with active disease who have normal levels of plasma ACTH (Yalow, 1979; Torstensson et al., 1980). The presence of elevated plasma ACTH in a significant number of patients with chronic obstructive pulmonary disease (Yalow, 1979) may be an early indicator of metaplastic changes, but this will require careful prospective clinical study for verfication.

Comparison of plasma ACTH levels in patients with different types of lung cancer have failed to demonstrate a correlation with histologic type

(Torstensson et al., 1980) or with the subtypes of small cell anaplastic carcinoma (Hansen et al., 1980).

At the present time it appears that the frequency of both elevated plasma ACTH in the absence of confirmed neoplastic disease and normal ACTH in the presence of active tumor growth contraindicate the use of plasma ACTH as a screening or diagnostic tool. Studies to correlate serial changes in plasma ACTH with changes in clinical evaluation of tumor size are needed to further understand the relationship and also to ascertain the effect of various forms of therapy on ACTH levels. Studies of synthesis and turnover of big ACTH under various conditions are also needed to evaluate the role of this hormone as a tumor marker for the monitoring of therapy.

3.2. Lipotropin (LPH)

The ectopic production by lung tumors of beta-melanocyte-stimulating hormone (β-MSH) has been closely associated with ectopic production of ACTH (Rees et al., 1974; Coscia et al., 1977). Recent studies have demontrated that β-MSH is a fragment of LPH produced during the isolation procedure (Bloomfield et al., 1974), but fortunately the radioimmunoassay developed for the fragment cross-reacts in parallel with the native hormone (Bachelot et al., 1977).

In a study of 107 patients presenting with an abnormal chest X-ray and hospitalized for diagnostic evaluation, plasma LPH was quantitated on each patient before the diagnosis was known (Odell et al., 1979). Of the 74 patients with histologically confirmed primary lung cancer, 28 (36%) had elevated LPH whereas only 2 (7%) of the 33 patients with benign lung disease had LPH above the 95% confidence limits of normal subjects. Repeated evaluation of the elevated values confirmed the reliability of the testing.

Despite the frequent association of ACTH and β-MSH in tumors with demonstrable ectopic hormone production, quantitation of both hormones in the same patients showed the frequency of elevated ACTH to be much higher in patients with squamous cell carcinoma and adenocarcinoma, while being about the same in patients with oat cell carcinoma (Odell et al., 1979).

Plasma LPH has been quantitated in 100 patients with chronic obstructive pulmonary disease (COPD), who were then closely followed for 2 years. Initial results showed 13 patients with elevated and 87 with normal LPH. During the followup period, three of the patients (23%) with elevated LPH developed lung cancer, while four with a normal level (5%) developed lung cancer (Odell et al., 1979). It was not reported whether elevated LPH values continued to rise during the followup, but it was, nevertheless, promising that this test might provide some aid in selecting individuals at high risk for development of lung cancer.

3.3. Calcitonin (CT)

The first demonstration of calcitonin synthesis by a nonthyroid cancer associated with elevated plasma levels of hormone was published by Silva and coworkers (1973) in a patient with small cell carcinoma. There was an increased venous CT concentration in veins draining the tumor and a rapid fall in plasma CT as the tumor responded to chemotherapy. Subsequent studies of small cell carcinoma patients ranged from finding elevated CT in the majority (Silva et al., 1974; Milhaud et al., 1974; Coombes et al., 1974; Hansen and Hummer, 1979) to finding normal CT in all (Abeloff et al., 1976) of ten patients. This variation may occur because there are several immunochemical forms of calcitonin with different molecular sizes that also differ in antigenicity (Singer and Habener, 1974; Sizemore and Heath, 1975). Evidence suggests that the CT associated with medullary carcinoma of the thyroid (MTC) is physically and antigenically distinguishable from the CT ectopically produced in patients with lung cancer (Becker et al., 1978, 1979). The antisera to one of the forms may react poorly with the other forms, thereby necessitating the use of two assays for measuring CT in both MTC and nonthyroid tumors.

There is evidence that many nonthyroid tumors are capable of CT synthesis. In addition, the work of Silva et al. (1979) has suggested that some patients with elevated serum CT may have tumors that secrete a substance that stimulates excess thyroid CT production.

The development of tests that specifically measure nonthyroid CT without cross-reactivity with CT of thyroid origin, and vice versa, will aid the clarification of the role of CT in the management of lung cancer patients. Careful prospective studies that attempt to correlate serum CT with clinical observations of tumor change will provide insight into which patients, if any, are appropriate for serial followup with hormone measurements to evaluate the effectiveness of therapy. Additionally, this might help identify a subset of lung cancers, where CT may be an aid to early diagnosis.

3.4. Human Chorionic Gonadotropin (HCG)

The development of a sensitive quantitative immunoassay for HCG that detects the specific determinants on the beta subunit (Vaitukaitis et al., 1972) has confirmed the virtual absence of this hormone in the circulation of healthy men and nonpregnant women (Vaitukaitis and Ross, 1972) despite the fact that it has now been recognized that normal tissues other than placenta can be responsible for the synthesis of HCG (Braunstein et al., 1975; Chen et al., 1976). In addition to the early recognition of HCG in association with gestational and nongestational trophoblastic neoplasms, there have been many reports of HCG production by nontrophoblastic tumors, many of which were primary lung tumors (Fusco and Rosen, 1966; Sussman et al., 1974; Muggia et al., 1975).

Utilizing sensitive radioimmunoassays, retrospective analysis of sera from patients with lung cancer have demonstrated 5–15% with elevated values of HCG (Braunstein et al., 1973; Goldstein el al., 1974; Gailani et al., 1976; McIntire and Princler, 1978); these values are almost all less than 10 ng/mL in assays where the upper limit of normal is 1 ng/mL. A recent study, measuring the beta subunit (Blackman et al., 1980) found values exceeding the 95th percentile in 41% of men and 16% of women with lung cancer. These low-level elevations for lung cancer can be contrasted with trophoblastic neoplasms, where HCG values greater than 1000 ng/mL are commonly seen. Careful studies have not yet been reported to correlate HCG serum levels with the stage or extent of tumor, and there is insufficient evidence to indicate how frequently HCG is elevated in early or small tumors. A single case has been reported where gynecomastia led to the finding of elevated serum HCG in a man 13 months before a squamous cell carcinoma of the lung became clinically evident (Rosen et al., 1968). There has been no evidence presented that HCG synthesis by lung cancers is of prognostic or therapeutic significance. Several groups have utilized isotopically labeled antisera to HCG for the radioimmunodetection of small, metastatic lesions (Goldenberg et al., 1980; Bagshawe et al., 1980) and this might also be modified to provide an aid to therapy (Order et al., 1980).

Serial measurement of serum HCG during treatment of patients with lung cancer usually shows correlation with changes in those tumors that are ectopically producing HCG, but have demonstrated occasional discordance with falling HCG in the face of progressive tumor growth (Sussman et al., 1974; Muggia et al., 1975). Increasing values of HCG appear invariably to indicate tumor growth.

In addition to the beta subunit, HCG also contains an alpha subunit that is common to the other glycoprotein hormones: luteinizing hormone (LH), follicle-stimulating hormone (FSH), and thyroid-stimulating hormone (TSH). Immunoassays for the alpha subunit are unable to distinguish the various glycoprotein hormones (Vaitukaitis and Ross, 1972). Elevated levels of serum alpha subunit have been reported in occasional nonneoplastic diseases (Rosen and Weintraub, 1974) but "values above 20 ng/mL are virtually diagnostic of cancer" (Rosen and Weintraub, 1979). Since the association of FSH, LH, and TSH with neoplastic disease is exceedingly rare (Rosen and Weintraub, 1979), it would appear that the elevations of alpha subunit values are most likely related to HCG synthesis either in conjunction with the beta subunit or as a free alpha chain.

The free alpha subunit has been found elevated in 3–16% of patients with bronchogenic carcinoma (Rosen and Weintraub, 1974; Blackman et al., 1980) and has also shown a good correlation with clinical response to chemotherapy in at least one patient (Muggia et al., 1975).

3.5. Parathyroid Hormone (PTH)

The ectopic production of PTH by lung tumors and other neoplasms had been suggested by the syndrome of pseudohyperparathyroidism. With the development of sensitive radioimmunoassay methods, it has now been demonstrated that about 30% of patients with bronchogenic carcinoma have elevated serum levels of PTH (Berson and Yalow, 1966; Sherwood et al., 1967; Arnaud et al., 1971). There is preliminary evidence that much of the ectopic PTH is a larger molecule than that produced by the parathyroid (Benson et al., 1974) and may be an inactive precursor of the active hormone.

There are no studies to demonstrate a correlation between quantitative PTH serum levels and changes in tumor size with treatment, but an earlier report describes the laboratory findings of pseudohyperparathyroidism reverting to normal following successful treatment of bronchogenic carcinoma (Turkington and Goldman, 1966). Prospective studies are needed to document the quantitative change in PTH following surgical resection of lung cancer and serial followup to determine whether recurrent disease or development of metastases is preceded by rising serum PTH.

3.6. Arginine Vasopressin (AVP)

The association of AVP or antidiuretic hormone with primary lung cancer has been the subject of many individual case reports (Schwartz et al., 1957; Roberts, 1959; Ivy, 1961; Ross, 1963) in which the great majority of the tumors have been of the small cell anaplastic type. The ectopic production of the hormone by lung cancer cells, and the resultant clinical syndrome of inappropriate antidiuresis are the same as are found occasionally with nonmalignant pulmonary disease, and other benign diseases, as well as secondary to a variety of drugs (Robertson, 1978), which makes it necessary to interpret AVP elevations cautiously.

The criteria of ectopic hormone production has been satisfied for AVP in lung tumors, especially small cell anaplastic carcinoma, by extraction from the tumor, by radioimmunoassay values correlating with changes in tumor size, and by demonstration of its in vitro synthesis by tumor cells (Lipscomb et al., 1968; George et al., 1972).

Quantitation of AVP in the urine and plasma of patients with lung cancer has demonstrated elevated urinary levels in 33% (Haefliger et al., 1977) and elevated plasma levels in 41% (Odell and Wolfsen, 1978). Since this incidence appears greater than the incidence of impaired water excretion with hyponatremia, it suggests that the immunoassay might measure biologically inactive forms of AVP, such as a precursor hormone, which can nevertheless be utilized as a potential tumor marker for lung cancer patients. The most meaningful description of AVP levels is expressed as a function of plasma osmolality (Robertson, 1978), since AVP in healthy individuals is raised when plasma osmolality is high, but AVP production by tumor cells results in elevated levels despite low plasma osmolality.

Substitution of a water-loading test to detect disturbances in AVP secretion may provide an indication of the frequency of the clinical disorder of secretion of inappropriate antidiuretic hormone, but fails to document the frequency of immunoassay elevations of an AVP-like antigen in the circulation that can serve as a lung tumor marker. When patients were tested simultaneously for AVP levels and response to water loading, only 61% with abnormal water-load response had elevated AVP, while 11 of the 12 with elevated AVP had abnormal water load response (Comis et al., 1980).

Serum immunoreactive AVP may provide yet another hormonal marker to aid in the diagnosis and management of lung cancer.

3.7. Prolactin

Prolactin has been reported elevated in primary lung cancer (Turkington, 1971; Rees and Ratcliffe, 1974) in isolated cases, but minimal attempts to find other cases with abnormal serum prolactin levels have been unsuccessful. The fact that many physiologic conditions as well as stress can produce elevated serum prolactin indicates the need for great care in defining ectopic production by a tumor (Rosen and Weintraub, 1979).

Prolactin deserves further immunoassay study to define its incidence of elevation and the degree of correlation with change in tumor size. It may well find usefulness in the management of selected patients.

In an immunochemical study of lung tumor extracts for concentrations of multiple hormones, the small cell carcinomas had increased prolactin in 36% and the nonsmall cell cancers occasionally had abnormal prolactin; normal lung extracts had no demonstrable hormone (Podmore et al., 1979).

3.8. Placental Lactogen (PL)

Attempts to demonstrate the presence of PL, also known as chorionic somatomammotropin, in sera of nonpregnant healthy persons and patients with nonneoplastic disease have been unsuccessful (Weintraub and Rosen, 1971). Therefore the finding of PL in even 2% of patients with bronchogenic carcinoma (Rosen et al., 1975) may provide a significant marker for such a common neoplasm. Owing to the possibility that chemotherapy produces a discordance in a marker correlation with tumor size (Muggia et al., 1975), it has been suggested that simultaneous monitoring of several tumor markers may afford better correlation with the clinical status (Braunstein el al., 1973). The major difficulty at this time is in identifying or matching the appropriate patients with the available markers, such as placental lactogen or any of the others discussed in this chapter.

3.9. Growth Hormone (GH)

Several isolated case reports of elevated serum GH in patients with lung cancer (Steiner et al., 1968; Sparanaga et al., 1971), usually in association with osteoarthropathy, suggest the possibility of ectopic production of this hormone. In vitro synthesis and secretion of GH has been demonstrated for lung cancer cells (Greenberg et al., 1972) and elevated concentrations of GH have been measured in extracts of lung tumors, in 38% of small cell anaplastic carcinomas, and in a smaller percentage of nonsmall cell carcinoma (Podmore et al., 1979).

In a series of 109 patients with proven lung cancer, an elevated level of GH was seen in only one patient. Other studies with different immunoassays should be utilized to confirm the incidence of GH in the plasma of patients with lung cancer since tissue extracts provide some evidence that it should be higher than 1%.

Rosen and Weintraub (1979) have emphasized the importance of differentiating between GH and PL because of chemical and immunological similarities, and also indicated the need to document ectopic tumor production as opposed to the more common pituitary response to stress.

4. Serum Proteins

4.1. Immunoglobulins (Ig)

The synthesis and secretion of homogeneous immunoglobulins or their subunits is associated with most plasma cell neoplasms and by some tumors of the B lymphocyte, such as lymphomas and chronic lymphocytic leukemia. Only rarely has monoclonal immunoglobulin production been associated with a primary lung cancer. Various reports have indicated a general change in serum immunoglobulins (Hughes, 1971; Zeromski et al., 1975; Nash, 1979; Plesnicar and Rudolf, 1979), or even a change for a specific class of immunoglobulins (Krant et al., 1968; Mandel et al., 1973; LoGerfo and McLanahan, 1976), usually IgA.

In a study of patients suspected of having primary lung cancer where sera were obtained before the confirmatory workup, the mean serum IgA was significantly elevated over control values for all histologic types of lung cancer, and two-thirds were more than two standard deviations above the normal mean value (Nash et al., 1980). Interestingly, serum IgM was significantly decreased in these same early lung cancer patients, indicating that this determination might also be useful in aiding early detection. The pattern of simultaneously elevated IgA and depressed IgM could provide greater specificity than either protein by itself.

A study of 57 patients with nonmetastatic epidermoid carcinoma of the lung showed that all (100%) of those that lived longer than the mean survival time had elevated serum IgA, and of those patients with elevated

IgA, over two-thirds lived longer than the mean survival time (Plesnicar and Rudolf, 1979). In the same study, 38 patients with small cell anaplastic carcinoma, 15 who lived longer than the mean survival almost all had elevation of either serum IgG or IgM, and the corollary demonstration was that the majority of patients with either elevated IgG or IgM lived longer than the mean survival time (Plesnicar and Rudolf, 1979). Serial studies would be helpful to show any correlation between change in Ig levels and change in tumor size.

4.2. Ferritin

Ferritin, found in normal tissues and serum, is an iron-containing protein that has been found to be elevated in many tumor tissues and in the serum of patients with various tumors (Marcus et al., 1979). There are over 15 different isomeric forms of ferritin that probably arise from changes in amino acid composition, subunit size, glycosylation, and so on (Marcus et al., 1979). Organ-specific isoferritin patterns have been recognized (Drysdale, 1970) and a prevalence of acidic forms in fetal and tumor tissue was thought to be specific for these conditions (Alpert et al., 1973) until it was recognized that several normal adult tissues such as heart, kidney, and placenta also had increased amounts of acidic isoferritins (Drysdale and Singer, 1974).

Total serum ferritin, quantitated by various immunologic assays, has been elevated in a high percentage of patients with lung cancer (Gropp et al., 1978; Urushizaki et al., 1979; Ishitani et al., 1979; Maxim et al., 1980) and especially in patients with Stage I disease. There is also preliminary reporting of the correlation of serum ferritin changes with change in lung tumor size during treatment by either radiotherapy or chemotherapy (Urushizaki, et al., 1979).

Despite certain antigenic differences between the acidic and basic forms of isoferritin, it has been difficult to develop specific immunoassays for each (Marcus et al., 1979). With an assay more reactive for the acidic ferritins (Hazard et al., 1977), it has been shown that the measurable serum ferritin level in patients with cancer is several times greater than when quantitated by an immunoassay for the basic ferritins (Hazard and Drysdale, 1977). Specifically this was noted for lung cancer and indicates an area where investigation is needed to confirm the greater relative specificity of acidic isoferritins with lung cancer.

4.3. Ceruloplasmin

The quantitation of serum ceruloplasmin by immunoassay has indicated that 81% of 48 patients with lung cancer had elevated values (Linder, 1979b). Although 55% of controls with benign lung disease also had elevated ceruloplasmin, the values were not as great as in the malignant disease patients. The level of ceruloplasmin was highly correlated with the stage of lung cancer and still was elevated in two-thirds of those patients with early or Stage I disease (Linder, 1979b). Very preliminary data indicated that elevated serum ceruloplasmin levels reverted to normal when treatment was successful in providing remission.

In addition to quantitation as antigen, ceruloplasmin is also active as an oxidative enzyme involved in iron metabolism, and serum can be quantitated specifically for the enzyme activity. The measurement of ceruloplasmin oxidase in human sera corroborates the findings of ceruloplasmin protein in that elevations are associated with lung cancer, and are greater in magnitude and incidence with increasing disease stage (Linder, 1979a).

Since the synthesis of ceruloplasmin has not yet been demonstrated for tumor cells, it is most likely that the elevated serum levels reflect increased synthesis by the liver (Cohen et al., 1979) as a response to tumor growth. However, the possibility that ceruloplasmin is responding simply as a nonspecific acute phase reactant still needs to be ruled out by careful longitudinal studies covering a variety of stress situations in patients with lung cancer.

4.4. Alpha$_1$-Antitrypsin (α_1-AT)

The serum levels of α_1-AT have been shown to be elevated in about two-thirds of the patients with primary lung cancer (Harris et al., 1974; Micksche and Kokron, 1977) with the elevations evenly distributed among the various histologic types of lung cancer (Nash et al., 1980).

Because of the response of α_1-AT as an acute phase reactant, it is crucial to develop data showing the degree to which α_1-AT concentration correlates with change in tumor size and that it is independent of concurrent infection or other causes of increase in acute-phase reactants.

4.5. β$_2$-Microglobulin

The β$_2$-m related to the immunoglobulin and histocompatibility locus A (HLA) molecules is elevated in the circulation of patients with impaired renal function, and has also been shown to be elevated in many patients with neoplastic disease, including lung cancer (Kithier et al., 1974).

In a study of β$_2$-m levels in lung cancer, elevated values were found in 21% of 230 patients with confirmed lung cancer, but also in 11% of 237 control patients with nonmalignant pulmonary disease (Hallgren, 1980). Elevations were found in both small cell and nonsmall cell carcinoma and appeared to increase with increase in tumor size. Unfortunately, there was no decrease in β$_2$-m following surgical removal of the tumor (Hallgren, 1980). Lung cancer patients with normal serum β$_2$-m had a better prognosis than those with elevated levels.

4.6. Tissue Polypeptide Antigen (TPA)

The TPA, originally described by Bjorklund (1957, 1958), has been found in elevated amounts in sera from a majority of patients with cancer of various organ sites (including lung), but also in a high percent of patients with benign diseases, especially urinary tract infection (Holyoke and Chu, 1979).

Eighty percent of 35 patients with lung cancer had elevated serum TPA in a study by Manendez-Botet and Schwartz (1975). Holyoke and Chu (1979) have noted that TPA and CEA were equally elevated in a study of 21 patients with bronchogenic carcinoma (57%) and that almost all elevations were coincidental. In patients with elevated TPA, the level fell after surgical resection of the tumor (Chu, 1980).

Further studies are needed to determine the accuracy of TPA in monitoring the effect of therapy and for the early detection of recurrent tumor. Studies should also be directed at the coincidence of CEA and TPA to see whether this improves the reliability of both tests.

4.7. Circulating Immune Complexes (CIC)

The majority of studies of immune complexes in patients with cancer have dealt with the disadvantages and advantages of the complexes at the surface of malignant and normal cells and their filtration from the circulation by various organs (reviewed by Theofilopoulos and Dixon, 1979).

The detection and quantitation of CIC can be performed by several different methodologies that may give dissimilar results and that at the present time are not well understood. The methods and their interpretation are discussed by Theofilopoulos and Dixon (1979). It is accepted that the measurement of immune complexes is a nonspecific assay and is, therefore, a nonspecific cancer test since the antigen–antibody interaction can be the result of many different factors, some of which may be tumor-related or even tumor-specific. Identification of the component parts of the immune complexes requires further immunochemical determination. The different assays for CIC may detect different components, so that ideally a survey of lung cancer patents would utilize more than one assay.

Using the Raji cell assay, sera from 26% of 51 patients with lung cancer had elevated CIC, but this result was not significantly different from the 176 healthy controls (Theofilopoulos and Dixon 1979). The C1q binding assay for CIC has been used in several studies and also showed elevations in lung cancer, but similar elevations occur in patients with benign lung disease (Rossen et al., 1977; Baldwin et al., 1979; Dent et al., 1979). This C1q assay may have predictive value in that lung cancer patients with elevated CIC levels in the post-operative period have significantly shorter median survival (Dent, 1980).

4.8. Other Serum Proteins

Concentration of serum haptoglobin, orosomucoid protein, and C-reactive protein were measured by immunoassays in patients with lung cancer before and after radical resection of the primary tumor. The protein values correlated well with increasing tumor size; in those patients with higher than expected protein levels, there was a significantly shorter survival time, which was interpreted as an indication that these proteins might be indicators of undetected metastases (Bradwell et al., 1979).

5. Enzymes

5.1. Placental Alkaline Phosphatase

The Regan isoenzyme, a placental-type alkaline phosphatase, was originally detected in bronchogenic carcinoma (Fishman et al., 1968), but has been demonstrated to be elevated in many different forms of cancer (Stolbach et al., 1969). This isoenzyme is elevated in 6–14% of patients with lung cancer and the majority of these are minimal elevations. Placental alkaline phosphatase might yet be useful in a battery of tests, where it may corroborate other results despite the fact that by itself it has not yet proven to be of great value.

5.2. 5'-Nucleotide Phosphodiesterase Isozyme-V (5'-NPD-V)

This enzyme appears to be more specific for liver metastases from any primary tumor site than it is for any certain organ cancer. Nevertheless, in sera of 36 lung cancer patients, over 60% were positive for 5'-NPD-V while 14/40 (35%) of heavy smokers had positive sera (Tsou et al., 1980). The positives in lung cancer sera were found in all histological types, but were much more frequent in patients with liver metastases (87%) than in patients without (38%).

This represents another assay where quantitative capability will allow easier comparison of serial samples. If there is no correlation with changes in the tumor, determinations of the enzyme may simply be an aid in confirming metastases to the liver.

5.3. Amylase

Case reports of elevated serum amylase in patients with lung cancer have appeared sporadically for almost three decades (Weiss et al., 1951; McGeachin and Adams, 1957; Ende, 1961; Ammann et al., 1973; Yokoyama et al., 1977). The histological type most frequently associated with this condition is adenocarcinoma and there is evidence that the isoenzyme form is chemically different from that produced by the normal pancreas or salivary gland (Yokoyama et al., 1977).

In a study of the frequency of elevated serum amylase and characterization of the enzyme, it was found that the heat-labile form of amylase occurred in all patients with primary lung cancer, but not in those with benign lung disease or in healthy controls. The heat-labile form accounted for 12–70% of the total serum amylase; 55% of the lung cancer patients had elevated levels of total amylase (Sirsat et al., 1979). There was a rapid fall in the heat-labile amylase of three patients following surgical resection of their tumor.

Further studies are needed to define the correlation of the heat-labile isozyme of amylase with the histology and stage of cancer. An immunoassay specific for this form would facilitate such studies.

5.4. Creatine Kinase BB

The isoenzyme CK-BB has been found elevated in the serum of various patients with adenocarcinoma of different organ sites (Hoag et al., 1978) and this includes 40% of 32 patients with lung cancer, while none of the 56 patients with nonmalignant disease had elevated isoenzyme (Paris et al., 1980). Serum CK-BB has also been elevated in patients with small cell carcinoma of the lung (Coolen, 1976).

With the development of a sensitive radioimmunoassay for CK-BB (Silverman et al., 1979), it is now possible to determine the frequency in a larger series of patients with lung cancer and to test for a correlation with change in clinical status. The definite advantage of the immunoassay is that it no longer requires the isoenzyme to retain biologic activity to enable identification and quantitation; even native, inactive forms (such as proenzyme), if they exist, might be measurable as a useful tumor marker (Silverman et al., 1979).

6. Other Substances

Tennessee Antigen (TA)

This tumor-associated antigen has been studied exclusively by a single group. While TA has some similarities to CEA, it is antigenically distinctive from CEA and several other known tumor-associated antigens, but has not been definitively compared with many others (Jordan et al., 1979).

Positive TA assays have been reported in the sera of two-thirds of patients with lung cancer and one-third of patients with benign lung disease (Potter et al., 1979). Improvement in the methods of quantitation of TA may be helpful in discriminating benign from malignant disease. Serial studies to demonstrate TA correlation with change in tumor size would be useful in deciding whether this glycoprotein will be of value in the management of therapy in patients with lung cancer.

Acknowledgment

I wish to thank Mr. Louis P. Greenberg for editorial assistance and Ms. Kathryn Telfer for preparing the manuscript.

References

Abeloff, M. D., D. S. Ettinger, S. B. Baylin, and T. Hazra (1976), *Cancer* **38**, 1394.

Alexander, J. C., N. A. Silverman, and P. B. Chretien (1976), *J. Amer. Med. Assoc.* **235**, 1975.

Alpert, E., R. L. Coston, and J. W. Drysdale (1973), *Nature* **242**, 194.

Ammann, R. W., J. E. Berk, L. Fridhandler, M. Ueda, and W. Wegmann (1973), *Ann. Int. Med.* **78**, 521.

Arnaud, C. D., H. S. Tsao, and T. Littledike (1971), *J. Clin. Invest.* **50**, 21.

Bachelot, I., A. R. Wolfsen, and W. D. Odell (1977), *J. Clin. Endocrin. Metab.* **44**, 939.

Bagshawe, K. D., F. Searle, J. Lewis, P. Brown, and P. Keep (1980), *Cancer Res.* **40**, 3016.

Baldwin, R. W., M. V. Pimm, P. B. Iles, and R. J. Webb (1979), in *Compendium of Assays for Immunodiagnosis of Cancer* (R. B. Herberman, ed.), Elsevier/North Holland, New York, p. 325.

Banwo, O., J. Versey, and J. R. Hobbs (1974), *Lancet* **1**, 643.

Becker, K. L., D. R. Nash, O. L. Silva, R. H. Snider and C. F. Moore (1980) AMA **243**, 670.

Becker, K. L., R. H. Snider, O. L. Silva, and C. F. Moore (1978), *Acta Endocrin.* **89**, 89.

Benson, R. C., Jr., B. L. Riggs, B. M. Pickard, and C. D. Arnaud (1974), *J. Clin. Invest.* **54**, 175.

Berson, S. A., and R. S. Yalow (1966), *Science* **154**, 907.

Bjorklund, B., and V. Bjorklund (1957), *Int. Arch. Allergy* **10**, 153.

Bjorklund, B., G. Lundblad, and V. Bjorklund (1958), *Int. Arch. Allergy* **12**, 241.

Blackman, M. R., B. D. Weintraub, S. W. Rosen, I. A. Kourides, K. Steinwascher, and M. H. Gail (1980), *J. Natl. Cancer Inst.* **65**, 81.

Bloomfield, G. A., A. P. Scott, and P. J. Lowry (1974), *Nature* **252**, 492.

Braunstein, G. D., K. R. McIntire, and T. A. Waldmann (1973), *Cancer* **31**, 1065.

Braunstein, G. D., J. Rasor, and M. E. Wade (1975), *New Engl. J. Med.* **293**, 1339.

Braunstein, G. D., J. L. Vaitukaitis, P. P. Carbone, and G. T. Ross (1973), *Ann. Int. Med.* **78,** 39.

Brown, W. H. (1928), *Lancet* **2,** 1022.

Chen, H. C., G. D. Hodgen, S. Matsuura, L. J. Lin, E. Gross, L. E. Reichert, Jr., S. Birken, R. E. Canfield, and G. T. Ross (1976), *Proc. Natl. Acad. Sci. USA* **73,** 2885.

Chretien, P. B., J. F. Weiss, D. Chiuten, and H. H. Hansen (1979), in *Lung Cancer: Progress in Therapeutic Research* (F. M. Muggia and M. Rozencweig, eds.), Raven Press, New York, p. 179.

Chu, T. M. (1980), personal communication.

Cohen, D. I., B. Illowsky, and M. C. Linder (1979), *Am. J. Physiol.* **236,** E309.

Comis, R. L., M. Miller, and S. J. Ginsberg (1980), *Cancer* **45,** 2414.

Concannon, J. P., M. H. Dalbow, S. E. Hodsson, J. J. Headings, E. Markopoulos, J. Mitchell, W. J. Cushins, and G. A. Liebler (1978), *Cancer* **42,** 1477.

Concannon, J. P., M. H. Dalbow, G. A. Liebler, K. E. Blake, C. S. Weil, and J. W. Cooper (1974), *Cancer* **34,** 184.

Coolen, R. B. (1976), *Clin. Chem.* **22,** 1174.

Coombes, R. C., P. B. Greenberg, C. Hillyard, and I. MacIntyre (1974), *Lancet* **1,** 1080.

Corlin, R. F., and R. K. Tompkins (1972), *Digest. Diseases* **17,** 553.

Coscia, M., R. D. Brown, and M. Miller (1977), *Am. J. Med.* **62,** 303.

Cullen, K. J., D. P. Stevens, M. A. Frost, and I. R. Mackay (1976), *Austral. N. Z. J. Med.* **6,** 279.

Dent, P. B. (1980), *Cancer* **45,** 130.

Dent, P. B. and P. B. McCulloch (1979), in *Compendium of Assays for Immunodiagnosis of Human Cancer* (R. B. Herberman, ed.), Elsevier/North Holland, New York, p. 273.

Dent, P. B., P. B. McCulloch, J. A. Louis, and J.-C. Cerottini (1979), *in Compendium of Assays for Immunodiagnosis of Cancer* (R. B. Herberman, ed.), Elsevier/North Holland, New York, p. 329.

Drysdale, J. W. (1970), *Biochim. Biophys. Acta* **207,** 256.

Drysdale, J. W., and R. M. Singer (1974), *Cancer Res.* **34,** 3352.

Ende, N. (1961), *Cancer* **14,** 1109.

Fishman, W. H., N. R. Inglis, L. L. Stolbach, and M. J. Krant (1968), *Cancer Res.* **28,** 150.

Ford, C. H., C. E. Newman, and I. G. Anderson (1979), *in Carcino-Embryonic Proteins,* vol. 2, (F.-G. Lehmann, ed.), Elsevier/North Holland, Amsterdam. p. 169.

Fusco, F. D., and S. W. Rosen (1966), *New Engl. J. Med.* **275,** 507.

Gailani, S., T. M. Chu, A. Nussbaum, M. Ostrander, and N. Christoff (1976), *Cancer* **38,** 1684.

Gelder, F. B., C. Reese, A. R. Moossa, and R. L. Hunter (1979), in *Immunodiagnosis of Cancer* (R. B. Herberman and K. R. McIntire, eds.), Dekker, New York, p. 357

George, J. M., C. C. Capen, and A. S. Phillips (1972), *J. Clin.. Invest.* **51,** 141.

Gewirtz, G., and R. S. Yalow (1974), *J. Clin. Invest.* **53,** 1022.

Gilby, E. D., L. H. Rees, and P. K. Bondy (1975), *Excerpta Med.* **375,** 132.

Gold, P., and S. O. Freedman (1965a), *J. Exptl. Med.* **121,** 439.

Gold, P., and S. O. Freedman (1965b), *J. Exptl. Med.* **122,** 467.

Gold, D. A., and D. M. Goldenberg (1980), in *Cancer Markers* (S. Sell, ed.), Humana, Clifton, New Jersey, p. 329.

Goldenberg, D. M., F. DeLand, E. Kim, S. Bennett, F. J. Primus, J. R. Van Nagell, Jr., N. Estes, P. DeSimone, and P. Rayburn (1978), *New Engl. J. Med.* **298,** 1384.

Goldenberg, D. M., E.. E. Kim, F. H. DeLand, J. R. Van Nagell, Jr., and N. Javadpour (1980), *Science* **208,** 1284.

Goldstein, D. P., T. S. Kosasa, and A. T. Skarin (1974), *Surg. Gynecol. Obstet.* **138,** 747.

Goslin, R. H., A. T. Skarin, J. MacIntyre, and N. Zamcheck (1981), submitted for publication.

Greenberg, P. B., T. J. Martin, C. Beck, and H. G. Burger (1972), *Lancet* **1,** 350.

Gropp, C., K. Havemann, and F. G. Lehmann (1978), *Cancer* **42,** 2802.

Gropp, C., K. Havemann, A. Scheuer, and R. Grun (1979), *Protides Biol. Fluids Proc. Colloq.* **27,** 331.

Haefliger, J. M., M. C. Dubied, and M. B. Vallotton (1977), *Schweiz. Med. Wochenschr.* **107,** 726.

Hallgren, R., E. Nou, and G. Lundquist (1980), *Cancer* **45,** 780.

Hansen, M., H. H. Hansen, F. R. Hirsch, J. Arends, J. D. Christensen, J. M. Christensen, L. Hummer, and C. Kuhl (1980), *Cancer* **45,** 1432.

Hansen, M., and L. Hummer (1979), in *Lung Cancer: Progress in Therapeutic Research* (F. Muggia and M. Rozencweig, eds.), Raven Press, New York, p. 199.

Hansen, H. J., L. J. Snyder, E. Miller, J. P. Vandervoorde, O. N. Miller, L. R. Hines, and J. J. Burns (1974), *J. Human Path.* **5,** 139.

Harris, C. C., A. Primack, and M. H. Cohen (1974), *Cancer* **34,** 280.

Hazard, J. T., and J. W. Drysdale (1977), *Nature* **265,** 755.

Hazard, J. T., M. Yokota, P. Arosio, and J. W. Drysdale (1977), *Blood* **49,** 139.

Hoag, G. N., C. R. Franks, and W. E. DeCoteau (1978), *Clin. Chem.* **24,** 1654.

Holyoke, D., and T. M. Chu (1979), in *Immunodiagnosis of Cancer* (R. B. Herberman and K. R. McIntire, eds.), Dekker, New York. p. 513.

Hughes, N. R. (1971), *J. Natl. Cancer Inst.* **46,** 1015.

Ishitani, K., Y. Niitsu, N. Watanabe, J. Koseki, J. Oikawa, Y. Kadono, T. Ishii, Y. Goto, Y. Onodera, and I. Urushizaki (1979), in *Carcino-Embryonic Proteins,* vol. 1 (F.-G. Lehmann, ed.), Elsevier/North Holland, Amsterdam. p. 279.

Ivy, H. K. (1961), *Arch. Int. Med.* **108,** 115.

Jordan, T. A., T. P. Potter, J. D. Jordan, K. Johnston, and H. A. Lasater (1979), *Protides Biol. Fluids Proc. Colloq.* **27,** 95.

Katoh, Y., G. D. Stoner, K. R. McIntire, T. A. Hill, R. Anthony, E. M. McDowell, B. F. Trump, and C. C. Harris (1979). *J. Natl. Cancer Inst.* **62,** 1177.

Kelly, B. S., and J. G. Levy (1980), *Brit. J. Cancer* **41,** 388.

Kithier, K., J. Cejka, J. Belamaric, M. Al-Sarraf, W. D. Peterson, Jr., V. K. Vaitkevicius, and M. D. Poulik (1974), *Clin. Chim. Acta* **52,** 293.

Krant, M. J., G. Manskopf, C. S. Brandrup, and M. A. Madoff (1968), *Cancer* **21**, 623.
Linder, M. C. (1979a), in *Compendium of Assays for Immunodiagnosis of Human Cancer* (R. B. Herberman, ed.), Elsevier/North Holland, New York, p. 305.
Linder, M. C. (1979b), in *Compendium of Assays for Immunodiagnosis of Human Cancer* (R. B. Herberman, ed.), Elsevier/North Holland, New York. p. 311.
Lipscomb, H. S., C. Wilson, K. Retiene, F. Matsen, and D. N. Ward (1968), *Cancer Res.* **28**, 378.
LoGerfo, P., J. Krupey, and H. J. Hansen (1971), *New Engl. J. Med.* **285**, 138.
LoGerfo, P., and J. McLanahan (1976), *J. Surg. Res.* **20**, 481.
Mandel, M. A., K. Dvorak, and J. J. DeCosse (1973), *Cancer* **31**, 1408.
Manendez-Botet, C. V., H. F. Oettgen, C. M. Pinsky, and M. K. Schwartz (1978), *Clin. Chem.* **24**, 868.
Marcus, D. M., N. Zinberg, and I. Listowsky (1979), in *Immunodiagnosis of Cancer* (R. B. Herberman and K. R. McIntire, eds.), Dekker, New York, p. 473.
Maxim, P. E., J. R. Prather, and R. W. Veltri (1980), *Fed. Proc.* **39**, (3, part 1), 413.
McGeachin, R. L., and M. R Adams (1957), *Cancer* **10**, 497.
McIntire, K. R. (1979), in *Compendium of Assays for Immunodiagnosis of Human Cancer* (R. B. Herberman, ed.), Elsevier/North Holland, New York. p. 259.
McIntire, K. R., R. Masseyeff, and H. Breuer (1979), in *Carcino-Embryonic Proteins*, vol. 1 (F.-G. Lehmann, ed.), Elsevier/North Holland, Amsterdam. p. 517.
McIntire, K. R., and Princler, G. L. (1978), unpublished data.
Micksche, M., and O. Kokron (1977), *Osterr. Z. Onkol.* **3**, 116.
Milhaud, G., C. Calmette, J. Taboulet, A. Juliene, and M. S. Moukhtar (1974), *Lancet* **1**, 462.
Muggia, F. M., S. W. Rosen, B. D. Weintraub, and H. H. Hansen (1975), *Cancer* **36**, 1327.
Nash, D. R. (1979), *Ann. Clin. Res.* **11**, 78.
Nash, D. R., J. W. McLarty, and N. G. Fortson (1980), *J. Natl. Cancer Inst.* **64**, 721.
Odell, W. D., and A. R. Wolfsen (1978), *Ann. Rev. Med.* **29**, 379.
Odell, W. D., A. R. Wolfsen, I. Bachelot, and F. M. Hirose (1979), *Am. J. Med.* **66**, 631.
Odell, W., A. R. Wolfsen, Y. Yoshimoto, R. Weltzman, D. Fisher, and F. Hirose (1977), *Trans. Assoc. Am. Phys.* **90**, 204.
Order, S. E., J. L. Klein, D. Ettinger, P. Olderson, S. Siegelman, and P. Leichner (1980), *Cancer Res.* **40**, 3001.
Paris, M., P. Leclerc, B. Lebeau, J. Rochemaure, and M. Leclerc (1980), *Sem. Hop. Paris* **56**, 329.
Pearse, A. G. E., and J. M. Polak (1974), *Med. Biol.* **52**, 3.
Plesnicar, S., and Z. Rudolf (1979), *Neoplasma* **26**, 721.
Plow, E. F., and T. S. Edgington (1979), in *Immunodiagnosis of Cancer* (R. B. Herberman and K. R. McIntire, eds.), Dekker, New York, p. 181.

Podmore, J., B. Wilson, E. A. Cowden, G. H. Beastall, and J. G. Ratcliffe (1979), in *Carcino-Embryonic Proteins*, vol. 1 (F.-G. Lehmann, ed.), Elsevier/North Holland, Amsterdam, p. 457.

Potter, Jr., T. P., J. D. Jordan, and T. A. Jordan (1979), in *Compendium of Assays for Immunodiagnosis of Human Cancer* (R. B. Herberman, ed.), Elsevier/North Holland, New York, p. 217.

Primack, A. (1974), *Semin. Oncol.* **1**, 235.

Rees, L. H., G. A. Bloomfield, G. M. Rees, B. Corrin, L. M. Franks, and J. G. Ratcliffe (1974), *J. Clin. Endocrin. Metab.* **38**, 1090.

Rees, L. H., and J. G. Ratcliffe (1974), *Clin. Endocrin. (Oxford)* **3**, 263.

Reynoso, G., T. M. Chu, D. Holyoke, E. Cohen, T. Nemoto, J. J. Wang, J. Chuang, P. Guinan, and G. Murphy (1972), *J. Amer. Med. Assoc.* **220**, 361.

Roberts, H. J. (1959), *Ann. Int. Med.* **51**, 1420.

Robertson, G. L. (1978), in *Biological Markers of Neoplasia* (R. W. Ruddon, ed.), Elsevier/North Holland, New York, p. 277.

Rosen, S. W., C. W. Becker, S. Schlaff, J. Easton, and M. C. Gluck (1968), *New Engl. J. Med.* **279**, 640.

Rosen, S. W., B. D. Weinstein, J. L. Vaitukaitis, H. H. Sussman, J. M. Hershman, and F. M. Muggia (1975), *Ann. Int. Med.* **82**, 71.

Rosen, S. W., and B. D. Weintraub (1974), *New Engl. J. Med.* **290**, 1441.

Rosen, S. W., and B. D. Weintraub (1979), in *Immunodiagnosis of Cancer* (R. B. Herberman and K. R. McIntire, eds.), Dekker, New York, p. 420.

Ross, E. J. (1963), *Quart. J. Med.* **32**, 297.

Rossen, R. D., M. A. Reisberg, E. M. Hersh, and J. U. Gutterman (1977), *J. Natl. Cancer Inst.* **58**, 1205.

Schwartz, W.. B., W. Bennett, S. Curelop, and F. C. Bartter (1957), *Am. J. Med.* **23**, 529.

Sherwood, L. M., J. L. H. O'Riordan, G. D. Aurbach, and J. T. Potts, Jr. (1967), *J. Clin. Endocrin. Metab.* **27**, 140.

Silva, O., K. Becker, A. Primack, J. Doppman, and R. Snider (1973), *Lancet* **2**, 317.

Silva, O. L., K. L. Becker, A. Primack, J. L. Doppman, and R. H. Snider (1974), *New Engl. J. Med.* **290**, 1122.

Silva, O. L., L. E. Broder, J. L. Doppman, R. H. Snider, C. F. Moore, M. H. Cohen, and K. L. Becker (1979), *Cancer* **44**, 680.

Silverman, L. M., G. B. Dermer, M. H. Zweig, A. C. VanSteirteghem, and Z. A. Tokes (1979), *Clin. Chem.* **25**, 1432.

Singer, F. R., and J. F. Habener (1974), *Biochem. Biophys. Res. Commun.* **61**, 710.

Sirsat, A. V., R. V. Talavdekar, A. K. Jain, and J. J. Vyas (1979), *Indian J. Cancer* **16**, 37.

Sizemore, G. W., and H. Heath, III (1975), *J. Clin. Invest.* **55**, 1111.

Sparanga, M., G. Phillips, C. Hoffman, and L. Kucera (1971), *Metab.* **20**, 730.

Steiner, H., O. Dahlback, and J. Waldenstrom (1968), *Lancet* **1**, 783.

Sternberger, L. A. (1979), in *Immunocytochemistry*, Wiley, New York, p. 82.

Stolbach, L. L., J. J. Krant, and W. H. Fishman (1969), *New Engl. J. Med.* **281**, 757.

Sussman, H. H., B. D. Weintraub, and S. W. Rosen (1974), *Cancer* **33**, 820.

Theofilopoulos, A. N. (1979), in *Compendium of Assays for Immunodiagnosis of Human Cancer* (R. B. Herberman, ed.), Elsevier/North Holland, New York, p. 113.

Theofilopoulos, A. N., and F. J. Dixon (1979), in *Immunodiagnosis of Cancer* (R. B. Herberman and K. R. McIntire, eds.), Dekker, New York, p. 896.

Thomson, D. M. P., J. Krupey, S. O. Freedman, and P. Gold (1969), *Proc. Natl. Acad. Sci.* **64**, 161.

Torstensson, S., M. Thoren, and K. Hall (1980), *Acta Medica Scand.* **207**, 353.

Tsou, K. C., K. W. Lo, R. B. Herberman, A. J. Schutt, and V. L. Go (1980), *J. Clin. Hematol. Oncol.* **10**, 1.

Turkington, R. W. (1971), *New Engl. J. Med.* **285**, 1455.

Turkington, R. W., and J. K. Goldman (1966), *Cancer* **19**, 406.

Urushizaki, I., N. Yoshiro, and K. Ishitani (1979), in *Compendium of Assays for Immunodiagnosis of Human Cancer* (R. B. Herberman, ed.), Elsevier/North Holland, New York, p. 199.

Vaitukaitis, J. L., G. D. Braunstein, and G. T. Ross (1972), *Am. J. Obstet. Gyn.* **113**, 751.

Vaitukaitis, J. L., and G. T. Ross (1972), in *Gonadotropins* (B. Saxena, H. Gandy, and C. Beling, eds.), Wiley, New York, p. 435.

Veltri, R. W., H. F. Mengoli, P. E. Maxim, S. Westfall, J. M. Gopo, C. W. Huang, and P. M. Sprinkle (1977), *Cancer Res.* **37**, 1313.

Vincent, R. G., and T. M. Chu (1973), *J. Thoracic Cardiovasc. Surg.* **66**, 320.

Vincent, R. G., T. M. Chu, T. B. Fergen, and M. Ostrander (1975), *Cancer* **36**, 2069.

Vincent, R. G., T. M. Chu, W. W. Lane, A. C. Gutierrez, P. J. Stegemann, and S. Madajewicz (1979), in *Lung Cancer: Progress in Therapeutic Research* (F. Muggia and M. Rozencweig, eds.), Raven Press, New York, p. 191.

Waalkes, T. P., M. D. Abeloff, K. B. Woo, D. S. Ettinger, R. W. Ruddon, and P. Aldenderfer (1980), *Cancer Res.* **40**, 4420.

Waldmann, T. A., and K. R. McIntire (1974), *Cancer* **34**, 1510.

Weintraub, B. D., andd S. W. Rosen (1971), *J. Clin. Endocrin. Metab.* **32**, 94.

Weiss, M. J., H. A. Edmondson, and M. Wertman (1951), *Am. J. Clin. Pathol.* **21**, 1057.

Weiss, J. F., S. M. Milulski, and P. B. Chretien (1979), in *Lung Cancer: Progress in Therapeutic Research* (F. M. Muggia and M. Rozencweig, eds.), Raven Press, New York, p. 227.

Wolfson, A. R., and W. D. Odell (1979), *Am. J. Med.* **66**, 765.

Yalow, R. S. (1979), in *Lung Cancer: Progress in Therapeutic Research* (F. M. Muggia and M. Rozencweig, eds.), Raven Press, New York, P. 209.

Yalow, R. S., and S. A. Berson (1971), *Biochem. Biophys. Res. Commun.* **44**, 439.

Yokoyama, M., T. Natsuizaka, Y. Ishii, S. Onshima, A. Kasagi, and S. Tateno (1977), *Cancer* **40**, 766.

Zeromski, J., M. K. Gorny, M. Wruk, and J. Sapula (1975), *Int. Arch. Allergy Appl. Immunol.* **49**, 548.

16

Central Nervous System Tumor Markers

Trevor R. Jones and Darell D. Bigner

Department of Pathology, Duke University Medical Center, Durham, North Carolina

1. Introduction

Tumors of the human central nervous system (CNS) can be divided into two large groups: primary and metastatic. Although primary CNS tumors are less common than metastatic tumors, primary tumors are seen at a rate of about 10,000–15,000 per year or 0.5–2/100,000 population. This is a higher incidence than is seen in Hodgkin's disease. Primary CNS tumors are also the most common solid tumors of childhood (Jellinger, 1978; Posner et al., 1979). Although a large number of systems for the classification of primary CNS neoplasia has been generated during the last century, primary intracranial tumors are now categorized using one of a small number of systems. The most common primary CNS tumors of adults are of glial origin, including astrocytomas, glioblastomas, oligodendrogliomas, and ependymomas. Other tumors are of questioned origin. Included here are medulloblastoma, a tumor of childhood, and hemangioblastoma, a tumor classically described as being of blood vessel origin; that concept is, however, now under scrutiny. Several types of meningiomas develop from the tissues covering the brain, the leptomeninges. The adenohypophysis is the source of four types of pituitary adenomas; some of these benign tumors secrete pituitary hormones. A discussion of CNS tumor morphology and classification is outside the limits of this review and if the reader wishes a comprehensive treatment of this subject, he is referred to Burger and Vogel (1976) and Russell and Rubinstein (1977).

In 1964, Aronson and colleagues found intracranial metastases in approximately 18% (67,000) of all cancer patients coming to autopsy. Posner et al. (1979) cited a 30% incidence of metastases to the brain and noted that a majority of these patients had CNS symptoms during life. They also postulated that as chemotherapeutic treatment for systemic cancers improves, the number of patients dying from CNS metastases will increase. Tumors originating in the lung and breast are the most frequent primary lesions in cases of secondary CNS neoplasia. Other common extracranial tumors metastasizing to the brain are melanoma, choriocarcinoma, renal cell carcinoma, and carcinomas of the gastrointestinal tract (Posner et al., 1979).

Even this cursory list of primary and metastatic CNS tumors indicates the great variety of tumors, many of which are of questioned or unknown origin, that can afflict the CNS. Because of the great cellular heterogeneity of normal brain tissues, much effort over the years has been applied to discovering characteristics useful in identifying the various normal cell subpopulations. The search for markers useful in detecting, identifying, and monitoring CNS tumors has, quite naturally, sprung from and become inexorably entwined with this study of normal CNS cell subpopulations. It would, therefore, be difficult to discuss sensibly brain tumor markers without also discussing markers of normal brain tissue and this review will reflect that view.

Although recent reviews discussing brain tumor markers are available, they are either brief (Bock, 1978; Hamprecht, 1978) or they are focused on one particular area such as CSF markers (Seidenfeld and Marton, 1979; Schold and Bullard, 1980), biochemical markers (Wollemann, 1974; Herschman, 1978; Kleihues and Bigner, 1981), and immunologic markers and characteristics (Goridis and Schachner, 1978; Wikstrand and Bigner, 1980). In this review we are attempting to provide a concise yet comprehensive study of all significant, potentially useful CNS tumor markers.

The markers of primary intracranial tumors have been divided into four groups in this review. Those markers that have been discovered or defined by immunologic reagents have been collected under the heading of "Markers Detected by Immunochemical Methods." All enzymes, regardless of the methods used to detect them, have been grouped together, and other markers not fitting in either of the first two sections have been placed in a third section. The pituitary hormones make up the fourth group. Although the criteria used to place the markers in groups may seem arbitrary, it is difficult to group them by a relevant biologic characteristic such as function. Although their distributions have been studied, the function of many of the markers is unknown. Glial fibrillary acidic protein (GFAP) is often described as a cytoskeletal protein, but the specific function it performs in astrocytes, the only cells containing it, is unknown. The function of S-100 protein is undetermined and although the specific reactions catalyzed by the enzymes are well understood, the significance of their presence or absence in a particular cell or tissue type is far from clear. Although the biologic basis for the restriction of expression of these markers has not been discovered, the fact that expression is restricted clearly suggests, however, that the markers perform a function important to the cell or tissue types that express them. Even with their functions unknown, these markers are still of great use to both the neurobiologist and the clinician. Once the distribution of a given marker has been described, it may be of use to the clinician in one of two ways. It may help in (1) the diagnosis of tumors of questioned origin, and (2) it may be of use in the detection of cancer and in the monitoring of tumor burden during chemotherapy and radiotherapy regimens.

When considering this second type of marker, one useful in the detection and monitoring of tumor, one finds that the search for such markers has centered around the CSF. Tumors of the CNS are unique in the sense that they are near or in contact with the subarachnoid space or ventricular system, a compartment relatively isolated from the rest of the body and filled with only about 130 mL of a dilute, protein-poor fluid. Because proteins pass with ease between the ventricular system and the brain parenchyma via the spaces between ependymal cells (Brightman, 1968), it seems reasonable that large amounts of any tumor product could easily accumulate in the adjacent CSF. Another reason for searching the CSF rather than the serum has been the concern that brain tumor products may not readily gain access to the blood because of the blood–brain barrier. The cerebral capillary endothelia are tightly bound to one another by pentalaminar "tight" junctions thereby making transcapillary transit difficult except for compounds with high lipid solubility. Although most studies have involved blood to brain transit of compounds, Brightman and Reese (1969) showed that proteins in the brain substance were blocked from entering the blood by the same barrier. Within the past few years, however, evidence has been produced showing that the blood–brain barrier in brain tumor vasculature is frequently breached. Discontinuous and fenestrated endothelia are common, especially in the more anaplastic tumors, and blood channels lined with both the remnants of endothelial cells and tumor cells have been noted (Vick et al., 1977). Even if brain tumor products do have easy access to the blood via any incomplete capillaries that may be present, the CSF remains superior to serum as a brain tumor marker "reservoir" owing to its small size, its proximity to the tumor, and its isolation from other organ systems.

The primary disadvantage to CSF studies is that a lumbar puncture is potentially life threatening in patients with space occupying lesions because of the possibility that perturbations in CSF pressure can lead to intracranial herniation. Nevertheless, in most clinical settings, experienced neurologists and neurosurgeons aided by computerized axial tomography can safely obtain CSF, but should do so only if the information gained is of sufficient value to outweigh the discomfort and potential danger involved in lumbar puncture.

2. Markers of Primary Intracranial Tumors

2.1. Markers Detected by Immunochemical Methods

2.1.1. Glial Fibrillary Acidic Protein

Glial fibrillary acidic protein (GFAP) is an intracellular protein first described by two independent groups. Mori and colleagues (1968) isolated an acidic protein from brain tissue taken from Tay-Sachs disease patients and showed through immunofluorescence its specificity for fibrillary astrocytes. They called this protein "astroprotein." Eng et al. (1971), working with fibrous astrocyte-rich multiple sclerosis plaques and postleukotomy scars, also isolated an acidic protein that they called glial fibrillary acidic protein. GFAP isolated from multiple sclerosis plaques migrated as two bands with molecular weights of 47,000 and 41,000 daltons, while that from normal brain gave one 47,000 dalton band by SDS gel electrophoresis (Eng and Bigbee, 1978). Mori et al. (1975b) found their anti-astroprotein serum and Eng's anti-GFAP serum to have immunologically identical specificity, as demonstrated by immunodiffusion and immunoelectrophoresis. Bignami et al. (1972) showed by immunofluorescence the localization of GFAP within astrocytes seen in sectioned brain and Antanitus and coworkers (1975) studied in vitro GFAP expression in human fetal cerebrum explants. Cells judged neuronal in origin by silver stain positivity and the presence of 20–25 nm microtubules under electron microscopy were negative for GFAP on immunofluorescence; on the other hand, cells judged to be astroglial on morphological grounds (large nuclei, large broad cytoplasmic processes, and bundles of 6–9 nm filaments seen in the electron microscope) showed fluorescence-positive fibrils sweeping through the cytoplasm.

Because of the astroglial localization of GFAP, it has been considered a potential marker for the astroglial component of gliomas. A quantitative immunoelectrophoretic study of 20 tumors showed that viable glioblastoma had between two and six times more GFAP than did normal brain. Necrotic tumors had less GFAP than normal brain. Three metastatic tumors showed small amounts of GFAP, but the authors felt this owed to contamination with brain parenchyma. Six meningiomas were GFAP negative (Dittman et al., 1977). Jacque et al. (1978) found that glioblastomas had the lowest amount of GFAP of all astrocytomas. They found a positive correlation between cellular differentiation and GFAP content and an inverse correlation between GFAP content on the one hand and cellular anaplasia, increased number of mitotic figures, and abnormal and giant cells on the other. Two hemangioblastomas and one choroid plexus papilloma were strongly positive and four acoustic neurinomas were totally negative. GFAP positivity in some of the cells in hemangioblastoma and the presence of S-100 protein in a cell line derived from a hemangioblastoma have led to the questioning of the concept that hemangioblastoma is a tumor solely of vascular origin. Cellular subpopulations seen within some hemangioblastomas show CNS markers (GFAP and S-100 protein) and may be neoplastic (Kepes et al., 1979a; Bigner et al., 1980; Rasmussen et al., 1980). Several other types of tumors studied by Jacque et al. (1978) were found to contain trace levels of GFAP, but the authors admitted that in these cases (ependymoma, craniopharyngiomas, meningiomas, and metastatic lesions), contamination with tissue from surrounding areas of gliosis was postulated as the basis for GFAP positivity. Unlike Dittmann et al. (1977) and Delpech et al. (1978), they found no correlation between GFAP concentration and necrosis or hemorrhage. In a recent study employing rocket immunoelectrophoresis, Rasmussen et al. (1980) quantitated levels of GFAP in a variety of CNS tumors and found GFAP in all astrocytomas, glioblastomas, ependymomas, oligodendrogliomas, hemangioblastomas, and medulloblastomas tested. Unlike Jacque et al. (1978), they found no correlation between GFAP concentration and malignancy within the group of astroglial tumors. One craniopharyngioma was GFAP positive, but no GFAP was found in a collection of neurinomas, meningiomas, and pituitary adenomas.

Eng and Rubinstein (1978), van der Meulen et al. (1978), and Velasco et al. (1980) have all used immunohistochemical techniques to study GFAP expression in brain tumors. All found GFAP in tumors of astrocytic origin (astrocytomas, astroblastomas, glioblastomas, and subependymomas). van der Meulen et al. (1978) found that in grade I and II astrocytomas, nearly all cells were GFAP positive in all tumors. All grade III astrocytomas were also positive but a variable number of GFAP negative cells were present. Most grade IV astrocytomas were GFAP negative and those that were positive (four of 17) could not be distinguished from the negative ones by any routine diagnostic criteria. The three studies were not, however, in total agreement. van der Meulen et al. (1978) found all medulloblastomas GFAP negative, while Eng and Rubinstein (1978) and Velasco et al. (1980) found areas within these tumors that were GFAP positive; the differentiation of the pluripotent medulloblastoma cells into cells with astrocytic characteristics was given by the authors as the basis for this GFAP positivity. Two other inconsistencies exist in regard to these studies. van der Meulen et al. (1978) found three of 21 oligodendrogliomas to be GFAP positive while both Eng and Rubinstein (1978) and Velasco et al. (1980) found all oligodendrogliomas studied to be GFAP negative and ependymomas to be GFAP positive. Although normal ependymal cells were found to be either GFAP negative or weakly positive, cells derived from an ependymoma maintained in organ culture generated glial fibrils after three weeks in culture and were intensely GFAP positive (Vraa-Jensen et al., 1976). This suggests that ependymoma cells have sufficient plasticity to express GFAP. These data do not agree with those of van der Meulen et al. (1978) who found four of four ependymomas to contain no GFAP.

Although sections and homogenates of tumors have been the most intensively studied (Fig. 1), the most unequivocal demonstrations of the expression of GFAP in neoplastic astrocytes have been performed on cells grown in culture and in nude mice. Bigner et al. (1981) have reported that two of fifteen cell lines derived from human anaplastic gliomas were positive for GFAP (Fig. 2), while Jones et al. (1980) demonstrated GFAP posi-

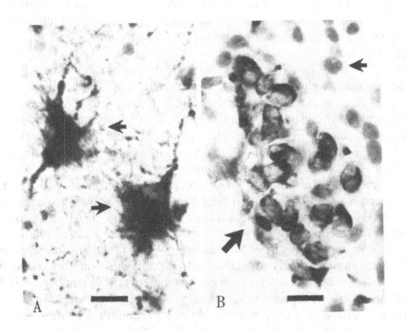

Fig. 1. A. Two astrocytes (arrows) in the reactive zone surrounding an anaplastic glioma stain positively for GFAP using peroxidase–antiperoxidase technique. Hematoxylin counterstain. Bar equals 20 μm. B. A nest of GFAP positive cells (large arrow) in this anaplastic glioma is indistinguishable by conventional staining techniques from the GFAP negative cells (small arrow) surrounding it. Hematoxylin counterstain. Photographs courtesy of Dr. R. D. McComb of this laboratory and anti-GFAP serum courtesy of Dr. L. F. Eng. Bar equals 20 μm.

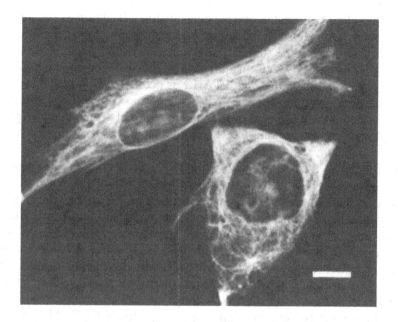

Fig. 2. Immunofluorescent localization of GFAP in a cell line derived from an anaplastic glioma (U-251 MG) demonstrates the fibrillar nature of GFAP. Anti-GFAP serum courtesy of Dr. L. F. Eng. Bar equals 20 μm.

tivity in seven of eight anaplastic gliomas grown in athymic "nude" mice. GFAP positivity in these in vitro systems convincingly shows that neoplastic glia can synthesize GFAP because reactive, nontransformed astrocytes, often present in surgical specimens, are absent in these in vitro systems because nontransformed cells are incapable of both immortal replication in culture and tumor generation in athymic "nude" mice.

One problem encountered in the use of anti-GFAP sera is contamination with antitubulin activities. The hydroxyapatite method for GFAP isolation from whole brain (Dahl, 1976; Dahl and Bignami, 1976) was found to give a product contaminated with tubulin (Bignami et al., 1977; Rueger et al., 1978a). Liem and Shelanski (1978) studied this purification procedure and found that only traces of GFAP were obtained; the bulk of the protein isolated was tubulin. These authors feel that multiple sclerosis plaques remain the best source of GFAP. These findings help explain Bignami and Dahl's (1977) detection of GFAP in peripheral nerve. Tubulin-free GFAP preparations are now being prepared by immunoaffinity chromatography (Rueger et al., 1978b).

Because of the astroglial specificity of GFAP, it has been used in clinical settings to demonstrate the astrocytic nature of primitive or highly anaplastic tumors and in gliomas metastasizing to or invading leptomeninges and extraneural locations (Eng and Rubinstein, 1978). GFAP staining can also help identify the astrocytic elements within mixed tumors such as gliosarcomas (Duffy et al., 1977; Eng and Rubinstein, 1978). Deck et al. (1978) felt that GFAP staining was superior to phosphotungstic acid–hematoxylin (PTAH). No unequivocal astrocyte failed to show GFAP even in sarcoma-like areas, but PTAH was occasionally negative in questionable areas of tumor where GFAP staining was positive. Demonstration of GFAP content in one type of uncommon tumor of disputed origin (pleomorphic xanthoastrocytoma) has shown this tumor to be astroglial rather than mesenchymal in origin (Kepes et al., 1979b).

Studies of astroprotein (GFAP) in the cerebrospinal fluid of patients with neurologic disease have shown elevated GFAP levels in a variety of disorders including both primary and secondary CNS tumors, aneurysms, meningitis, hydrocephalus, epilepsy, hematomas, and acute intracerebral hemorrhage (Mori et al., 1975a, 1978; Hayakawa et al., 1979). No specific disorder showed consistently increased CSF astroprotein levels, but the only tumors to show CSF levels of astroprotein greater than 500 ng/mL were glioblastomas and an anaplastic astrocytoma (Hayakawa et al., 1980).

In the future, use of highly specific antisera to GFAP, such as monoclonal antibody, or the measurement of GFAP subunits may provide more specific correlations with disease states. Presently, however, GFAP is already successfully being used in the diagnosis and classification of tumors of questioned origin and is rapidly replacing older histochemical techniques used to stain glial fibrils. Care must be exercised, however, in interpreting all GFAP-positive cells in tumors as neoplastic since (1) reactive astrocytes can be trapped in the tumors and (2) normal cells that may have phagocytized GFAP also can be easily confused with neoplastic cells expressing GFAP.

2.1.2. S-100 Protein

S-100 protein, named for is solubility in saturated ammonium sulfate at pH 7.1, was first isolated in 1965 (Moore; Moore and MacGregor). S-100 protein, in bovine brain at least, is not a single protein, but consists of at least two highly acidic, phenylalanine-rich proteins, one of which (PAP I-b) has been found to be a dimer of two identical polypeptide chains each containing 91 amino acid residues and weighing 10,507 daltons (Isobe et al., 1977, 1978). PAP I-b has also been sequenced (Isobe and Okuyama, 1978).

Hyden and McElven (1966) showed that S-100 protein was localized mostly in astrocytes, but was also seen in lesser amounts in the perinuclear cytoplasm of oligodendroglia and within the nuclei of neurons, indicating that S-100 protein might be specific to the CNS, but not specific to any particular cell type. This view was strengthened when S-100 protein was found in nitrosoethylurea-induced mouse tumors of putative neuronal origin (Schubert et al., 1974). Levels of S-100 protein were measured in thalamic nuclei undergoing retrograde cell degeneration after appropriate lesions were made in the cerebral cortex and in the optic nerve after enucleation and a rise in S-100 protein levels was found to parallel gliosis in both cases (Cicero et al., 1970; Perez et al., 1970). This suggests a predominantly, though not exclusive, glial distribution for S-100 protein. Recent work, however, has shown the presence of S-100 protein in cultures derived from melanomas, tumors of neural crest origin (Bigner et al., 1981). This finding indicates S-100 protein expression is not as limited as once thought.

Studies of S-100 protein expression in human brain tumors have shown that both astrocytomas and glioblastomas express S-100 protein (Haglid et al., 1973a, 1973b; Dittmann et al., 1977) but levels of S-100 protein do not correlate well with either histologic cell type or patient survival (Dohan et al., 1977). Oligodendrogliomas were found by Haglid et al. (1973a) and Dohan et al. (1977) to contain detectable amounts of S-100 protein while ependymomas contained little or none (Haglid et al., 1973a, 1973b). Meningiomas had either very small amounts of S-100 protein (Haglid et al., 1973a) or none (Haglid et al., 1973b; Dittmann et al., 1977; Dohan et al., 1977). Acoustic neurinoma, a tumor of disputed origin, was shown by Pfeiffer and coworkers (1972) to contain S-100 protein. Fifteen of these tumors were studied and all were S-100 protein positive. Haglid et al. (1973a) and Dohan et al. (1977) have corroborated this observation, thus lending evidence to the theory of the neural crest origin of human acoustic neurinomas.

2.1.3 Alphafetoprotein

Alphafetoprotein (AFP) is an oncofetal antigen seen not only in the serum of patients with hepatocellular carcinoma, but also in fetal and regenerating liver and in cases of hepatitis.

AFP is also produced by some germ cell tumors and by measuring both CSF AFP and CSF β-human chorionic gonadotropin (βHCG), it may be possible to differentiate between tumor types. In a study of six patients with histologically verified primary intracranial germ cell tumors, the two patients with embryonal cell carcinoma were both AFP and βHCG positive; the two patients with choriocarcinoma were βHCG positive and AFP negative; the two patients with dysgerminomas were negative for both (Allen et al., 1979). Nørgaard-Pedersen et al. (1978) described a primary intracranial germ cell tumor that showed elevated serum AFP and HCG before surgery. The levels dropped to normal after surgery. Slight AFP and marked HCG immunofluorescence staining was seen in the tumor. The diagnosis of teratocarcinoma was made. In ten cases of pediatric primary intracranial tumors including four medulloblastomas, two astrocytomas, and four germ cell tumors, only one tumor, an embryonal cell carcinoma, showed increased AFP levels (Shinomiya et al., 1979).

Although the number of patients in these AFP studies is small, the results indicate that AFP levels, especially if monitored in conjunction with βHCG levels, may be a useful marker for the monitoring of chemotherapy and radiotherapy regimens in patients bearing CNS germ cell tumors.

2.1.4. Myelin Basic Protein

Myelin basic protein (MBP) is a component of the myelin sheath. Human MBP has 169 amino acid residues, 24 of which are basic; it weighs 18,300 daltons (Braun and Brostoff, 1977). Although considerable attention has been paid to MBP in connection with experimental allergic encephalomyelitis and multiple sclerosis, few studies have been done to detail its distribution in CNS tumors.

In 1972, Pfeiffer and Wechsler assayed an ethylnitrosourea-induced rat schwannoma and detected a protein immunologically and biochemically similar to MBP. Volpe et al. (1975) ran C6 rat glioma cell membrane fractions on electrophoretic gels and found two bands that migrated to positions corresponding to MBP. McDermott and Smith (1978), however, were unable to duplicate this observation. Acid extracts of cells from C6, two other rat glioma lines, a rat schwannoma line, and primary cell cultures derived from a human oligodendroglioma and an astrocytoma were assayed for MBP using a radioimmunoassay; all showed no MBP within assay sensitivity. Although this inconsistency is difficult to explain, the work of Sheffield and Kim (1977) suggests that cell growth phase may be directly related to MBP expression in vitro. They found that in fetal mouse spinal cord cultures, no MBP was detectable by RIA until day seven in vitro. The appearance of MBP paralleled the appearance of myelination, as seen by light microscopy and an increase in CNPase levels; without visible myelination, MBP could not be detected.

CSF has been assayed for the presence of MBP. In a study of nonneoplastic disease states (Trotter et al., 1978), the only positive samples came from patients with multiple sclerosis, stroke, or encephalitis. Whitaker et al. (1980) found the CSF of patients with a variety of brain tumors to contain no MBP. One glioma patient was CSF MBP positive, but an intratumoral hemorrhage had occurred before lumbar puncture. Elevated CSF MBP was detected most commonly in cases involving strokes and multiple sclerosis.

2.1.5. Fibronectin

Fibronectin (FN) is a cell membrane associated glycoprotein first isolated from chick embryo fibroblasts by Ruoslahti et al. (1973) and shown to be almost identical to and immunologically indistinguishable from a serum glycoprotein, cold insoluble globulin, first isolated by Morrison et al. (1948). Although this 220,000 dalton molecule is seen on the membranes of a variety of cells, mostly mesodermal in origin, it has been found associated, under certain circumstances, with glia. In 1976, Vaheri and coworkers detected, via radioimmunoassay, FN in the culture medium of normal glia and of cell lines derived from anaplastic gliomas. All normal glial cultures were FN positive by immunofluorescence and radioimmunoassay, although two of five cell lines derived from anaplastic gliomas were FN positive by immunofluorescence and all had FN in their spent culture media samples. On the other hand, Schachner et al. (1978) used immunocytochemical electron microscopic methods and found no FN in either the glia or neurons seen in brain sections taken from a variety of nonprimate animals. Although these observations may appear to conflict, one must bear in mind that very different systems were studied. FN has been implicated in cell adhesion and motility phenomena (Yamada et al., 1976; Singer, 1979) and it may be necessary, in some systems, for the completion of cytokinesis (Orly and Sato, 1979). This suggests that FN may be synthesized and expressed by glia only during periods of growth and replication, while in steady-state, there may be no need for FN expression by glia. The fact that FN is demonstrable by immunofluorescence in cultures of nontransformed glia, but is rarely noted in cultures of cells derived from gliomas is not unusual considering the transformation sensitivity of FN. In several cell culture systems, FN production has dropped and FN expression ceased after transformation (Yamada and Olden, 1978).

The question of FN expression in human gliomas has been difficult to attack. Because of breaches in the blood–brain barrier, any FN revealed in tumor sections by immunofluorescence could easily be cold insoluble globulin, which has leached in from the plasma. By studying human gliomas grown subcutaneously in athymic "nude" mice, the problem of leaching FN is bypassed by using anti-FN serum rendered specific for human FN by exhaustive absorption with mouse FN and mouse serum proteins. Jones and coworkers (1980) have, by such methods, found FN in seven of eight human anaplastic gliomas and both GFAP and FN in six of eight. We also have shown the simultaneous expression of FN and GFAP in the same cultured cell (Jones et al., manuscript in preparation.) Whether the GFAP positive cell is actually synthesizing the FN it is expressing is unclear. It is possible that other GFAP negative cells in the culture are producing and exporting the FN, which is then absorbed to the surface of or engulfed by the GFAP positive cells.

Once cells have been shown to be of glial origin by means such as GFAP or glutamine synthetase expression, FN may prove to be a useful indicator of glial growth and replication.

2.1.6. Alpha-2 Glycoprotein

In 1967, Warecka and Bauer isolated a brain glycoprotein with $\alpha2$ mobility in electrophoretic gels and serum $\alpha2$-glycoprotein was unable to ablate antibody acitivity against the brain $\alpha2$-glycoprotein. Warecka and coworkers (1972) found that $\alpha2$ glycoprotein predominates in hemispheric white matter with only trace amounts seen in myelin poor areas. It appears at 24–28 weeks of fetal age; this is when oligodendroglia are first seen. Crude neuron-rich and glia-rich preparations showed $\alpha2$-glycoprotein greatly concentrated in the glial preparation. Using immuno-electrophoresis, Warecka (1975) found $\alpha2$-glycoprotein in all astrocytomas tested; glioblastomas and oligodendrogliomas were, however, negative.

2.1.7. Antigens Defined by Monoclonal Antibody

The recent developments in monoclonal antibody production by murine hybridoma methods are likely to revolutionize immunological detection of antigenic markers of normal and neoplastic CNS cells (see Chapter 1). The hybridoma technique is a probe potentially capable both of producing monospecific antibodies against partially purified proteins and of examining different antigenic determinants in heterogeneous substances such as glial fibrillary acidic protein and S-100 protein. Monoclonal antibody may also be useful in detecting unknown or insufficiently studied membrane antigens that may be expressed in extremely small amounts, yet which have the high degree of specificity characteristic of good markers. In general, the use of hybridoma-produced monospecific antibodies allows the use of reagents of exquisite specificity because the antibodies are directed against individual determinants, are homogeneous in regard to immunoglobulin class and affinity, and can be produced in virtually unlimited amounts. If they are generated against already known antigens such as carcinoembryonic antigen and hormones and are made widely available, they will act as standardized reagents and may reduce the variations seen in data generated in different laboratories.

Koprowski and coworkers (1978) have generated monoclonal antibody against cultured human melanoma cells. They isolated hybridoma clones producing antibody that reacted only with melanomas and others that reacted with melanomas, colorectal carcinoma, and normal human cells. Our laboratory has also screened these antibodies; the first failed to react with cell lines derived from glioblastomas, neuroblastomas, carcinomas, and sarcomas and with normal fibroblasts. The latter antibodies did, however, react with cultured brain, an osteogenic sarcoma-derived cell line and two of five cell lines derived from glioblastomas. Ballou et al. (1979) have used radioactive iodine-labeled monoclonal antibody and external gamma-ray scintigraphy to localize murine teratocarcinomas in the mouse host.

Monoclonal antibody has also been made against several normal CNS antigens: nicotinic acetylcholine receptors (Gomez et al., 1979; Moshly-Rosen et al., 1979), substance P, a peptide of putative neurotransmitter function (Cuello et al., 1979), and a chick embryo retinal cell plasma membrane antigen tentatively described as a complex ganglioside (Eisenbarth et al., 1979).

Kennett and Gilbert (1979) immunized mice with a cultured human neuroblastoma (IMR6) and used the spleen cells from those mice to produce hybridomas. Two clones were isolated that had antineuroblastoma activity. One (PI 153/3) reacted with normal fetal brain and cell lines derived from six neuroblastomas, one of two cell lines derived from retinoblastomas, and one cell line derived from a glioblastoma. Our laboratory has also screened this antibody using a ^{14}C-nicotinamide complement-dependent antibody-mediated cell lysis assay; the antibody reacted with three neuroblastoma-derived cell lines (IMR-32, SK-N-SH, SK-N-MC) and did not react with cell lines derived from nine glioblastomas, two melanomas, one medulloblastoma, one osteogenic sarcoma, and fetal brain. Kennett et al. (1980) have recently reported that the antibody also reacts with four of six null-cell acute lymphocytic leukemia cell lines, one B cell acute lymphocytic leukemia cell line, and samples of peripheral blood from two of three B cell chronic lymphocytic leukemia patients. It failed to react with a cell line derived from a T cell acute lymphocytic leukemia or a peripheral blood sample from a T cell chronic lymphocytic leukemia patient.

Eisenbarth and coworkers' monoclonal antibody directed against a plasma membrane component of chick embryo retinal cells has recently been shown to react with neuroblastoma. Studies are now underway in which the Kennett and Eisenbarth monoclonal antibodies are being used to detect immunohistochemically individual metastatic neuroblastoma cells in bone marrow aspirates. These cells would ordinarily be undetectable by standard light and electron microscopic methods (personal communication).

Hybridoma-produced immunoglobulin will have a significant effect on the search for brain tumor markers not only because of its exquisite specificity and sensitivity, but also because of its versatility. Monoclonal antibody can be incorporated into a radioimmunoassay to quantitate amounts of a specific antigen or it can be used in electron microscopic immunoperoxidase techniques to localize the antigen at cellular and subcellular levels.

The development of monoclonal antibodies against human glioblastoma multiforme-associated antigens is in its infancy, but in Nicolas de Tribolet's laboratory in Lausanne and in our laboratory, monoclonal antibody reactive with permanent cell lines derived from human gliomas has already been raised.

2.2. Enzymatic Markers

2.2.1. CNPase

2',3'-Cyclic nucleotide 3'-phosphohydrolase (CNPase) catalyzes the hydrolysis of 2',3'-cyclic nucleotides to form 2'-nucleotides (Drummond et al., 1962; Sims and Carnegie, 1976). Study of bovine tissues has shown the greatest amounts of CNPase activity to be localized in the spinal cord and the substance of the brain. Very low activities were found in the major organs, muscle, plasma, red blood cells, adrenal gland, and gut (Drummond et al., 1962). When red blood cells were studied (Sudo et al., 1972), CNPase was found to be selectively attached to the cell membrane. Kurihara and Tsukada (1967) showed that white matter had ten times the concentration of CNPase found in gray matter and determined that the CNPase was localized in the myelin sheath or intimately associated structures. Kurihara and coworkers (1971) studied myelin deficient Jimpy mice and found CNPase to be present in the membranes of oligodendroglia. They felt CNPase was a part of the oligodendroglial membrane and was seen in such great amounts in myelin only because it was concentrated by the folding of the cell membranes during the generation of the myelin sheath. Poduslo's work (1975) seems to support this thesis. She found high concentrations of CNPase in bulk prepared bovine brain myelin, but also found significant levels in the fraction containing oligodendroglial membranes. C6, a well-described rat glioma cell line, has relatively high levels of specific CNPase activity (Zanetta et al., 1972; Volpe et al., 1975; Sims et al., 1979), but no myelin basic protein was detectable by radioimmunoassay (Sims et al., 1979). These data suggest that CNPase expression is not totally tied to myelin synthesis and that CNPase should be considered as a glial rather than an oligodendroglial marker. A recent study by Parker and coworkers (1980) has emphasized this point. Studying early (21–26) and late (82–88) passage C6 rat glioma cells, they found that CNPase levels were initially high, but dropped with increased passage level. As CNPase levels dropped, levels of glutamine synthetase, an astrocyte marker discussed later in this review, rose. The authors suggest "transdifferentiation," the ability of a cell to lose one characteristic and acquire another, as the basis for this phenomenon. Bigner et al. (1981) studied CNPase levels in 15 permanent cell lines derived from human gliomas and found a wide range in activity from undetectable to 12.8 ± 1.5 μmol 2'AMP formed/h/mg protein. The observed range was as great for nonneural cell lines as for glioma-derived cell lines, and there was a low CNPase level of 3.5 ± 0.2 μmol 2'AMP for one of the lines expressing GFAP.

Dohan and coworkers (1977) detected CNPase in all astrocytomas and glioblastomas tested and, as with S-100 protein, CNPase levels correlated poorly with patient survival. They also found CNPase in a choroid plexus papilloma, in two oligodendrogliomas and in two acoustic neurinomas. Pfeiffer et al. (1979) also detected CNPase in acoustic neurinomas (22 of 24 studied) and these data, combined with the S-100 protein studies already discussed, make a powerful case for the neural crest nature of acoustic neurinomas. Kurihara et al. (1974) compared CNPase levels measured in a variety of CNS tumors and found oligodendrogliomas to have the highest levels, but these were only 1/20th of the levels found in normal white matter. Neurinomas and astrocytomas had the next highest levels of CNPase followed by undifferentiated gliomas and glioblastomas, then medulloblastomas, and finally meningiomas. The study, however, contained only eleven tumors and whereas the detection and measurement of CNPase constitute valid observations, the number of tumors is too small to allow any generalizations to be made concerning comparative CNPase levels. Moreover, in such tumor analysis studies, it is impossible to be sure that the CNPase detected was in neoplastic cells and not in trapped normal brain or myelin.

2.2.2. Lactate Dehydrogenase

Lactate dehydrogenase (LDH), a glycolytic enzyme that signals tissue injury when serum levels are elevated, has been measured in the CSF of patients with primary and secondary CNS tumors. The early studies measured total LDH, not comparative levels of the five LDH isozymes, and results achieved were not entirely consistent. Wroblewski et al. (1957) found significant elevations of CSF LDH only in metastatic tumors, whereas Fleisher et al. (1957) found no significant elevations; Wroblewski (1959) and Niebroj-Dobosz and Hetnarska (1969) did find elevations, but these were usually small and sporadic. Green et al. (1958, 1959), however, found CSF LDH titers elevated in all CNS tumor bearing patients studied. Hildebrand (1973) found 50% and Dharker et al. (1976) 90% of brain tumor patients to have elevated CSF LDH levels. Green et al. (1959) felt they noted some correlation between CSF LDH levels and degree of malignancy. Fleisher et al. (1957) and Dharker et al. (1976), on the other hand, could find no correlation between CSF LDH titer and tumor malignancy, and Buckell and Robertson (1965) could not distinguish between primary and metastatic lesions from CSF LDH studies. Hildebrand (1973) also noted that elevations in CSF LDH parallel elevations in CSF protein and found large increases in CSF LDH in cases of meningitis and cerebrovascular accidents. The inconsistent data generated in studies of total LDH in the CSF of tumor patients and the demonstrated nonspecificity of elevated CSF LDH for CNS tumors led other investigators to study the levels of LDH isozymes both in the CSF and in the tumors themselves.

Gerhardt et al. (1963), Haglid et al. (1970), and Rabow and Kristensson (1977) measured LDH isozyme levels in homogenized normal brain and gliomas. Compared to normal tissue, grade I and II astrocytomas had isozyme patterns that were shifted toward isozymes one and two while grade III and IV astrocytomas were skewed in the other direction, toward isozymes four and five. While no isozyme pattern change was specific to one tumor type, the authors felt LDH isozyme shifts as measured in homogenized tumor biopsy samples could be of some use in determining degree of malignancy. Rabow and Kristensson (1977) also studied blood and CSF levels of LDH isozymes and found that they produced little if any useful information.

2.2.3. Glutamic–Oxaloacetic Transaminase

Glutamic–oxaloacetic transaminase (GOT) is one of the several transaminases involved in amino acid synthesis. As with LDH, results from CSF GOT studies are not consistent. Green et al. (1957), Katzman et al. (1957), Miyazaki (1958), Green et al. (1958), Mann et al. (1960) and Hildebrand (1973) found that most CNS tumor patients tested had normal CSF GOT levels. Green et al. (1957) noted that in several cases, CSF GOT levels remained normal even in the face of abnormally high CSF protein. However, Myerson et al. (1957) found slightly to moderately elevated CSF GOT levels in half of the tumor patients they studied. The study contained patients with both primary and metastatic lesions. Fleisher et al. (1957) found statistically significant elevations of CSF GOT in some but not all tumors studied and Mellick and Bassett (1964) found significant elevations only in cases of glioblastoma. Dharker et al. (1976) felt that CSF GOT levels could help differentiate between benign and malignant tumors.

Because elevated CSF GOT levels can be seen in hydrocephalus, brain abscesses (Dharker et al., 1976), subarachnoid hemorrhage (Katzman et al., 1957), head injury, CNS degenerative diseases, and convulsive disorders (Fleisher et al., 1957), CSF GOT is both an insensitive and nonspecific monitor for the presence of brain tumors and is therefore of little value.

2.2.4. Beta-Glucuronidase

Beta-glucuronidase (BG) catalyzes the hydrolysis of β glucuronides to yield various aglycans and free glucuronic acid. High activities are usually found in spleen, liver, kidney, and neoplastic tissue (Levvy and Conchie, 1966). In the brain, BG is richest in white matter and histochemical and electron microscopic studies suggest the enzyme is localized in lysosomes in neuronal perikarya. A slight amount of activity was noted in glia (Allen, 1972). Fishman and Hayashi (1962) found that in rat brain the most intensively BG-positive cells were the Purkinje cells of the cerebellum.

When tissue samples of 32 primary and three metastatic human CNS tumors were tested for BG levels, all malignant tumors showed BG levels that far exceeded those found in normal brain, but because the range of BG levels found in benign tumors overlapped with the range found in malignant ones, BG levels were not useful in separating tumors on the basis of their benign or malignant nature. For example, medulloblastoma had lower levels than ependymoma and the highest levels of BG were seen in a choroid plexus papilloma. Within a single histologic tumor type, BG levels sometimes paralleled anaplasia; this was the case in astroglial tumors. Low-grade astrocytomas had the lowest levels, while glioblastomas had the highest. In the ependymoma series, however, no correlation between BG levels and anaplasia was noted (Allen, 1961). Tumor tissue sections stained for BG gave results that corroborated Allen's data (1961). In the astrocytoma series, BG activity increased with increasing anaplasia, and medulloblastoma, which had showed only moderate levels in Allen's study (1961), was positive only in perivascular areas and in regions of meningeal infiltration (Schiffer et al., 1969).

Cerebrospinal fluid levels of BG were approximately doubled in glioblastoma patients as compared to control CSF levels, but the two groups overlapped (Anylan and Starr, 1952). Two other CSF studies were able to demonstrate elevated BG CSF levels only in patients with intraspinal tumors (Allen and Reagen, 1964; Allen, 1972).

Elevated CSF BG is not restricted to primary brain tumors. Leptomeningeal carcinomatosis and bacterial, viral, and fungal meningitides will also increase CSF BG titers (Schold et al., 1980). Although CSF BG does not appear promising as a tool in primary intracranial tumor diagnosis, it may be of use in the diagnosis of leptomeningeal carcinomatosis and shows some promise as a tumor burden monitor for this disease.

2.2.5. Glycerol Phosphate Dehydrogenase

Glycerol phosphate dehydrogenase (GPDH) is an NAD^+ dependent enzyme which catalyzes the conversion of dihydroxyacetone phosphate to glycerol phosphate in the glycerol phosphate shuttle system (de Vellis and Brooker, 1973). Two forms of the enzyme, one detected in muscle, the second in brain, are identical by immunodiffusion and polyacrylamide gel electrophoresis analyses and have the same molecular weight of 70,000 daltons (McGinnis and de Vellis, 1977). In 1968, de Vellis and Inglish found that hypophysectomy or adrenalectomy decreased GPDH levels in adult rat brains and appropriate hormone supplements (ACTH or cortisol for the former, cortisol for the latter) returned GPDH activity to normal. Muscle GPDH levels are not inducible, however, suggesting that the muscle and brain enzymes may differ not in structure but in the mechanisms that control them. Breen and de Vellis (1975) found that in fetal rat brain explants, hydrocortisone increased by ten times total and specific activity of cytoplasmic GPDH. Hydrocortisone had no effect on total or soluble protein, protein synthesis or LDH activity. Hydrocortisone was continuously required to keep GPDH levels elevated, and tests with DNA and RNA inhibitors indicated protein and RNA synthesis were required for GPDH induction; DNA synthesis was not.

Cell lines derived from G-26, a transplantable glioma from C57B1/6 mice, did not increase GPDH production under hydrocortisone or cortisol induction (Sundarraj et al., 1975) while C6, a rat glioma line, did (de Vellis and Brooker, 1973; Sundarraj et al., 1975). Although GPDH has not yet been shown specific for any histologic tumor type, it is accepted as a glial marker and has been shown by light and electron microscopic peroxidase techniques to be localized only in oligodendroglia and not in neurons or astrocytes (de Vellis et al., 1977).

2.2.6. Enolase

Moore and Perez (1968) described a protein that they called 14-3-2 and found it to be 100–200 times more concentrated in the CNS than in other organs tested. Through Wallerian degeneration experiments on rabbit optic nerve and rat thalamic nuclei, a neuronal localization of 14-3-2 was strongly suggested (Perez et al., 1970; Cicero et al., 1970) and Herschman and Lerner (1973) and Augusti-Tocco et al. (1973) found that human and mouse neuroblastomas produced it. In 1975, Bock and Dissing showed that 14-3-2 was identical to the enzyme enolase (2-phospho-D-glycerate hydrolase). Pickel et al. (1976) and Grasso et al. (1977), using immunohistochemistry and immunocytochemical electron microscopy, localized enolase to neurons. None was found in astrocytes or oligodendroglia.

Two enolase isoenzymes have been isolated; the one having neuron specificity is synonymous with 14-3-2 and is called neuron specific enolase (NSE). Nonneuronal enolase (NNE) is found in glia and blood vessels, but not in neurons. Each isoenzyme is made up of two subunits with NSE having two λ chains (39,000 daltons each) whereas NNE has two α' (43,000 daltons each) chains and is analogous with, but not yet shown to be identical to, the liver enolase. An $\alpha'\lambda$ hybrid also exists (Marangos et al., 1978b; Schmechel et al., 1978).

Schubert and coworkers (1974) studied S-100 and 14-3-2 expression in a collection of clonal cell lines derived from rat CNS tumor lines, but were unable to divide the tumors into either glial or neuronal groups. Some cell lines expressed both, some only one, and some neither. They suggested the failure to distinguish between tumor types owed to the lack of glial specificity on the part of S-100 protein. Haglid et al. (1973a) found 14-3-2 in glioblastomas, astrocytomas, acoustic neurinomas, choroid plexus papillomas, in some oligodendrogliomas and, curiously, in chromophobe pituitary adenomas. None was found in areas of tumor necrosis, meningiomas, or metastatic lesions. If the 14-3-2 levels detected were produced by the tumor cells and not by neurons lying within or on the periphery of the tumor, then 14-3-2 (NSE) cannot be considered specific for tumors of putative neuronal origin. Marangos et al. (1978a) studied cell lines derived from both human (IMR-32) and mouse (N-18) neuroblastomas and found very low levels of NSE compared to those found in normal brain homogenate. Total enolase levels were equal; the preponderance of enolase in the lines was NNE. Treatment with db-cAMP caused NSE levels in N-18 to rise. The low NSE and high NNE levels in these cultures could owe to either the fact that while neuroblastomas are of putative neuronal origin, they are not CNS tumors, or it could owe to transformation-induced phenotype changes. The latter is suggested by the db-cAMP treatment-induced increase in NSE levels in N-18.

2.2.7. Glutamine Synthetase

Glutamate is a putative amino acid transmitter and glutamine synthetase catalyzes the synthesis of glutamine from glutamate (Hamberger et al., 1977; Hertz, 1977). Martinez-Hernandez et al. (1977) and Norenberg (1979) found by light microscopic immunohistochemistry that glutamine synthetase was localized in glia. Neurons, endothelial cells, and choroid plexus cells were negative and only a trace of reaction product was seen in ependymal cells. Electron microscopic immunohistochemistry further localized the reaction product to astrocytic glia. No glutamine synthetase was detected in any other cell within the brain (Norenberg and Martinez-Hernandez, 1979).

Any studies attempting to localize glutamine synthetase by studying bulk prepared neurons, glia, and neuronal synaptosomes (Weiler et al., 1979) should be viewed with caution. Cell injury during processing can result in enzyme leakage and identification of the isolated cells is usually done by morphology alone. Neuronal synaptosome preparations can also be heavily contaminated, with "synaptosomes" of glial origin (Henn et al., 1976).

Although no work has been published on the distribution of glutamine synthetase in CNS tumors, it holds promise as a putative astrocytoma cell marker.

2.2.8. Aldolase C

The three aldolase isozymes are glycolytic enzymes that cleave fructose 1,6-diphosphate to glyceraldehyde 3-phosphate and dihydroxyacetone phosphate. Aldolase A is found in most tissues, aldolase B in kidney and liver, and aldolase C predominantly in the brain, but variably in heart, spleen, and other tissues (Penhoet et al., 1966; Lebherz and Rutter, 1969). All three isozymes have a molecular weight of 160,000 daltons and can be dissociated into subunits of about 40,000 daltons. This subunit structure explains the existence of three hybrids when two of the isozymes are found in the same tissue. Brain, for example, shows five aldolases: A, C and the three hybrids possible by combining A and C subunits (Sugimura et al.,

1969; Bodansky, 1975). Sato and coworkers (1971) found that nearly all gliomas studied had A, C and all hybrids and that the pattern was nearly identical to that of normal brain. However, Kumanishi et al. (1970) found that while both A and C isozymes were present in astrocytomas and malignant gliomas, their relative concentrations were not identical with normal brain. Astrocytomas had the greatest amount of C found in any of the tumors analyzed and this caused the electrophoretic pattern to be skewed toward C. Malignant gliomas, on the other hand, were skewed toward A. Acoustic neurinomas were also skewed toward A. Both Kumanishi et al. (1970) and Sato et al. (1971) agreed that meningiomas had little or no C isozyme.

2.2.9. Carbonic Anhydrase

Carbonic anhydrase (CA), an enzyme accelerating the reaction $CO_2 + H_2O \rightleftharpoons H_2CO_3$ in both directions, was first localized to glia by Giacobini (1961, 1962). He dissected the glia from the neurons of Deiter's nucleus and used a Cartesian diver to test a single cell's ability to generate CO_2 from $NaHCO_3$. Red blood cells and choroid plexus cells were also tested and had three and two times, respectively, the amount of carbonic anhydrase found in glia while the glia themselves had 120 times more of the enzyme than did neurons.

There are three isozymes of carbonic anhydrase. Isozyme A is extensively different from B and C in terms of catalytic efficiency, amino acid composition, molecular weight, and tissue distribution (Holmes, 1977). Carbonic anhydrase C (also called carbonic anhydrase II) is the isozyme that has been localized to glia, but whether it is found in astrocytes or oligodendroglia is unclear. Sensenbrenner et al. (1977) found both carbonic anhydrase C and glycerol phosphate dehydrogenase in "astroblasts" cultured from disassociated newborn rat brains. Both the appearance of glial filaments and the production of GFAP increased over time and addition of cAMP caused a more "astrocytic" appearance in these cells. Kimelberg et al., (1977a, 1977b) also found carbonic anhydrase C in astrocyte-like cells derived from newborn rat brain cultures and noted that 36% of the enzyme was found in membrane fractions. On the other hand, Delaunoy et al. (1977), Mandel et al. (1977), and Spicer et al. (1979) stained rat and mouse CNS histologic sections with fluorescent antibody and immunoperoxidase methods and found staining only in cells they identified by light microscopy as oligodendroglia and in areas of myelin deposition.

Carbonic anhydrase C was also found in myelin fractions isolated from homogenized rat brain (Sapirstein and Lees, 1977). Mandel and coworkers (1977) also used light microscopic immunohistochemistry to localize carbonic anhydrase C to oligodendroglia and myelin sheaths. In a study of both Jimpy mice (deficient in oligodendroglia and myelin) and normal mice, however, they found that Jimpy mice contain half the normal amount of carbonic anhydrase C and they concluded that this did not correlate well with the severe oligodendroglia deficiency seen in the mutant mice. This suggested to the authors that carbonic anhydrase C may also be present in astrocytes.

No comprehensive study has yet been done to study the distribution of carbonic anhydrase C in CNS tumors.

2.2.10. Lysozyme

Lysozyme is a lysosomal enzyme with nonspecific antibacterial activities and has been studied as a potential CSF monitor of brain tumors. Although baseline levels of CSF lysozyme are disputed (Newman et al., 1974; Hansen et al., 1977), there is general agreement that the highest levels of CSF lysozyme are found in infectious diseases, especially bacterial meningitis (Newman et al., 1974; Reitamo and Klockars, 1976; Hansen et al., 1977). Elevated levels were also found in cases of fungal meningitis (Reitamo and Klockars, 1976), multiple sclerosis (Hansen et al., 1977) and neurosarcoidosis and CNS syphilis (Mason and Roberts-Thomson, 1974). In both small (Constantopoulos et al., 1976) and large studies (Newman et al., 1974; Hansen et al., 1977), elevated levels of lysozyme were found in the CSF of tumor patients but the levels often overlapped with normal controls and in immunoperoxidase staining, no lysozyme could be found within tumors. The source of the enzyme was postulated to be the reactive zone surrounding the tumor. DiLorenzo and Palma (1976), Reitamo and Klockars (1976), and DiLorenzo and coworkers (1977) found that CSF lysozyme correlated with CSF leukocytes and protein levels. Even in patients with demonstrated CNS tumors, unusual lysozyme levels were not seen until after protein and/or leukocyte levels became elevated.

Because CNS disorders other than tumors elevate CSF lysozyme levels and because CSF protein and leukocyte levels parallel rises in lysozyme, it is both nonspecific and redundant as CNS tumor marker and, hence, is of no use in the diagnosis of CNS neoplasia.

2.3. Other Markers

2.3.1. Polyamines

The polyamines are side-products of RNA synthesis and are generated in increased amounts when a cell shifts into growth phase (Russell, 1973; Russell and Durie, 1978). In 1971, Russell and Russell et al. found increased levels of three polyamines (putrescine, spermidine, and spermine) in the urine of patients bearing solid tumors. Only four CNS tumor patients were studied and urinary polyamine levels were increased two to six times.

In the last decade, several studies have examined CSF polyamine levels as a potential monitor of human CNS tumor burden. In three studies, glioblastoma patients showed statistically significant increases in CSF putrescine (Marton et al., 1974b; Marton et al., 1976); in one study (Marton et al., 1974a), six of six glioblastoma patients showed levels above the highest putrescine level found in the nonneoplastic neurologic disease controls. All three studies also found CSF spermidine levels to be increased, but not with the consistency of putrescine. Patients with astrocytomas also had increased CSF levels of both putrescine and spermidine, but the levels did not consistently exceed the control group. In medulloblastoma patients, significantly increased putrescine levels were noted in the CSF, and in cases where the tumor failed to remit, putrescine, and often spermidine levels, remained high (Marton et al., 1974b; Marton et al., 1976). CSF polyamine levels dropped in cases where therapy was judged by conventional clinical means to be successful. In one half of the cases of tumor recurrence, CSF polyamine levels predicted tumor regrowth weeks or months ahead of routine clinical tests (Marton et al., 1979).

Tumor tissue homogenization studies have shown that all astrocytomas have putrescine levels in excess of the range found in normal brain, and astrocytoma grade IV (glioblastoma) had levels statistically higher than astrocytoma grade II or III. Spermidine and spermine varied over a wide range. Benign CNS tumors (meningioma, chordoma, neurofibroma, and schwannoma) had putrescine levels lower than normal brain tissue (Harik and Sutton, 1979).

Terabayashi (1976), in a study of blood polyamine levels in patients with CNS tumors, found that 14 of 21 glioma patients exceeded the upper limit of the control group and that polyamine concentration paralleled anaplasia. All levels were normal in the benign tumors tested and in hemangioblastoma.

2.3.2. Desmosterol

Desmosterol (24-dehydrocholesterol) is a precursor of cholesterol in the cholesterol synthetic pathway. Saturation of the double bond at position 24 of desmosterol results in the creation of cholesterol, but this conversion can be inhibited by triparanol, a drug that blocks the action of 24,25-reductase. Triparanol does not affect normal adult brain, but a single dose led to an increase in tumor desmosterol levels in transplantable G26C (glioblastoma) and ZE (ependymoma) mouse tumors (Fumagalli et al., 1964, 1966). They also noted that in triparanol-treated brain tumor patients, desmosterol made up 6% of all brain tumor sterols and 12% of all blood sterols.

When nonneoplastic neurologic disease controls are given triparanol, fewer than half have measurable desmosterol in the CSF and all the samples that were positive showed levels less than 0.1 µg/mL. In patients bearing a wide variety of CNS tumors, administration of triparanol causes CSF desmosterol levels to increase from an average of 0.06 to 0.204 μg/mL. Not all patients, however, responded equally to triparanol treatment. Twenty-eight of 30 showed increased CSF desmosterol titers, but only 17 of 30 showed levels above 0.1 μg/mL (the highest level found in a triparanol-treated control) (Paoletti et al., 1969). Weiss and coworkers (1972) and Ransohoff and Weiss (1977) obtained similar results in triparanol-treated glioma patients with 60% of the patients showing CSF desmosterol levels of greater than 0.1 μg/mL.

CSF desmosterol levels greater than 0.3 μg/mL were found in patients bearing neurinomas, meningiomas, ependymomas, glioblastomas, medulloblastomas, and tumors of the third ventricle. CSF desmosterol levels greater than 0.1 μg/mL and a desmosterol × 100/cholesterol ratio >3 were used as tumor indicators and Paoletti et al. (1977) identified tumor presence in all cases of medulloblastoma and third ventricle tumors, in 81.5% of the cases of glioblastoma, 62.5% of all metastatic carcinomas, and 25% of all low grade astrocytomas. On the average, CSF desmosterol tests predicted correctly in 77% of the cases, incorrectly in 8%, and were uncertain in 15%.

Paoletti et al. (1969) found no correlation between CSF desmosterol titers and malignancy or proximity of the tumor to the ventricular system. Fumagalli and Paoletti (1971), on the other hand, felt they saw some correlation between CSF desmosterol levels and malignancy, but thought the correlation incomplete because proximity to the ventricular system did indeed seem to be leading to higher desmosterol levels.

No comprehensive studies have been done to determine if CSF desmosterol levels may be of use in following the efficacy of therapy. The two studies performed (Weiss et al., 1972; Fumagalli et al., 1976) were too small to produce any conclusive results.

Although the triparanol-induced accumulations of desmosterol in the CSF of brain tumor patients is an interesting observation, its inconsistency does not make it useful as a marker. It is not as sensitive as the conventional diagnostic tests now in use. Another problem with this technique is that triparanol is toxic. Some of its side effects include alopecia, leukopenia, diminished libido, and cataracts (Paoletti et al., 1972). Marton et al. (1973) attempted to measure CSF desmosterol both in brain tumor patients and in patients free of neoplastic disease without first administering triparanol. Desmosterol was not found in any of the CSF taken from the brain tumor patients or the controls. The authors claim their gas chromatographic system for analysis (a different system than the one used by the Paoletti, Fumagalli group) was capable of detecting low nanogram quantities of desmosterol in test standards. These data conflict with those of Paoletti et al. (1969) who were able to detect, by their methods, desmosterol in seven of 22 patients who had histologically verified intracranial tumors, but had not been treated with triparanol.

2.4. Hormonal Markers

2.4.1. Prolactin

Schroeder and coworkers (1976) studied CSF prolactin levels in 33 patients with pituitary disease, three pregnant women and 30 controls. Forty percent of the controls had CSF prolactin levels below the level of detectability (1.0 ng/mL) with the control mean equaling 7.0 ng/mL. All three pregnant women showed elevated CSF prolactin levels whereas all 15 patients with empty sella syndrome had normal levels. Among the tumor patients, only two of 18 had CSF prolactin levels that exceeded plasma levels. The authors felt that CSF prolactin levels were probably merely a reflection of plasma levels, but they did not rule out the possibility of direct secretion of prolactin into the CSF. Login and MacLeod (1977) found that five of five patients with pituitary adenomas had increased CSF prolactin levels, even though only one patient had suprasellar extension (SSE). The SSE patient did, however, have CSF prolactin levels about ten times greater than the other tumor patients. Assies et al. (1978) found that plasma prolactin levels rather than the presence or absence of SSE was the best predictor of CSF prolactin levels.

Balagura et al. (1979) measured serum prolactin levels in 205 neurologic disease patients, including 70 with pituitary adenomas. They found that absence of elevated serum prolactin titers did not rule out pituitary pathology. Thirty-three percent of the adenoma patients had normal prolactin levels. Three of seven acromegalics and 43 of 61 adenoma patients had elevated serum prolactin levels. The authors felt that once drug-induced hyperprolactinemia was excluded, elevated serum prolactin levels accurately predicted the presence of hypothalamic–hypophyseal region pathology including conditions other than pituitary adenoma (parasellar meningioma and aneurysms projecting into the pituitary fossa).

2.4.2. Adrenocorticotrophic Hormone

In 1972, Kleerekoper and coworkers reported elevated CSF adrenocorticotrophic hormone (ACTH) in patients who had had tumor following bilateral adrenalectomy (Nelson's syndrome). Compared to control patients, the three adrenalectomized patients studied showed both increased plasma and CSF ACTH levels and the one patient with suprasellar extension (SSE) of the pituitary tumor had the highest CSF ACTH levels. This led the authors to suggest that only SSE could produce CSF ACTH levels that greatly deviated from normal levels.

Allen et al. (1974b) found no correlation between plasma and CSF ACTH levels measured in the same patient. This suggests that CSF ACTH levels are independent of plasma CSF levels, perhaps because of an inability of ACTH to cross readily from the blood to the CSF. Even in patients with extremely elevated plasma ACTH levels, low CSF ACTH levels were noted. The one patient studied who had SSE had a higher CSF ACTH level than plasma level. Another report from the same laboratory (Allen et al., 1974a) stated that in one Nelson's syndrome patient without SSE, CSF ACTH levels were low but in the other Nelson's syndrome patient, CSF ACTH levels were higher than plasma levels and SSE was present. Jordan et al. (1976), also from the same laboratory, failed, in a study of three cases of Nelson's syndrome, to find any correlation between plasma and CSF ACTH levels.

2.4.3. Human Growth Hormone

Wright et al. (1969) measured plasma human growth hormone (HGH) levels in 84 cases of untreated acromegaly and found a correlation between serum HGH levels and pituitary size. Linfoot et al. (1970) were the first to study via radioimmunoassay HGH levels in the CSF of untreated acromegalics. They found a fivefold increase in CSF HGH and a 16-fold increase in plasma HGH. Those patients with SSE had CSF HGH levels 140–800 times higher than those found in normal controls. There was no correlation between CSF HGH and either plasma HGH or CSF protein. Thomas et al. (1972) and Allen et al. (1974a) corroborated some of these data when they found HGH in the CSF of acromegalics and particularly high titers in patients with SSE. Unlike Wright et al. (1969), however, Thomas et al. (1972) were unable to find a correlation between plasma HGH levels and tumor size. Schaub et al. (1977) studied ten acromegaly patients, but could find no correlation between SSE and CSF HGH levels.

3. Markers of Metastatic Intracranial Tumors

3.1. Human Chorionic Gonadotropin

Human chorionic gonadotropin (HCG) is a hormone produced by the trophoblastic cells of the placenta. Because it can be produced by some types of neoplastic tissue, its presence in the urine, blood, or CSF of men and nonpregnant females is a specific indicator of the presence of a tumor. HCG consists of two subunits, alpha and beta, and while the α subunit is common among other glycoprotein hormones such as luteinizing hormone, the β subunit is HCG specific and it should be used as the immunogen for the generation of HCG-reactive antisera (Vaitukaitis et al., 1972).

Early studies not using the HCG specific detection methods gave results similar to those generated later when βHCG levels were measured. Bagshawe et al. (1968) studied women with trophoblastic disease but without CNS metastases and found a close correlation between plasma and CSF concentrations. The mean plasma/CSF ratio was 177:1. Rushworth et al. (1968) measured HCG concentrations in the plasma and CSF of trophoblastic tumor patients with and without CNS metastatic disease. These authors felt that HCG plasma/CSF ratio greater than 100/1 suggested the absence of a CNS metastatic lesion, while an HCG plasma/CSF ratio less than 35/1 indicated the likelihood of a CNS lesion.

The first study where βHCG was measured directly was done in 1973 by Braunstein and coworkers. They found, via RIA, low levels of βHCG in the serum of patients with tumors of the gastrointestinal tract.

Although the early cases they studied were monitored for HCG, not βHCG, Bagshawe and Harland (1976) found in a study of HCG levels in 73 patients with gestational choriocarcinoma that the HCG plasma/CSF ratio in cases without CNS metastasis was 208, while those patients with CNS metastatic lesions averaged 22.4. Using an HCG plasma/CSF ratio of 60 as an indicator for the presence of CNS lesions, they were able to predict the presence of CNS involvement in 13 of 17 cases one to 20 weeks before any confirming diagnostic signs were presented. In all cases where a positive plasma/CSF ratio was noted, metastatic lesions were eventually found. Bagshawe (1977) feels that the basis for these CSF HCG concentration shifts lies in the fact that HCG does not easily enter the CSF from the blood, and with no brain metastases the plasma/CSF ratio is greater than 200. If the ratio falls below 60, CNS involvement is indicated and if the CNS lesion mass is high in relation to the systemic tumor burden, CSF HCG levels may even exceed plasma levels.

In a study of teratocarcinoma patients whose tumors apparently contained a subpopulation of βHCG secreting cells, Kaye et al. (1979) found a correlation between serum βHCG titers and the likelihood of brain metastases. In 47 patients, 37 of whom had stage 4 disease and peak βHCG levels greater than 10^4 IU/L, there was a 26% incidence of CNS metastatic disease. In the group of patients whose serum βHCG levels never exceeded 10^4 IU/L, the incidence of CNS lesions was only 1.8%.

βHCG levels in the serum and in the CSF constitute a marker capable of both predicting the likelihood and detecting the presence of βHCG producing intracranial tumors. Once a CNS metastasis has been detected, βHCG can continue to be of use. Because choriocarcinoma is becoming more manageable through chemotherapy, a sensitive tumor burden monitor like βHCG allows the clinician to treat the marker level and hence the disease.

3.2. Carcinoembryonic Antigen

Gold and Freedman (1965a, 1965b) generated an antiserum that reacted with human colon adenocarcinoma cells and at first thought it to be tumor specific. Carcinoembryonic antigen (CEA) has since been found in varying numbers of cases of carcinoma of the breast, stomach, gut, and bladder and in nonneoplastic states such as hepatic cirrhosis, emphysema, intestinal inflammation, and in subjects who smoke (Shively and Todd, 1978).

CEA was found in the CSF of most but not all patients suffering from metastatic lesions. The most common tumors carried by these patients were carcinomas of the breast and lung. CSF samples from patients with primary intracranial tumors were usually CEA negative (Snitzer and McKinney, 1976; Kido et al., 1976; Yap et al., 1978). Because CSF CEA levels might be a reflection of plasma CEA levels, these levels were compared but no correlation was found. A drop in CSF CEA levels was noted without a change in plasma levels (Snitzer et al., 1975) and CSF CEA levels did not correlate with CSF RBC count or CSF protein, suggesting that CEA in the CSF of CNS tumor patients is not hematogenous in origin, but rather is produced by the CNS tumor itself (Yap et al., 1978; Hill et al., 1979).

In cases where a patient is known to have a CEA-secreting tumor metastatic to the brain, CSF CEA may be of use in following tumor burden changes during the course of the treatment.

4. Conclusion

Cell or tissue-associated markers have been most intensely studied in normal tissues but even the normal distributions of most are not yet clear. Fifteen years of study, for instance, have not been sufficient to show with absolute confidence that S-100 protein is a good marker for distinguishing cells of neuroectodermal origin. Only GFAP has documented astroglial specificity and GPDH, although less studied, is the best candidate for an oligodendroglial marker (Table 1).

Once one shifts from normal to neoplastic tissue, especially in a clinical environment, the picture becomes even more unclear. GPDH expression in normal brain is restricted to oligodendroglia, but in neoplastic tissue, no such restriction has been demonstrated and GPDH remains only glioma-associated. Other potential brain tumor markers such as MBP, aldolase C, and carbonic anhydrase have been insufficiently studied in tumors to allow their distributions to be well documented. On the bright side, GFAP has already been put into use in a clinical setting and has provided new information about several types of primary CNS tumors (Eng and Rubinstein, 1978; Kepes et al., 1979b; Velasco et al., 1980).

Considerable evidence exists to support a theory of clonal evolution within tumor cell populations (Nowell, 1976). Such evolution would help to explain the variation that exists both among brain tumors of one diagnostic category and among cell populations within a given tumor. Fifteen cell lines derived from anaplastic human gliomas that were studied in this laboratory were divided into four groups on the basis of morphology, had different chromosomal patterns and modal numbers and gave widely varying results when parameters such as GFAP positivity, CNPase activity, re-

Table 1

Cells or tissues expressing marker

Marker	Tumor	Normal	References
GFAP		Astrocytes	Mori et al., 1968
			Antanitus et al., 1975
			Jacque et al., 1978
	Astrocytomas		Eng and Rubinstein, 1978
			van der Meulen et al., 1978
			Rasmussen et al., 1980
			Dittmann et al., 1977
	Glioblastomas		Rasmussen et al., 1980
			van der Meulen et al., 1978
			Velasco et al., 1980
	Ependymomas		Rasmussen et al., 1980
			Eng and Rubinstein, 1978
			Velasco et al., 1980
	Oligodendrogliomas		van der Meulen, 1978
	Hemangioblastomas		Jacque et al., 1978
			Rasmussen et al., 1980
			Kepes et al., 1979a
	Medulloblastomas		Rasmussen et al., 1980
			Eng and Rubinstein, 1978
			Velasco et al., 1980

Marker	Cell/Tumor	Reference
S-100	Astrocytes	Hyden and McElven, 1966
	Neurons	Cicero et al., 1970
		Perez et al., 1970
		Hyden and McElven, 1966
	Astrocytomas	Haglid et al., 1973a
		Haglid et al., 1973b
		Dittmann et al., 1977
	Glioblastomas	Haglid et al., 1973a
		Haglid et al., 1973b
		Dittman et al., 1977
	Oligodendrogliomas	Haglid et al., 1973a
		Dohan et al., 1977
	Acoustic neurinomas	Pfeiffer et al., 1972
		Haglid et al., 1973a
		Dohan et al., 1977
CNPase	Oligodendroglia	Bigner et al., 1981
	Melanomas	Kurihara et al., 1971
	Astrocytomas	Dohan et al., 1977
	Glioblastomas	Kurihara et al., 1974
		Dohan et al., 1977
	Oligodendrogliomas	Kurihara et al., 1974
		Kurihara et al., 1974
		Dohan et al., 1977
	Neurinomas	Pfeiffer et al., 1979
Glutamine synthetase	Astrocytes	Norenberg & Martinez-Hernandez, 1979

(continued)

Table 1 *(continued)*

Marker	Cells or tissues expressing marker		References
	Tumor	Normal	
Enolase		Neurons	Pickel et al., 1976
			Grasso et al., 1977
	Glioblastomas		Haglid et al., 1973a
	Astrocytomas		Haglid et al., 1973a
	Acoustic neurinomas		Haglid et al., 1973a
	Choroid plexus papillomas		Haglid et al., 1973a
	Oligodendrogliomas		Haglid et al., 1973a
	Pituitary adenomas		Haglid et al., 1973a
GPDH		Oligodendroglia	de Vellis et al., 1977
Carbonic anhydrase		Glia	Sensenbrenner et al., 1977
			Kimelberg et al., 1977a, b
			Delaunoy et al., 1977
			Mandel et al., 1977
			Spicer et al., 1979
Aldolase C		Brain	Sugimura et al., 1969
			Bodansky, 1975
	Gliomas		Sato et al., 1971
	Acoustic neurinomas		Kumanishi et al., 1970
			Kumanishi et al., 1970
Alpha-2-glycoprotein		White matter	Warecka et al., 1972
	Astrocytomas		Warecka, 1975

sponse to db-cAMP, and fibronectin synthesis were measured (Bigner et al., 1981). Shapiro et al. (1979) found that human gliosarcomas grown in athymic "nude" mice responded differently to chemotherapeutic agents and that each tumor required a drug regimen tailored to fit its own sensitivities. If one looks at the expression of just one marker (GFAP) detectable in surgical biopsies, one finds variations in degree of expression between different glioblastomas (Jacque et al., 1978) and within a single glioblastoma (van der Meulen et al., 1978). Because of this heterogeneity in marker expression and because the absence of any given marker is meaningless, evaluation of several markers within each tumor may be necessary to allow accurate predictions to be made concerning the behavior of the tumor.

Although several molecules have been investigated as potentially useful markers in the initial diagnosis of CNS cancer, none has shown much promise. Seidenfeld and Marton (1979) reviewed the literature on several potential CNS cancer markers tested for use as diagnostic tools. They used four parameters to evaluate the usefulness of the markers: (1) sensitivity was defined as the fraction of tumor-bearing patients giving positive results, (2) specificity was defined as the fraction of tumor-free patients giving negative results, (3) predictive value was defined as the fraction of positive results that were true positives, and (4) efficiency was defined as the fraction of all correct results. The authors added that disease incidence is also important. A test having 95% sensitivity and specificity would have a 68% value when disease incidence was one in ten, but only a two percent predictive value when disease incidence was one in 100. Because of the low incidence of CNS neoplasia within the general population, a screening test would be useless unless based on a marker with 100 percent sensitivity and specificity. If the test group were limited to those patients who have CNS symptoms, it is conceivable that a screening test might be of some use. The authors concluded that while some marker candidates appeared useless for cancer detection and others were insufficiently studied to allow conclusions, several appeared to have potential as tumor burden monitors.

A few other markers of use or possible use in a clinical setting should also be mentioned. The use of GFAP in determining the astrocytic origin of tumors has already been discussed. CSF titers of both βHCG and alpha-fetoprotein can help in both the diagnosis and monitoring of primary and metastatic germ cell tumors while CEA titers may be of use in following tumor burden in those patients with demonstrated CNS metastatic lesions which secrete CEA. Pituitary hormones are also useful in the diagnosis of pituitary adenomas.

Most of the markers discussed in this review are not yet ready for clinical application; many may never be. But if more markers can be used in the future to monitor tumor burden, rapidly and easily gained information indicating chemotherapy and radiation therapy regimen efficacy would give the clinician the ability to quickly modify treatment schedules to fit the behavior of the tumor.

5. Future Prospects

None of the CNS tumor markers discussed is ideal; each gives some information about a certain aspect of the biology of brain tumors, but none provides all the information that both the clinician and the basic researcher wish. An ideal CNS tumor marker is specific to the disease; positivity accurately predicts the presence of neoplasia and negativity its absence. This type of specificity is extremely rare with human chorionic gonadotropin in testicular germ cell tumors and myeloma proteins in multiple myeloma as the closest examples. Consistency of expression is another ideal characteristic but, as mentioned earlier, a common, almost universal, phenomenon seen in tumor cells is the loss of differentiated characteristics including those useful as markers. An ideal marker should be found in highly accessible body fluids, for example, blood and urine, so the clinician can monitor markers levels easily and repeatedly. It appears, however, that in the case of CNS cancer, the most likely target for assay will be the CSF. Although not as accessible as blood or urine, the CSF can still be sampled with relative ease and the significance of a useful CNS tumor marker to the regulation of treatment might outweigh the trauma incurred by repeated lumbar punctures.

If a marker possessing the ideal characteristics already described were found, a system for quickly and precisely measuring it would be required. Presently, the most accurate and versatile detection system is based on monospecific antibody. A wide variety of assays including radioimmunoassay, enzyme-linked immunosorbent assay, and complement fixation assays give sensitive ways to quantitate marker titers, while fluorescent antibody and ferritin or peroxidase-linked antibody allow accurate tissue, cellular, and subcellular localization. There is, however, an inherent danger in the use of antibody-based assay systems. The worth of the data received from such techniques rests entirely on the specificity of the antibody. It must be directed against the marker and only against the marker. The generation and testing of antisera are often difficult tasks and one must be fully conversant in both the theory and techniques of antigen isolation and antiserum testing. Once a marker is established as clinically useful, a large number of clinicians will most likely be using antibody against it. If they are inexperienced in the methods of antibody generation and purification, contaminated, polyspecific antisera may be used and spurious, confusing data generated.

No ideal marker has yet been found and one probably does not exist, but there are several putative markers that may be of use in more limited situations. Glutamine synthetase is specific to astrocytic glia in normal tissue, but its cellular distribution within tumors and its relationship to the CSF in tumor patients are unknown. GPDH, MBP, aldolase C, and carbonic anhydrase are also of interest because they have not yet been fully investigated, especially in regard to their levels in the CSF and their use as tumor burden monitors.

Another area of great potential, but one that has not been heavily investigated in glia, is cell membrane receptors. The brain is a tissue engaged in intense chemical and electrical activity. For cells to communicate via chemical transmitters, the cells involved must carry receptors capable of detecting the presence of the chemical messenger. A vast quantity of work has been done over the years describing normal neuronal receptors such as those binding acetylcholine and opiates, but less work has been done with transformed cells. The bulk of the work done with transformed cells involves a tumor of putative neuronal origin, but one found almost exclusively in extracranial sites, the neuroblastoma. It is becoming clear that glia are not static cells that exist solely to provide structural support for neurons. Their apparent part in amino acid neurotransmitter metabolism suggests the presence of receptors that may be of considerable use in cell-type classification, in both normal and neoplastic tissues.

Perhaps the most exciting and versatile system at present is the hybridoma antibody. It has the potential to detect and make possible the isolation of antigens hitherto unknown. Because hybridoma antibody is monoclonal, it can be used as a highly specific probe in the demonstration of marker expression. Because of its specificity, it is vastly superior to antibody raised by conventional animal immunization techniques and should reduce the possibility of, as mentioned before, incorrect data being generated through the use of polyspecific antibody.

Acknowledgments

The authors thank Ms. Candiss Weaver for the rapid and accurate preparation of the manuscript and Mr. William Boyarsky for the preparation of the photographs. This work was supported by USPHS grants CA-11898 and CA-22790 from the National Cancer Institute and by grant IM-150 from the American Cancer Society.

This review covers the literature published prior to August, 1980.

References

Allen, J. C., J. Nisselbaum, F. Epstein, G. Rosen, and M. K. Schwartz (1979), *J. Neurosurg.* **51**, 368.

Allen, J. P., J. W. Kendall, R. McGilvra, T. L. Lamorena, and A. Castro (1974a), *Arch. Neurol.* **31**, 325.

Allen, J. P., J. W. Kendall, R. McGilvra, and C. Vancura (1974b), *J. Clin. Endo. Metab.* **31**, 586.

Allen, N. (1961), *Neurol.* **11**, 578.

Allen, N. (1972), *Prog. Exptl. Tumor Res.* **17**, 291.

Allen, N., and E. Reagan (1964), *Arch. Neurol.* **11**, 144.

Anlyan, A. J., and A. Starr (1952), *Cancer* **5**, 578.

Antanitus, D. S., B. H. Choi, and L. W. Lapham (1975), *Brain Res.* **89**, 363.

Aronson, S. M., J. H. Garcia, and B. E. Aronson (1964), *Cancer* **17**, 558.

Assies, J., A. P. M. Schellekins, and J. L. Touber (1978), *J. Clin. Endo. Metab.* **46**, 576.

Augusti-Tocco, G., L. Casola, and A. Grasso (1973), *Cell Diff.* **2**, 157.

Bagshawe, K. D. (1977), in *Tumor Markers* (K. Griffiths, A. M. Neville, and C. G. Pierrepont, eds.), University Park Press, Baltimore, pp. 90–100.

Bagshawe, K. D., and S. Harland (1976), *Cancer* **38**, 112.

Bagshawe, K. D., A. H. Orr, and A. G. J. Rushworth (1968), *Nature* **217**, 950.

Balagura, S., A. G. Frantz, E. M. Housepian, and P. W. Carmel (1979), *J. Neurosurg.* **51**, 42.

Ballou, B., G. Levine, T. R. Hakala, and D. Solter (1979), *Science* **206**, 844.

Bignami, A., and D. Dahl (1977), *J. Histochem. Cytochem.* **25**, 466.

Bignami, A., L. F. Eng, D. Dahl, and C. T. Uyeda (1972), *Brain Res.* **43**, 429.

Bignami, A., D. Dahl, and D. C. Rueger (1977), in *Mechanisms, Regulation and Special Functions of Protein Synthesis in the Brain* (S. Roberts, A. Lajtha, and W. H. Gispen, eds.), Elsevier/North Holland, Amsterdam, pp. 153–160.

Bigner, D. D., S. H. Bigner, J. Pontén, B. Westermark, E. Ruoslahti, H. Herschman, and C. J. Wikstrand (1981), *J. Neuropath. Exptl. Neurol.*, **40**, 201.

Bigner, S. H., T. R. Jones, R. D. Serano, H. R. Hershman, and D. D. Bigner (1980), *J. Neuropath. Exptl. Neurol.* **39**, 341.

Bock, E. (1978), *J. Neurochem.* **30**, 7.

Bock, E., and J. Dissing (1975), *Scand. J. Immunol. Suppl.* **2**, 31.

Bodansky, O. (1975), *Biochemistry of Human Cancer* Academic Press, New York, p. 657.

Braun, P. E., and S. W. Brostoff (1977), in *Myelin* (P. Morrell, ed.), Plenum, New York, pp. 201–232.

Braunstein, G. D., J. L. Vaitukaitis, P. P. Carbone, and G. T. Ross (1973), *Ann. Int. Med.* **78**, 39.

Breen, G. A. M., and J. de Vellis (1975), *Exptl. Cell Res.* **91**, 159.

Brightman, M. W. (1968), *Prog. Brain Res.* **29**, 19.

Brightman, M. W., and T. S. Reese (1969), *J. Cell Biol.* **40**, 648.

Buckell, M., and M. C. Robertson (1965), *Brit. J. Cancer* **19**, 83.

Burger, P. C., and F. S. Vogel (1976), *Surgical Pathology of the Nervous System and its Coverings*, Wiley, New York, pp. 623.

Cicero, T. J., W. M. Cowan, B. W. Moore, and V. Suntzelf (1970), *Brain Res.* **18**, 25.

Constantopoulos, A., K. Antonakakis, N. Matsaniotis, and Z. Kapsalakis (1976), *Neurochir.* **19**, 169.

Cuello, A. C., G. Galfre, and C. Milstein (1979), *Proc. Natl. Acad. Sci. USA* **76**, 3532.

Dahl, D. (1976), *Biochim. Biophy. Acta* **420**, 142.

Dahl, D., and A. Bignami (1976), *Brain Res.* **116**, 150.

Deck, J. H. N., L. F. Eng. J. Bigbee, and S. M. Woodcock (1978), *Acta Neuropath.* **42**, 183.

Delaunoy, J.-P., G. Roussel, and P. Mandel (1977), *CR Acad. Sci. Paris* **285**, 801.

Delpech, B., A. Delpech, M. N. Vidard, N. Girard, J. Tayot, J. C. Clement, and P. Creissard (1978), *Brit. J. Cancer* **37**, 33.

de Vellis, J., and G. Brooker (1973), in *Tissue Culture of the Nervous System* (G. Sato, ed.), Plenum, New York, pp. 231–245.

de Vellis, J., and D. Inglish (1968), *J. Neurochem.* **15**, 1061.

de Vellis, J., J. F. McGinnis, G. A. M. Breen, P. LeVeille, K. Bennett, and K. McCarthy (1977), in *Cell, Tissue and Organ Cultures in Neurobiology* (S. Federoff and L. Hertz, eds.), Academic Press, New York, pp. 485–511.

Dharker, S. R., R. S. Dharker, and B. D. Chaurasia (1976), *J. Neurol. Neurosurg. Psych.* **39**, 1081.

DiLorenzo, N., and L. Palma (1976), *Lancet* **1**, 1077.

DiLorenzo, N., L. Palma, and L. Ferrante (1977), *Neurochir.* **20**, 19.

Dittman, L., N. H. Axelsen, B. Nørgaard-Pedersen, and E. Bock (1977), *Brit. J. Cancer* **35**, 135.

Dohan, F. C., P. L. Kornblith, G. R. Wellum, S. E. Pfeiffer, and L. Levine (1977), *Acta Neuropath.* **40**, 123.

Drummond, G. I., N. T. Iyer, and J. Keith (1962), *J. Biol. Chem.* **237**, 3535.

Duffy, P. E., L. Graff, and M. M. Rapport (1977), *J. Neuropath. Exptl. Neurol.* **36**, 645.

Eisenbarth, G. S., F. S. Walsh, and M. Nirenberg (1979), *Proc. Natl. Acad. Sci. USA* **76**, 4913.

Eng, L. F., and J. W. Bigbee (1978), *Adv. Neurochem.* **3**, 43.

Eng. L. F., and L. J. Rubinstein (1978), *J. Histochem. Cytochem.* **26**, 513.

Eng. L. F., J. J. Vanderhaeghen, A. Bignami, and B. Gerstl (1971), *Brain Res.* **28**, 351.

Fishman, J. S., and M. Hayashi (1962), *J. Histochem. Cytochem.* **10**, 515.

Fleisher, G. A., K. G. Wakim, and N. P. Goldstein (1957), *Proc. Staff Meetings Mayo Clinic* **32**, 188.

Fumagalli, R., and P. Paoletti (1971), *Neurol.* **21**, 1149.

Fumagalli, R., E. Grossi, P. Paoletti, and R. Paoletti (1964), *J. Neurochem.* **11**, 561.

Fumagalli, R., E. Grossi-Paoletti, P. Paoletti, and R. Paoletti (1966), *J. Neurochem.* **13**, 1005.

Fumagalli, R., S. Pezzotta, A. R. Racca, and P. Paoletti (1976), *Pharm. Res. Comm.* **8,** 127.

Gerhardt, W., J. Clausen, E. Christensen, and J. Riisheda (1963), *Acta Neurol. Scand.* **39,** 85.

Giacobini, E. (1961), *Science* **134,** 1524.

Giacobini, E. (1962), *J. Neurochem.* **9,** 169.

Gold, P., and S. O. Freedman (1965a), *J. Exptl. Med.* **121,** 439.

Gold, P., and S. O. Freedman (1965b), *J. Exptl. Med.* **122,** 467.

Gomez, C. M., D. P. Richman, P. W. Berman, S. A. Burres, B. G. W. Arnason, and F. W. Fitch (1979), *Biochem. Biophys. Res. Comm.* **88,** 575.

Goridis, C., and M. Schachner (1978), in *Biology of Brain Tumors* (O.D. Laerum, D. D. Bigner, and M. F. Rajewsky, eds.), International Union Against Cancer, Geneva, pp. 158–171.

Grasso, A., K. G. Haglid, H.-A. Hansson, L. Persson, and L. Ronnback (1977), *Brain Res.* **122,** 582.

Green, J. B., H. A. Oldewurtel, D. S. O'Doherty, F. M. Forster, and L. P. Sanchez-Longo (1957), *Neurol.* **7,** 313.

Green, J. B., H. A. Oldewurtel, D. S. O'Doherty, and F. M. Forster (1958), *Arch. Neurol. Psych.* **80,** 148.

Green, J. B., H. A. Oldewurtel, and F. M. Forster (1959), *Neurol.* **9,** 540.

Haglid, K., C.-A. Carlsson, and C.-A. Thulin (1970), *Neurochir.* **13,** 19.

Haglid, K., C.-A. Carlsson, and D. Stavrou (1973a), *Acta Neuropath.* **24,** 187.

Haglid, K. G., D. Stavrou, L. Ronnback, C.-A. Carlsson, and W. Weidenbach (1973b), *J. Neurol. Sci.* **20,** 103.

Hamberger, A., C. W. Cotman, A. Sellstrom, and C. T. Weiler (1977), in *Dynamic Properties of Glia Cells* (E. Schoffeniels, G. Franck, L. Hertz, and D. B. Tower, eds.), Pergamon, Oxford, pp. 163–172.

Hamprecht, B. (1978), in *Biology of Brain Tumors* (O. D. Laerum, D. D. Bigner, and M. F. Rajewsky, eds.), International Union Against Cancer, Geneva, pp. 143–157.

Hansen, N. E., H. Karle, A. Jensen, and E. Bock (1977), *Acta Neurol. Scand.* **55,** 418.

Harik, S. I., and C. H. Sutton (1979), *Cancer Res.* **39,** 5010.

Hayakawa, T., Y. Ushio, T. Mori, N. Arita, T. Yoshimine, Y. Maeda, K. Shimizu, and A. Myoga (1979), *Stroke* **10,** 685.

Hayakawa, T., K. Morimoto, Y. Ushio, T. Mori, T. Yoshimine, A. Myoga, and H. Mogami (1980), *J. Neurosurg.* **52,** 229.

Henn, F. A., D. J. Anderson, and D. G. Rustand (1976), *Brain Res.* **101,** 341.

Herschman, H. R. (1978), in *Biology of Brain Tumors* (O. D. Laerum, D. D. Bigner, and M. F. Rajewsky, eds.), International Union Against Cancer, Geneva pp. 172–183.

Herschman, H. R., and M. P. Lerner (1973), *Nature New Biol.* **241,** 242.

Hertz, L. (1977), in *Cell, Tissue and Organ Cultures in Neurobiology* (S. Fedoroff and L. Hertz, eds.), Academic Press, New York, pp. 39–71.

Hildebrand, J. (1973), *Eur. J. Cancer* **9,** 621.

Hill, S. A., E. C. Ellison, and E. W. Martin (1979), in *Immunodiagnosis of Human Cancer* (R. B. Herberman, ed.), Elsevier/North Holland, New York, p. 33.

Holmes, R. S. (1977), *Eur. J. Biochem.* **78,** 511.

Hydén, H., and B. McElven (1966), *Proc. Natl. Acad. Sci. USA* **55**, 354.

Isobe, T., and T. Okuyama (1978), *Eur. J. Biochem.* **89**, 379.

Isobe, T., T. Nakajima, and T. Okuyama (1977), *Biochim. Biophys. Acta* **494**, 222.

Isobe, T., A. Tsugita, and T. Okuyama (1978), *J. Neurochem.* **30**, 921.

Jacque, C. M., C. Vinner, M. Kujas, M. Raoul, J. Racadot, and N. A. Baumann (1978), *J. Neurol. Sci.* **35**, 147.

Jellinger, K. (1978), *Acta Neurochir.* **42**, 5.

Jones, T. R., E. Ruoslahti, S. C. Schold, L. F. Eng, and D. D. Bigner (1980), *J. Neuropath. Exptl. Neurol.* **39**, 365.

Jordan, R. M., J. W. Kendall, J. L. Seaich, J. P. Allen, C. A. Paulsen, C. W. Kerber, and W. P. Vanderlaan (1976), *Ann. Int. Med.* **85**, 49.

Katzman, R., R. A. Fishman, and E. S. Goldensohn (1957), *Neurol.* **7**, 853.

Kaye, S. B., K. D. Bagshawe, T. J. McElwain, and M. J. Peckham (1979), *Brit. J. Cancer* **39**, 217.

Kennett, R. H., and F. Gilbert (1979), *Science* **203**, 1120.

Kennett, R. H., Z. Jonak, and K. B. Bechtol (1980), *Prog. Cancer Res. Therapy* **12**, 209.

Kepes, J. J., S. S. Rengachary, and S. H. Lee (1979a), *Acta Neuropath.* **47**, 99.

Kepes, J. J., L. J. Rubinstein, and L. F. Eng (1979b), *Cancer* **44**, 1839.

Kido, D. K., B. J. Dyce, B. J. Haverback, and C. L. Rumbaugh (1976), *Bull. L. A. Neurol. Soc.* **41**, 47.

Kimelberg, H. K., S. Narumi, S. Biddlecome, and R. S. Bourke (1977a), in *Dynamic Properties of Glia Cells* (E. Schoffeniels, G. Franck, L. Hertz, and D. B. Tower, eds.), Pergamon, Oxford, pp. 347–358.

Kimelberg, H. K., S. Narumi, S. Biddlecome, and R. S. Bourke (1977b), *Trans. Am. Soc. Neurochem.* **8**, 89.

Kleerekoper, M., R. A. Donald, and S. Posen (1972), *Lancet* **1**, 74.

Kleihues, P., and D. D. Bigner (1981), in *The Molecular Basis of Neuropathology* (R. H. S. Thompson and A. N. Davison, eds.), in press.

Köhler, G., and C. Milstein (1975), *Nature* **256**, 495.

Köhler, G., and C. Milstein (1976), *Eur. J. Immunol.* **6**, 511.

Koprowski, H., Z. Steplewski, D. Herlyn, and M. Herlyn (1978), *Proc. Natl. Acad. Sci. USA* **75**, 3405.

Kumanishi, T., F. Ikuta, and T. Yamamoto (1970), *Acta Neuropath.* **16**, 220.

Kurihara, T., and Y. Tsukada (1967), *J. Neurochem.* **14**, 1167.

Kurihara, T., J. L. Nussbaum, and P. Mandel (1971), *Life Sci.* **10**(II), 421.

Kurihara, T., S. Kawakami, K. Ueki, and Y. Takahashi (1974), *J. Neurochem.* **22**, 1143.

Lebherz, H. G., and W. J. Rutter (1969), *Biochem.* **8**, 109.

Levvy, G. A., and J. Conchie (1966), in *Glucuronic Acid Free and Combined* (G. J. Dutton, ed.), Academic Press, New York, pp. 301–364.

Liem, R. K. H., and M. L. Shelanski (1978), *Brain Res.* **145**, 196.

Linfoot, J. A., J. F. Garcia, W. Wei, R. Fink, R. Sarin, J. L. Born, and J. H. Lawrence (1970), *J. Clin. Endo. Metab.* **31**, 230.

Login, I. S., and R. M. MacLeod (1977), *Brain Res.* **132**, 477.

Mandel, P., G. Roussel, J.-P. Delaunoy, and J.-L. Nussbaum (1977), in *Dynamic Properties of Glia Cells* (E. Schoffeniels, G. Franck, L. Hertz, and D. B. Tower, eds.) Pergamon, Oxford, pp. 267–274.

Mann, S. H., N. DePasquale, and R. Paterson (1960), *Neurol.* **10**, 381.

Marangos, P. J., F. K. Goodwin, A. Parma, C. Lauter, and E. Trams (1978a), *Brain Res.* **145**, 49.

Marangos, P. J., A. M. Parma, and F. K. Goodwin (1978b), *J. Neurochem.* **39**, 727.

Martinez-Hernandez, A., K. P. Bell, and M. D. Norenberg (1977), *Science* **195**, 1356.

Marton, L. J., G. S. Gordon, M. Barker, C. B. Wilson, and W. Lubich (1973), *Arch. Neurol.* **28**, 137.

Marton, L. J., O. Heby, and C. B. Wilson (1974a), *Int. J. Cancer* **14**, 731.

Marton, L. J., O. Heby, C. B. Wilson, and P. L. Y. Lee (1974b), *FEBS Letters* **46**, 305.

Marton, L. J., O. Heby, V. A. Levin, W. P. Lubich, D. C. Crafts, and C. B. Wilson (1976), *Cancer Res.* **36**, 973.

Marton, L. J., M. S. Edwards, V. A. Levin, W. P. Lubich, and C. B. Wilson (1979), *Cancer Res.* **39**, 993.

Mason, D. Y., and P. Roberts-Thomson (1974), *Lancet* **2**, 952.

McDermott, J. R., and A. R. Smith (1978), *J. Neurochem.* **30**, 1637.

McGinnis, J. F., and J. de Vellis (1977), *Arch. Biochem. Biophys.* **179**, 682.

Mellick, R. S., and R. L. Bassett (1964), *Lancet* **1**, 904.

Miyazaki, M. (1958), *J. Nerv. Ment. Dis.* **126**, 169.

Moore, B. W. (1965), *Biochem. Biophys. Res. Comm.* **19**, 739.

Moore, B. W., and D. J. MacGregor (1965), *J. Biol. Chem.* **240**, 1647.

Moore, B. W., and V. J. Perez (1968), in *Physiological and Biochemical Aspects of Neurons in Integration* (F. D. Carlson, ed.), Prentice-Hall, Englewood Cliffs, New Jersey, pp. 343–359.

Mori, T., H. Mogami, P. F. Benda, and W. H. Sweet (1968), *Neurol. Med. Chir.* **10**, 103.

Mori, T., K. Morimoto, Y. Ushio, T. Hayakawa, and H. Mogami (1975a), *Neurol. Med. Chir.* **15**, 23.

Mori, T., K. Morimoto, Y. Ushio, and H. Mogami (1975b), *Igaku-No-Ayumi* **18**, 16.

Mori, T., K. Morimoto, T. Hayakawa, Y. Ushio, H. Mogami, and K. Sekiguchi (1978), *Neurol. Med. Chir.* **18**, 25.

Morrison, P., J. Edsall, and S. Miller (1948), *J. Amer. Chem. Soc.* **70**, 3103.

Moshly-Rosen, D., S. Fuchs, and Z. Eshhar (1979), *FEBS Letters* **106**, 389.

Myerson, R. M., J. K. Hurwitz, and T. Sall (1957), *New Engl. J. Med.* **257**, 273.

Newman, J., A. S. Josephson, A. Cacatian, and A. Tsang (1974), *Lancet* **2**, 756.

Niebroj-Dobosz, I., and L. Hetnarska (1969), *Polish Med. J.* **8**, 451.

Norenberg, M. D. (1979), *J. Histochem. Cytochem.* **27**, 756.

Norenberg, M. D., and A. Martinez-Hernandez (1979), *Brain Res.* **161**, 303.

Nørgaard-Pedersen, B., J. Lindholm, R. Albrechtsen, J. Arends, N. H. Diemer, and J. Riishede (1978), *Cancer* **41**, 2315.

Nowell, P. C. (1976), *Science* **194**, 23.

Orly, J., and G. Sato (1979), *Cell* **17**, 295.

Paoletti, P., F. A. Vandenheuvel, R. Fumagalli, and R. Paoletti (1969), *Neurol.* **19**, 190.

Paoletti, P., R. Fumagalli, E. Grossi-Paoletti (1972), in *The Experimental Biology of Brain Tumors* (W. M. Kirsch, E. Grossi-Paoletti, and P. Paoletti, eds.), Charles C Thomas, Springfield, Illinois, pp. 457–479.

Paoletti, P., R. Fumagalli, F. J. Weiss, and S. Pezzotta (1977), *Surg. Neurol.* **8,** 399.

Parker, K. K., M. D. Norenberg, and A. Vernadakis (1980), *Science* **208,** 179.

Penhoet, E., T. Rajkumar, and W. J. Rutter (1966), *Proc. Natl. Acad. Sci. USA* **56,** 1275.

Perez, V. J., J. W. Olney, T. J. Cicero, B. W. Moore, and B. A. Bahn (1970), *J. Neurochem.* **17,** 511.

Pfeiffer, S. E., and W. Wechsler (1972), *Proc. Natl. Acad. Sci. USA* **69,** 2885.

Pfeiffer, S. E., P. L. Kornblith, H. L. Cares, J. Seals, and L. Levine (1972), *Brain Res.* **41,** 187.

Pfeiffer, S. E., N. Sundarraj, G. Dawson, and P. L. Kornblith (1979), *Acta Neuropath.* **47,** 27.

Pickel, V. M., D. J. Reis, P. J. Marangos, and C. Zomzely-Neurath (1976), *Brain Res.* **105,** 184.

Poduslo, S. E. (1975), *J. Neurochem.* **24,** 647.

Posner, J. B., D. D. Bigner, W. Shapiro, G. J. D'Angio, and M. D. Walker (1979), *National Institute of Neurological and Communicative Disorders and Stroke,* NIH publication, p. 224.

Rabow, L., and K. Kristensson (1977), *Acta Neurochir.* **36,** 71.

Ransohoff, J., and J. Weiss (1977), *Natl. Cancer Inst. Monographs* **46,** 119.

Rasmussen, S., E. Bock, K. Warecka, and G. Althage (1980), *Brit. J. Cancer* **41,** 113.

Reitamo, S., and M. Klockars (1976), *Acta Med. Scand.* **199,** 321.

Rueger, D. C., D. Dahl, and A. Bignami (1978a), *Brain Res.* **153,** 188.

Rueger, D. C., D. Dahl, and A. Bignami (1978b), *Anal. Biochem.* **89,** 360.

Ruoslahti, E., A. Vaheri, P. Kuusela, and E. Linder (1973), *Biochim. Biophys. Acta* **322,** 352.

Rushworth, A. G. J., A. H. Orr, and K. D. Bagshawe (1968), *Brit. J. Cancer* **22,** 253.

Russell, D. H. (1971), *Nature New Biol.* **233,** 144.

Russell, D. H. (1973), *Life Sci.* **13,** 1635.

Russell, D. H., and B. C. M. Durie (1978), *Progress in Cancer Research and Therapy,* Vol. 8, Raven, New York, p. 178.

Russell, D. H., C. C. Levy, S. C. Schimpff, and I. A. Hawk (1971), *Cancer Res.* **31,** 1555.

Russell, D. S., and L. J. Rubinstein (1977), *Pathology of Tumours of the Nervous System,* Williams and Wilkins, Baltimore, p. 448.

Sapirstein, V. S., and M. B. Lees (1977), *Trans. Am. Soc. Neurochem.* **8,** 245.

Sato, S., T. Sugimura, T. C. Chien, and K. Takakura (1971), *Cancer* **27,** 223.

Schachner, M., G. Schoonmaker, and H. O. Hynes (1978), *Brain Res.* **158,** 149.

Schaub, C., M. T. Bluet-Pajot, G. Szikla, C. Lornet, and J. Talairach (1977), *J. Neurol. Sci.* **31,** 123.

Schiffer, D., A. Fabiani, A. Cognazzo, and G. F. Monticone (1969), *Acta Neuropath.* **13,** 91.

Schmechal, D., P. J. Marangos, A. P. Zis, M. Brightman, and F. K. Goodwin (1978), *Science* **199**, 313.

Schold, S. C., and D. E. Bullard (1980), in *Neurobiology of Cerebrospinal Fluid* (J. N. Wood, ed.), Plenum, New York, pp. 549–559.

Schold, S. C., W. R. Wasserstrom, M. Fleisher, M. K. Schwartz, and J. B. Posner (1980), *Ann. Neurol.* **8**, 597.

Schroeder, L. L., J. C. Johnson, and W. B. Malarkey (1976), *J. Clin. E ndo. Metab.* **43**, 1255.

Schubert, D., S. Heineman, W. Carlisle, H. Tarikas, B. Kimes, J. Patrick, J. H. Steinbach, W. Culp, and B. L. Brandt (1974), *Nature* **249**, 224.

Seidenfeld, J., and L. J. Marton (1979), *J. Natl. Cancer Inst.* **63**, 919.

Sensenbrenner, M., G. Moonen, J. P. Delaunoy, E. Bock, P. Poindron, and P. Mandel (1977), *Trans. Am. Soc. Neurochem.* **8**, 82.

Shapiro, W. R., G. A. Basler, N. L. Chernik, and J. B. Posner (1979) *J. Natl. Cancer Inst.* **62**, 447.

Sheffield, W. D., and S. U. Kim (1977), *Brain Res.* **120**, 193.

Shinomiya, Y., S. Toya, T. Iwata, and Y. Hosoda (1979), *Child's Brain* **5**, 450.

Shively, J. E., and C. W. Todd (1978), *Scand. J. Immunol. Suppl.* **6**, 91.

Sims, N. R., and P. R. Carnegie (1976), *J. Neurochem.* **27**, 769.

Sims, N. R., L. B. Horvath, and P. R. Carnegie (1979), *Biochem. J.* **181**, 367.

Singer, I. (1979), *Cell* **16**, 675.

Snitzer, L. S., and E. C. McKinney (1976), *Proc. Amer. Assoc. Cancer Res. Amer. Soc. Clin. Oncol.* **17**, 249.

Snitzer, L. S., E. C. McKinney, F. Tejada, M. M. Sigel, N. L. Rosomoff, and C. G. Zubrod (1975), *New Engl. J. Med.* **293**, 1101.

Spicer, S. S., P. J. Stoward, and R. E. Tashian (1979), *J. Histochem. Cytochem.* **27**, 820.

Sudo, T., M. Kikuno, and T. Kurihara (1972), *Biochim. Biophys. Acta* **255**, 640.

Sugimura, T., S. Sato, S. Kawabe, N. Suzuki, T. C. Chein, and K. Takakura (1969), *Nature* **222**, 1070.

Sundarraj, N., M. Schachner, and S. E. Pfeiffer (1975), *Proc. Natl. Acad. Sci. USA* **72**, 1927.

Terabayashi, T. (1976) *Neurol. Med. Chir.* **16**, 43.

Thomas, F. J., H. M. Lloyd, and M. J. Thomas (1972), *J. Clin. Path.* **25**, 774.

Trotter, J. L., B. Huss, W. P. Blank, K. O'Connell, S. Hagan, W. T. Shearer, and H. C. Agrawal (1978), *Trans. Am. Soc. Neurochem.* **9**, 59.

Vaheri, A., E., Ruoslahti, B. Westermark, and J. Pontén (1976), *J. Exptl. Med.* **143**, 64.

Vaitukaitis, J. L., G. D. Braunstein, and G. T. Ross (1972), *Am. J. Obstet. Gynecol.* **113**, 751.

van der Meulen, J. D. M., H. J. Houthoff, and E. J. Ebels (1978), *Neuropath. Appl. Neurobiol.* **4**, 177.

Velasco, M. E., D. Dahl, U. Roessman, and P. Gambetti (1980), *Cancer* **45**, 484.

Vick, N. A., J. D. Khandekar, and D. D. Bigner (1977), *Arch. Neurol.* **34**, 523.

Volpe, J. J., K. Fujimoto, J. C. Marasa, and H. C. Agrawal (1975), *Biochem. J.* **152**, 701.

Vraa-Jensen, J., M. M. Herman, L. J. Rubinstein, and A. Bignami (1976), *Neuropath. Appl. Neurobiol.* **2**, 349.

Warecka, K. (1975), *J. Neuro. Sci.* **26**, 511.

Warecka, K., and H. Bauer (1967), *J. Neurochem.* **14**, 783.

Warecka, K., H. J. Moller, H.-M. Vogel, and I. Tripatzis (1972), *J. Neurochem.* **19**, 719.

Weiler, C. T., B. Nystrom, and A. Hamberger (1979), *Brain Res.* **160**, 539.

Weiss, J. F., J. Ransohoff, and H. J. Kayden (1972), *Neurol.* **22**, 187.

Whitaker, J. N., R. P. Lisak, R. M. Bashir, O. H. Fitch, J. M. Seyer, R. Krance, J. A. Lawrence, L. T. Ch'ien, and P. O'Sullivan (1980), *Ann. Neurol.* **7**, 58.

Wikstrand, C. J., and D. D. Bigner (1980), *Amer. J. Path.* **98**, 515.

Wollemann, M. (1974), *Biochemistry of Brain Tumors*, University Park Press, Baltimore, p. 194.

Wright, A. D., M. S. McLachlan, F. H. Doyle, and T. Fraser (1969), *Brit. Med. J.* **4**, 582.

Wroblewski, F. (1959), *Cancer* **12**, 27.

Wroblewski, F., B. Decker, and R. Wroblewski (1957), *Amer. J. Clin. Path.* **28**, 269.

Yamada, K., and K. Olden (1978), *Nature* **275**, 179.

Yamada, K., S. Yamada, and I. Pastan (1976), *Proc. Natl. Acad. Sci. USA* **73**, 1217.

Yap, B.-S., H.-Y. Yap, R. S. Benjamin, G. P. Bodey, and E. J. Freidreich (1978), *Proc. Amer. Assoc. Cancer Res. Amer. Soc. Clin. Oncol.* **19**, 98.

Zanetta, J. P., P. Benda, G. Gombos, and I. G. Morgan (1972), *J. Neurochem.* **19**, 881.

Note Added in Proof

Since the completion of this chapter, the field of monoclonal antibody-defined antigens has been as productive as predicted. Schnegg et al. (1981) reported the generation of three monoclonal antibodies against a glioma-derived cell line, LN-18. Two (BF7 and GE2) reacted only with gliomas, and one (CG 12), with 10/18 gliomas, 5/5 melanomas, normal adult brain, and fetal brain. Bourdon et al. (1981) have generated an anti-human glioma monoclonal antibody that recognizes an extracellular matrix antigen expressed by 4/4 gliomas, one sarcoma, and 2/2 kidneys, and 2/2 livers. The antigen appears unrelated to laminin, fibronectin, and collagen types 1, 3, and 4. Four studies describing anti-melanoma monoclonal antibodies (Dippold et al., 1980; Herlyn et al., 1980; Liao et al. 1981; and Imai et al., 1981) have also appeared; these antibodies displayed a wide range of reactive patterns including positive reactivity with glial tumors. The two monoclonal antibodies raised by Liao et al. (1981) are extensively reactive with tumors and tissues of neuroectodermal origin. Dippold et al. (1980) have isolated two membrane antigens recognized by antimelanoma monoclonal antibodies; both are glycoproteins and weigh 95,000 and 150,000 daltons. Both Seeger (1981) and Wikstrand et al. (1981) have produced monoclonal antibodies against human fetal brain; these immunizations resulted in antibodies that recognized not only surface antigens of tumors and fetal tissues of neuroectodermal origin, but also antigens present on the cell surfaces of some subpopulations of lymphoid cells. Seegar (1981) isolated an anti-human Thy-1 hybridoma from such a fusion, and Wikstrand et al. (1981) have four hybridomas which differentially describe antigens common to neuroectodermal, fetal, and lymphoid tissue.

The next step in the field of anti-CNS monoclonal antibodies will be the isolation aned characterization of cell and tissue-associated molecules that are at present not described and the further elucidation of already described molecules such as S-100 and GFAP. With this battery of potential tumor-associated markers increasing rapidly, the field of CNS tumors stands to be revolutionized within the next ten years.

References

Bourdon, M. A., C. J. Wikstrand, C. N. Pegram, and D. D. Bigner (1981), *Fed. Proc.* **40,** 821.

Carrel, S., R. S. Accolla, A. L. Carmagnola, and J. P. Mach (1980), *Cancer Res.* **40,** 2523.

Dippold, W. G., K. O. Lloyd, L. T. C. Li, H. Ideka, H. F. Oettgen, and L. J. Old (1980), *Proc. Natl. Acad. Sci. USA* **77,** 6114

Herlyn, M., W. H. Clark, M. J. Mastrangelo, D. Guerry, D. E. Elder, D. La Rossa, R. Hamilton, E. Bondi, R. Tuthill, Z. Steplewski, and H. Koprowski (1980), *Cancer Res.* **401,** 3602.

Imai, K., A. K. Ng, and S. Ferrone (1981), *J. Natl. Cancer Inst.* **66,** 489

Liao, S. K., B. J. Clarke, B. C. Gallie, and P. B. Dent (1981), *Eur. J. Cancer,* in press.

Schnegg, J. F., A. C. Diserenns, S. Carrel, R. S. Accolla, and N. de Triboet (1981), *Cancer Res.* **41,** 1290.

Seeger, R. C. (1981), in *Hybridomas in Cancer Diagnosis* (M. S. Mitchell and H. F. Oettgen, eds.), Raven Press, NY.

Wikstrand, C. J., C. N. Pegram, M. A. Bourdon, and D. D. Bigner (1981), *Proc. Amer. Assoc. Cancer Res.* **22,** 304.

Index